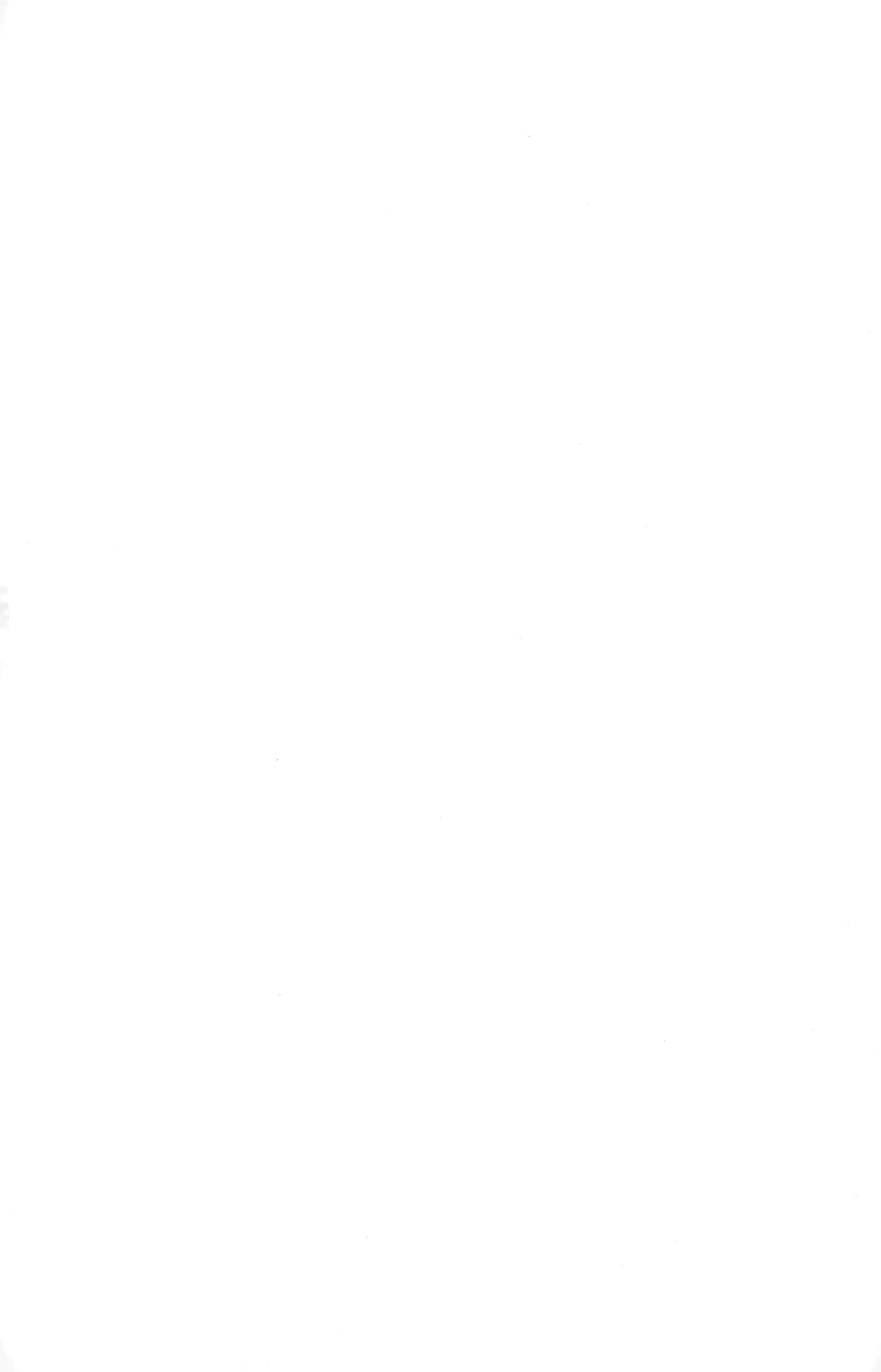

Orthopedics and Trauma in Children

Orthopedics and Trauma in Children

Editors

Axel A. Horsch
Maher A. Ghandour
Matthias Christoph M. Klotz

MDPI • Basel • Beijing • Wuhan • Barcelona • Belgrade • Manchester • Tokyo • Cluj • Tianjin

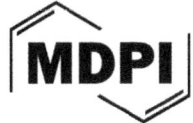

Editors
Axel A. Horsch
Orthopedic Department
Heidelberg University
Heidelberg
Germany

Maher A. Ghandour
Orthopedic Department
Heidelberg University
Heidelberg
Germany

Matthias Christoph M. Klotz
Orthopedics and
Trauma Surgery
Marienkrankenhaus
Soest
Germany

Editorial Office
MDPI
St. Alban-Anlage 66
4052 Basel, Switzerland

This is a reprint of articles from the Special Issue published online in the open access journal *Children* (ISSN 2227-9067) (available at: www.mdpi.com/journal/children/special_issues/Orthopedics_Trauma).

For citation purposes, cite each article independently as indicated on the article page online and as indicated below:

LastName, A.A.; LastName, B.B.; LastName, C.C. Article Title. *Journal Name* **Year**, *Volume Number*, Page Range.

ISBN 978-3-0365-7695-4 (Hbk)
ISBN 978-3-0365-7694-7 (PDF)

© 2023 by the authors. Articles in this book are Open Access and distributed under the Creative Commons Attribution (CC BY) license, which allows users to download, copy and build upon published articles, as long as the author and publisher are properly credited, which ensures maximum dissemination and a wider impact of our publications.

The book as a whole is distributed by MDPI under the terms and conditions of the Creative Commons license CC BY-NC-ND.

Contents

About the Editors ix

Preface to "Orthopedics and Trauma in Children" xi

Maher Ghandour, Matthias Klotz and Axel Horsch
Orthopedics and Trauma in Children: Key Problems and Future Insights
Reprinted from: *Children* **2023**, *10*, 119, doi:10.3390/children10010119 1

Axel Horsch, Svenja Gleichauf, Burkhard Lehner, Maher Ghandour, Julian Koch and Merkur Alimusaj et al.
Lower-Limb Amputation in Children and Adolescents—A Rare Encounter with Unique and Special Challenges
Reprinted from: *Children* **2022**, *9*, 1004, doi:10.3390/children9071004 5

Maher Ghandour, Burkhard Lehner, Matthias Klotz, Andreas Geisbüsch, Jakob Bollmann and Tobias Renkawitz et al.
Extraosseous Ewing Sarcoma in Children: A Systematic Review and Meta-Analysis of Clinicodemographic Characteristics
Reprinted from: *Children* **2022**, *9*, 1859, doi:10.3390/children9121859 17

Axel Horsch, Lara Petzinger, Maher Ghandour, Cornelia Putz, Tobias Renkawitz and Marco Götze
Defining Equinus Foot in Cerebral Palsy
Reprinted from: *Children* **2022**, *9*, 956, doi:10.3390/children9070956 31

Axel Horsch, Matthias Claus Michael Klotz, Hadrian Platzer, Svenja Elisabeth Seide and Maher Ghandour
Recurrence of Equinus Foot in Cerebral Palsy following Its Correction—A Meta-Analysis
Reprinted from: *Children* **2022**, *9*, 339, doi:10.3390/children9030339 43

Marja Perhomaa, Markus Stöckell, Tytti Pokka, Justus Lieber, Jaakko Niinimäki and Juha-Jaakko Sinikumpu
Clinical Follow-Up without Radiographs Is Sufficient after Most Nonoperatively Treated Distal Radius Fractures in Children
Reprinted from: *Children* **2023**, *10*, 339, doi:10.3390/children10020339 59

Domenic Grisch, Manuela Stäuble, Sandra Baumgartner, Hubertus J. A. van Hedel, Andreas Meyer-Heim and Thomas Dreher et al.
The Variable Influence of Orthotic Management on Hip and Pelvic Rotation in Children with Unilateral Neurogenic Equinus Deformity
Reprinted from: *Children* **2023**, *10*, 307, doi:10.3390/children10020307 69

Laura Zaccaria, Enno Stranzinger, Theodoros Xydias, Sabine Schaedelin, Kai Ziebarth and Mike Trück et al.
Partial Remodeling after Conservative Treatment of Trampoline Fractures in Children
Reprinted from: *Children* **2023**, *10*, 282, doi:10.3390/children10020282 79

Nikolaos Laliotis, Chrysanthos Chrysanthou and Panagiotis Konstandinidis
Concentric Circles: A New Ultrasonographic Sign for the Diagnosis of Normal Infantile Hip Development
Reprinted from: *Children* **2023**, *10*, 168, doi:10.3390/children10010168 91

Eetu N. Suominen and Antti J. Saarinen
Traumatic Hip Dislocation in Pediatric Patients: Clinical Case Series and a Narrative Review of the Literature with an Emphasis on Primary and Long-Term Complications
Reprinted from: *Children* **2023**, *10*, 107, doi:10.3390/children10010107 . . . . **99**

Filippo Migliorini, Nicola Maffulli, Andreas Bell and Marcel Betsch
Outcomes, Return to Sport, and Failures of MPFL Reconstruction Using Autografts in Children and Adolescents with Recurrent Patellofemoral Instability: A Systematic Review
Reprinted from: *Children* **2022**, *9*, 1892, doi:10.3390/children9121892 . . . . **105**

Julio J. Jauregui, Larysa P. Hlukha, Philip K. McClure, Dror Paley, Mordchai B. Shualy and Maya B. Goldberg et al.
Multiplier Method for Predicting the Sitting Height Growth at Maturity: A Database Analysis
Reprinted from: *Children* **2022**, *9*, 1763, doi:10.3390/children9111763 . . . . **115**

Tommi Yrjälä, Ilkka Helenius, Tiia Rissanen, Matti Ahonen, Markku Taittonen and Linda Helenius
The Extension of Surgery Predicts Acute Postoperative Pain, While Persistent Postoperative Pain Is Related to the Spinal Pathology in Adolescents Undergoing Posterior Spinal Fusion
Reprinted from: *Children* **2022**, *9*, 1729, doi:10.3390/children9111729 . . . . **125**

Sandra Trzcińska and Kamil Koszela
Retrospective Analysis of FED Method Treatment Results in 11–17-Year-Old Children with Idiopathic Scoliosis
Reprinted from: *Children* **2022**, *9*, 1513, doi:10.3390/children9101513 . . . . **135**

Thoralf Randolph Liebs, Alex Lorance, Steffen Michael Berger, Nadine Kaiser and Kai Ziebarth
Health-Related Quality of Life after Fractures of the Distal Forearm in Children and Adolescents—Results from a Center in Switzerland in 432 Patients
Reprinted from: *Children* **2022**, *9*, 1487, doi:10.3390/children9101487 . . . . **145**

Andreas Geisbüsch, Matthias C. M. Klotz, Cornelia Putz, Tobias Renkawitz and Axel Horsch
Mid-Term Results of Distal Femoral Extension and Shortening Osteotomy in Treating Flexed Knee Gait in Children with Cerebral Palsy
Reprinted from: *Children* **2022**, *9*, 1427, doi:10.3390/children9101427 . . . . **157**

Andrew W. Kuhn, Stockton C. Troyer and Jeffrey E. Martus
Pediatric Open Long-Bone Fracture and Subsequent Deep Infection Risk: The Importance of Early Hospital Care
Reprinted from: *Children* **2022**, *9*, 1243, doi:10.3390/children9081243 . . . . **169**

Kamal Jamil, Rostam Saharuddin, Ahmad Fazly Abd Rasid, Abdul Halim Abd Rashid and Sharaf Ibrahim
Outcome of Open Reduction Alone or with Concomitant Bony Procedures for Developmental Dysplasia of the Hip (DDH)
Reprinted from: *Children* **2022**, *9*, 1213, doi:10.3390/children9081213 . . . . **181**

Antti J. Saarinen, Eetu N. Suominen, Linda Helenius, Johanna Syvänen, Arimatias Raitio and Ilkka Helenius
Intraoperative 3D Imaging Reduces Pedicle Screw Related Complications and Reoperations in Adolescents Undergoing Posterior Spinal Fusion for Idiopathic Scoliosis: A Retrospective Study
Reprinted from: *Children* **2022**, *9*, 1129, doi:10.3390/children9081129 . . . . **191**

Katharina Susanne Gather, Ivan Mavrev, Simone Gantz, Thomas Dreher, Sébastien Hagmann and Nicholas Andreas Beckmann
Outcome Prognostic Factors in MRI during Spica Cast Therapy Treating Developmental Hip Dysplasia with Midterm Follow-Up
Reprinted from: *Children* **2022**, *9*, 1010, doi:10.3390/children9071010 201

Lorenz Pisecky, Gerhard Großbötzl, Stella Stevoska, Matthias Christoph Michael Klotz, Christina Haas and Tobias Gotterbarm et al.
Short Term Radiological Outcome of Combined Femoral and Ilium Osteotomy in Pelvic Reconstruction of the Child
Reprinted from: *Children* **2022**, *9*, 441, doi:10.3390/children9030441 215

Thoralf Randolph Liebs, Anna Meßling, Milan Milosevic, Steffen Michael Berger and Kai Ziebarth
Health-Related Quality of Life after Adolescent Fractures of the Femoral Shaft Stabilized by a Lateral Entry Femoral Nail
Reprinted from: *Children* **2022**, *9*, 327, doi:10.3390/children9030327 225

Ryszard Tomaszewski, Karol Pethe, Jacek Kler, Erich Rutz, Johannes Mayr and Jerzy Dajka
Supracondylar Fractures of the Humerus: Association of Neurovascular Lesions with Degree of Fracture Displacement in Children—A Retrospective Study
Reprinted from: *Children* **2022**, *9*, 308, doi:10.3390/children9030308 235

Lorenz Pisecky, Gerhard Großbötzl, Manuel Gahleitner, Christian Stadler, Stella Stevoska and Christina Haas et al.
Foam Splint versus Spica Cast—Early Mobilization after Hip Reconstructive Surgery in Children—Preliminary Data from a Prospective Randomized Clinical Trial
Reprinted from: *Children* **2022**, *9*, 288, doi:10.3390/children9020288 247

About the Editors

Axel A. Horsch

Dr. Axel Horsch has been a respected and esteemed doctor at the Department for Orthopedic and Trauma Surgery of Heidelberg University Hospital since 2015. His primary scientific focus centers around the study of the spastic equinus foot in cerebral palsy, and he has made substantial contributions to this field through his numerous published articles. Dr. Horsch currently holds the esteemed position of Senior Consultant at the Department of Orthopedics at Heidelberg University Hospital, where he continues to make significant advancements in orthopedic research and provide exceptional patient care.

Maher A. Ghandour

Dr. Maher Ghandour is a highly esteemed orthopedic surgeon and researcher, currently working as a Research Fellow at the University Hospital Heidelberg in Germany. His significant contributions to the field have earned him recognition, including being named the best International Resident Member of the Month by the American Academy of Orthopaedic Surgeons in September 2022. Dr. Ghandour's dedication to advancing orthopedic knowledge is demonstrated through his extensive research papers and publications. With two university diplomas in medical ethics and microsurgery, he possesses a diverse skill set that enhances his expertise. Additionally, he is currently pursuing his Orthopedic Surgery Residency at the Lebanese University, further expanding his knowledge and experience in the field. Dr. Ghandour's master's degree in health administration has also equipped him with valuable insights into healthcare management. Through his research, publications, and academic pursuits, Dr. Maher Ghandour continues to make significant strides in advancing orthopedic surgery and improving patient care.

Matthias Christoph M. Klotz

Dr. Matthias Klotz is a respected and accomplished orthopedic surgeon. He joined the Department for Orthopedic and Trauma Surgery of Heidelberg University Hospital in 2010, where he established himself as a dedicated professional. Throughout his tenure, Dr. Klotz has conducted notable biomechanical studies with a focus on gait analysis and assessing micromotions in total joint replacement. His commitment to research culminated in the successful completion of his PhD in 2018, solidifying his expertise in the field. Currently, Dr. Klotz holds the esteemed position of Head and Surgeon-in-Chief at the Orthopedic and Trauma Surgery Department of Marienkrankenhaus Soest and Mariannen-Hospital Werl in Germany. In this leadership role, he continues to provide exceptional orthopedic care, spearhead advancements in the field, and contribute to the growth of his department. Dr. Matthias Klotz's extensive experience and significant research contributions have established him as a highly respected figure in the field of orthopedic surgery.

Preface to "Orthopedics and Trauma in Children"

We are pleased to present this reprint book, which focuses on pediatric orthopedics and encompasses a wide range of topics related to pathophysiology, foot disorders, and musculoskeletal injuries in children. The field of pediatric orthopedics presents unique challenges due to the age-specific injury patterns and remarkable growth and remodeling capacity of children's bones. It demands specialized knowledge and expertise to accurately diagnose and effectively treat these conditions. The motivation behind compiling this reprint is to recognise the distinct nature of orthopedic issues in children. These issues can be congenital, developmental, or acquired, encompassing a broad spectrum that includes infectious, neuromuscular, nutritional, neoplastic, psychogenic, and traumatic conditions. The need for evidence-based recommendations to manage orthopedic deformities associated with various disorders is of paramount importance to ensure optimal patient care. The intended audience for this reprint includes orthopedic surgeons, pediatricians, rehabilitation specialists, and other healthcare professionals involved in the care of children with orthopedic conditions. It is our aim to provide comprehensive insights into the management approaches for different clinical scenarios, shedding light on the complexities involved in decision-making processes. By addressing these knowledge gaps, we hope to facilitate improved outcomes and enhanced quality of life for pediatric patients with orthopedic disorders.

We would like to express our gratitude to all the contributors who have generously shared their expertise and insights, filling the gaps in knowledge within this field. Their valuable contributions have made this reprint a comprehensive and authoritative resource for the study of pediatric orthopedics. We sincerely hope that this reprint book serves as a valuable reference and guide, aiding clinicians, researchers, and students in their pursuit of advancing knowledge and delivering the best possible care for children with orthopedic conditions.

Axel A. Horsch, Maher A. Ghandour, and Matthias Christoph M. Klotz
Editors

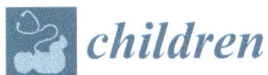

Editorial

Orthopedics and Trauma in Children: Key Problems and Future Insights

Maher Ghandour [1], Matthias Klotz [2] and Axel Horsch [1,*]

1. Department of Orthopedics, Heidelberg University Hospital, 69120 Heidelberg, Germany
2. Orthopedics and Trauma Surgery, Marienkrankenhaus Soest, 59494 Soest, Germany
* Correspondence: axel.horsch@med.uni-heidelberg.de

Orthopedic disorders among children are frequently encountered in clinical practice. The underlying causes of such issues can widely vary, including congenital diseases, developmental disorders, or acquired problems (i.e., infectious, neuromuscular, nutritional, neoplastic, psychogenic, or traumatic origin).

This special issue featured key research on some of the major disorders that affect the pediatric population, providing valuable insights into their diagnosis, treatment, clinical and radiologic outcomes, and prognosis predictors. The majority of articles reported original data on orthopedic issues and traumatic events that pediatric patients face in clinical settings, including developmental dysplasia of the hip (DDH), equinus foot deformity, idiopathic scoliosis, Ewing sarcoma, and bony fractures.

DDH, one of the most common skeletal abnormalities that affect children [1], was thoroughly investigated in this issue, with research reporting the clinical and radiologic outcomes following different therapeutic options, such as foam splint [2], Spica cast [2,3], or femoral and ileum osteotomy [4]. In addition, a systematic review highlighted some of the key prognostic factors of such outcomes in patients with DHD undergoing Spica cast therapy [3].

Other research papers have focused on one of the most critical problems that children with cerebral palsy (CP) face which is equinus foot deformity. Previous research highlighted the magnitude of equinus deformity in CP cases, with a prevalence rate ranging from 71 to 99% [5,6]. However, secondary to the absence of a standardized definition/diagnostic criteria, an accurate estimation cannot be reached. In this issue, key research proposed a definition criterion for equinus foot by using a cutoff value of $\leq 5°$ dorsiflexion. The authors also tackled one of the main problems that face orthopedic surgeons which is the recurrence of equinus foot following its surgical management in CP cases. The research indicated a rate of 5–18% for recurrence, varying widely according to the surgical method, being the highest in single-event multi-level surgery and lowest following the Illizarov procedure [7].

Bony fractures in children cover approximately one-fourth of all the accidents and injuries they experience, with distal radius fractures being the most frequent ones [8]. Upper and lower limb injuries have accounted for 1 out of 5 fracture cases among children. Open fractures, in particular, pose a significant risk for deep infection and subsequent morbidity and mortality. In this issue, Kuhn et al. [9] highlighted that the duration between fracture occurrence and hospital presentation is a significant determinant of deep infection, with the type of fracture not being associated with infection. Most orthopedic surgeons focus on the clinical and radiologic outcomes following the surgical management of fractures in children; however, patients' health-related quality of life (HR-QoL) is commonly neglected. Despite the very scarce data on HR-QoL, two of the published studies in this special issue assessed this outcome in children who have had fractures of the distal forearm and femur shaft and were treated surgically [10,11]. The extent of fractures correlated significantly with the resultant HR-QoL [10].

Citation: Ghandour, M.; Klotz, M.; Horsch, A. Orthopedics and Trauma in Children: Key Problems and Future Insights. *Children* **2023**, *10*, 119. https://doi.org/10.3390/children10010119

Received: 2 January 2023
Accepted: 4 January 2023
Published: 6 January 2023

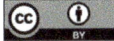

Copyright: © 2023 by the authors. Licensee MDPI, Basel, Switzerland. This article is an open access article distributed under the terms and conditions of the Creative Commons Attribution (CC BY) license (https://creativecommons.org/licenses/by/4.0/).

Idiopathic scoliosis, the most frequently reported 3-dimensional deformity of the spine, has a relatively low incidence. Based on a recent database analysis of records between 2011 and 2015, the incidence of idiopathic scoliosis was 0.497%, higher in females than males [12]. That being said, the management of idiopathic scoliosis poses a challenge for orthopedic surgeons. Research published in this issue denotes that 3D imaging can help reduce postoperative complications and/or reoperation rates in patients undergoing pedicle screw instrumentation [13]. Additionally, the implementation of the fixation, elongation, and de-rotation (FED) method can significantly improve most clinical parameters regardless of bone maturity or the size of scoliotic deformation [14]. Moreover, it has been shown that the extension of surgery can help predict the occurrence and longevity of acute postoperative pain in children undergoing posterior spinal fusion [15].

Ewing Sarcoma (ES), although rare, can occur among children and adults. It can originate from the bone or from the soft tissue around bones, referred to as extraosseous or extra-skeletal ES. To date, the clinical presentation, management strategies, clinical outcomes, and prognosis of extra-skeletal ES, particularly among children, have not been well-defined. The study of Ghandour et al. [16], which was published in this issue, is the first to provide valuable insights into the clinicodemographic characteristics of extra-skeletal ES in the pediatric population. That being said, future research should focus on the comparison between the adult and pediatric populations to determine any differences in their presentation patterns and clinical outcomes.

Children are a special population with very distinctive, yet widely variable, orthopedic issues and traumatic events. The presentation, management, and clinical outcomes in this population can differ from that of the adult population. Therefore, special care should be directed toward them. Therefore, articles within this special issue intend to contribute to the understanding of some of the most common orthopedic problems that face them with valuable insights into diagnosing and managing them.

Conflicts of Interest: The authors declare no conflict of interest.

References

1. Harsanyi, S.; Zamborsky, R.; Krajciova, L.; Kokavec, M.; Danisovic, L. Developmental Dysplasia of the Hip: A Review of Etiopathogenesis, Risk Factors, and Genetic Aspects. *Medicina* **2020**, *56*, 153. [CrossRef] [PubMed]
2. Pisecky, L.; Großbötzl, G.; Gahleitner, M.; Stadler, C.; Stevoska, S.; Haas, C.; Gotterbarm, T.; Klotz, M.C.M. Foam Splint versus Spica Cast—Early Mobilization after Hip Reconstructive Surgery in Children—Preliminary Data from a Prospective Randomized Clinical Trial. *Children* **2022**, *9*, 288. [CrossRef] [PubMed]
3. Gather, K.S.; Mavrev, I.; Gantz, S.; Dreher, T.; Hagmann, S.; Beckmann, N.A. Outcome Prognostic Factors in MRI during Spica Cast Therapy Treating Developmental Hip Dysplasia with Midterm Follow-Up. *Children* **2022**, *9*, 1010. [CrossRef] [PubMed]
4. Pisecky, L.; Großbötzl, G.; Stevoska, S.; Klotz, M.C.M.; Haas, C.; Gotterbarm, T.; Luger, M.; Gahleitner, M. Short Term Radiological Outcome of Combined Femoral and Ilium Osteotomy in Pelvic Reconstruction of the Child. *Children* **2022**, *9*, 441. [CrossRef] [PubMed]
5. Horsch, A.; Götze, M.; Geisbüsch, A.; Beckmann, N.; Tsitlakidis, S.; Berrsche, G.; Klotz, M. Prevalence and classification of equinus foot in bilateral spastic cerebral palsy. *World J. Pediatr.* **2019**, *15*, 276–280. [CrossRef] [PubMed]
6. Horsch, A.; Klotz, M.C.; Platzer, H.; Seide, S.; Zeaiter, N.; Ghandour, M. Is the prevalence of equinus foot in cerebral palsy overestimated? Results from a meta-analysis of 4814 feet. *J. Clin. Med.* **2021**, *10*, 4128. [CrossRef] [PubMed]
7. Horsch, A.; Klotz, M.C.M.; Platzer, H.; Seide, S.E.; Ghandour, M. Recurrence of Equinus Foot in Cerebral Palsy following Its Correction—A Meta-Analysis. *Children* **2022**, *9*, 339. [CrossRef] [PubMed]
8. Cooper, C.; Dennison, E.M.; Leufkens, H.G.; Bishop, N.; van Staa, T.P. Epidemiology of childhood fractures in Britain: A study using the general practice research database. *J. Bone Miner. Res.* **2004**, *19*, 1976–1981. [CrossRef] [PubMed]
9. Kuhn, A.W.; Troyer, S.C.; Martus, J.E. Pediatric Open Long-Bone Fracture and Subsequent Deep Infection Risk: The Importance of Early Hospital Care. *Children* **2022**, *9*, 1243. [CrossRef] [PubMed]
10. Liebs, T.R.; Lorance, A.; Berger, S.M.; Kaiser, N.; Ziebarth, K. Health-Related Quality of Life after Fractures of the Distal Forearm in Children and Adolescents—Results from a Center in Switzerland in 432 Patients. *Children* **2022**, *9*, 1487. [CrossRef] [PubMed]
11. Liebs, T.R.; Meßling, A.; Milosevic, M.; Berger, S.M.; Ziebarth, K. Health-Related Quality of Life after Adolescent Fractures of the Femoral Shaft Stabilized by a Lateral Entry Femoral Nail. *Children* **2022**, *9*, 327. [CrossRef] [PubMed]
12. Sung, S.; Chae, H.W.; Lee, H.S.; Kim, S.; Kwon, J.W.; Lee, S.B.; Moon, S.H.; Lee, H.M.; Lee, B.H. Incidence and Surgery Rate of Idiopathic Scoliosis: A Nationwide Database Study. *Int. J. Environ. Res. Public Health* **2021**, *18*, 8152. [CrossRef] [PubMed]

13. Saarinen, A.J.; Suominen, E.N.; Helenius, L.; Syvänen, J.; Raitio, A.; Helenius, I. Intraoperative 3D imaging reduces pedicle screw related complications and reoperations in adolescents undergoing posterior spinal fusion for idiopathic scoliosis: A retrospective study. *Children* **2022**, *9*, 1129. [CrossRef] [PubMed]
14. Trzcińska, S.; Koszela, K. Retrospective Analysis of FED Method Treatment Results in 11–17-Year-Old Children with Idiopathic Scoliosis. *Children* **2022**, *9*, 1513. [CrossRef] [PubMed]
15. Yrjälä, T.; Helenius, I.; Rissanen, T.; Ahonen, M.; Taittonen, M.; Helenius, L. The Extension of Surgery Predicts Acute Postoperative Pain, While Persistent Postoperative Pain Is Related to the Spinal Pathology in Adolescents Undergoing Posterior Spinal Fusion. *Children* **2022**, *9*, 1729. [CrossRef] [PubMed]
16. Ghandour, M.; Lehner, B.; Klotz, M.; Geisbüsch, A.; Bollmann, J.; Renkawitz, T.; Horsch, A. Extraosseous Ewing Sarcoma in Children: A Systematic Review and Meta-Analysis of Clinicodemographic Characteristics. *Children* **2022**, *9*, 1859. [CrossRef] [PubMed]

Disclaimer/Publisher's Note: The statements, opinions and data contained in all publications are solely those of the individual author(s) and contributor(s) and not of MDPI and/or the editor(s). MDPI and/or the editor(s) disclaim responsibility for any injury to people or property resulting from any ideas, methods, instructions or products referred to in the content.

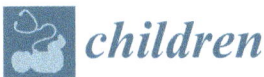

Article

Lower-Limb Amputation in Children and Adolescents—A Rare Encounter with Unique and Special Challenges

Axel Horsch *, Svenja Gleichauf, Burkhard Lehner, Maher Ghandour, Julian Koch, Merkur Alimusaj, Tobias Renkawitz and Cornelia Putz

Department of Orthopaedics, Heidelberg University Hospital, 69118 Heidelberg, Germany;
svenja.gleichauf@med.uni-heidelberg.de (S.G.); burkhard.lehner@med.uni-heidelberg.de (B.L.);
mghandourmd@gmail.com (M.G.); julian.koch@med.uni-heidelberg.de (J.K.);
merkur.alimusaj@med.uni-heidelberg.de (M.A.); tobias.renkawitz@med.uni-heidelberg.de (T.R.);
cornelia.putz@med.uni-heidelberg.de (C.P.)
* Correspondence: axel.horsch@med.uni-heidelberg.de

Abstract: Background/Aim: The pattern of lower-limb amputation, indications, complications, and revision in pediatric cases differs globally. Therefore, we conducted this study to describe the patterns of lower-limb amputation at our institution. Methods: During a set period between 2010 and 2020, adolescent patients undergoing lower-limb amputation within the orthopedic department of Heidelberg University Hospital were retrospectively collected and analyzed. The retrieved dataset included two parts: data on lower-limb amputations and data on subsequent complications and revision surgeries at the same time. Besides patients' general information (age, gender), the dataset included data regarding amputation patterns (number, indications, and level of amputation, complications, and revision surgeries and their indications). Results: Twenty-two patients undergoing lower-limb amputation were examined, of which the majority were males (63.6%) with a mean age of 12 (5.1) years. Tumor was the most common indication for amputation (72.7%), and transfemoral amputation was the most frequent level (68.2%). Complications occurred in 10 patients, mostly due to stump impalement or bony overgrowth. Of all recorded patients requiring revision, nine were regarding bone and one case regarding soft tissue. Conclusions: Lower-limb amputation in adolescents is a rare encounter and it is commonly indicated due to bone tumors. The thigh is the most common level of amputation. Postoperative complications are frequent, mainly secondary to bony overgrowth, and often require revision surgery.

Keywords: amputation; lower extremity; complications; children; adolescents

1. Introduction

Amputations of major limbs, especially in pediatric populations, are a rare encounter. In patients where amputation is necessary, the subsequent emotional and psychological impact is often detrimental to both the family and the affected child [1]. These major amputations of either the lower extremity or upper extremity lead to a substantial disfigurement of the amputated limb, carrying with it a fairly increased risk for postoperative morbidity and mortality, and especially children who suffer from limb amputation often perceive themselves as being incomplete [2]. In this context, creating a stump that is considered fit for a function-restoring prosthesis is essential for orthopedic surgeons.

The decision to amputate a limb follows at least one of several indications, including severe trauma, infection, tumors, congenital anomalies, and vascular abnormalities [1]. Evidence suggests that the reasons for amputations and their frequencies differ widely between countries. For instance, peripheral vascular affection is perceived as the leading cause of amputation in developed countries, while trauma, infection, and malignant tumors are reported as leading causes for major limb amputation in developing countries [3,4].

Although lower-limb amputations in pediatrics is rare, they are often associated with several complications, mostly being bone overgrowth regarding the amputated end of the limb and leading to permanent internal penetration of soft tissue under load, making prosthetic use impossible [5]. Another observed complication is the formation of a sharp-ended spur that potentially penetrates overlying soft tissue due to continuous growth, particularly in transfemoral (TF) and transtibial (TT) amputation. Addressing this, revision surgery may be considered, particularly to correct frequent growth abnormalities [6].

Due to the wide discrepancy in characteristics and outcome of pediatric patients undergoing major limb amputation within different countries, we conducted this research to study the pattern of lower-limb amputation in children and adolescents (<18 years of age), their indications, amputation levels, complications, and subsequent revision surgeries following amputation at our institution.

2. Materials and Methods

2.1. Study Population and Design

This research is based on a retrospective analysis of patient records containing lower-extremity amputations at the Orthopedic University Hospital Heidelberg (Figure 1). This retrospective analysis was based on two main datasets: (1) data of patients who underwent a lower-extremity amputation during the period from 2010 to February 2020 and (2) data on complications and revisions performed after amputation during the same period.

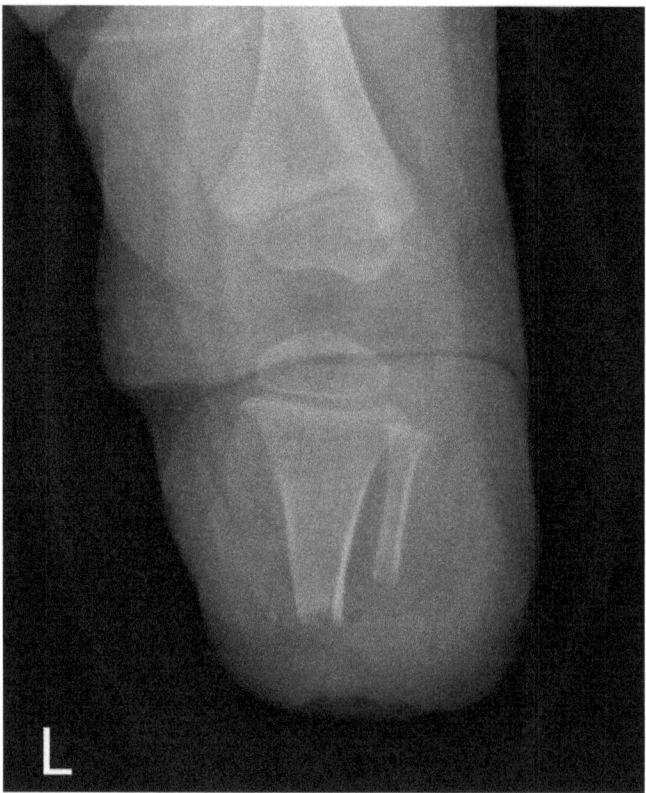

Figure 1. X-ray image of a patient included in our dataset.

To create the dataset, all surgical procedures with a corresponding code were selected from the internal procedure list. Then, a review of the collected data using the ICD-10 and the coding of the surgical procedures to determine complications and performed revisions was conducted. Retrieved data contained baseline characteristics of patients (age, gender) as well as clinical information (level and indication of amputation, complications, and revisions).

2.2. Inclusion and Exclusion Criteria for Amputations

Inclusion criteria were set to patients containing following variables: lower-extremity amputations, any sex, and less than 18 years of age, at time of amputation surgery. For dually listed patients, we considered whether the amputation was performed on the same extremity, thus changing only the level of amputation or whether amputations were performed on different extremities. In case of two separately conducted amputations of the same limb, scoring took place as one patient; otherwise, this patient counted as two cases.

Patients that underwent an amputation other than lower extremity, as well as patients undergoing nonprimary amputation surgery, were excluded from this study. Therefore, the patient collective contained 23 patients. Reviewing inclusion criteria, 22 patients were thereafter relevant for further analysis.

2.3. Inclusion and Exclusion Criteria for Complications

To determine whether complications occurred because of initially conducted amputations or independently, an examination was performed within the patient cohort undergoing amputation of the lower extremity. If this was not the case, the patient would be excluded. If multiple listing of patients was detected, it was checked whether complications were co- or independent. If a continuing complication was detected, it counted as one patient and was therefore flagged with "multiple necessary revisions". Independent complications were counted individually.

The patient population included a total of 10 patients, all of whom met the inclusion criteria and were therefore relevant for analysis.

2.4. Study Variables

Age, sex, cause of amputation, level of amputation, complications, and revisions performed were used as observation characteristics. A differentiated analysis of the above-mentioned characteristics was then considered.

The causes of amputation were divided into tumor, infection, dysmelia, and circulatory disorders. The amputation level was divided into TT amputation, TF amputation, hemipelvectomy (HP), and hip-disarticulation (HX). With regard to complications, only residual limb complications occurred in children and adolescents. Revisions were subdivided into soft-tissue and bony.

2.5. Statistical Analysis

Statistical analysis of the collected data was performed using Microsoft Excel 365 (Microsoft 2022, Redmond, Washington, DC, USA), and i.s.h.med (SAP Walldorf, Germany) to add missing information. Descriptive data were presented as means and standard deviations (SD) for continuous variables, while categorical and dichotomous variables were presented as numbers and frequencies.

3. Results
3.1. Demographic and Clinical Characteristics

The baseline characteristics of the retrieved records are summarized in Table 1. A total of 22 children/adolescents undergoing lower-extremity amputation were included in this analysis. The mean age was 12 (SD = 5.1) years, and 63.6% (14/22) of patients were males. The mean follow-up was 4.3 years (SD = 3.4).

Amputation was conducted in all 22 patients with tumor being the most common reason for amputation, accounting for 16 patients (72.7%), followed by dysmelia (13.6%) and circulation (9.1%), respectively. Of patients with tumor as indication for amputation, osteosarcoma was the most commonly reported cause (15/16 patients; 93.8%), while Ewing's sarcoma was reported in one case. TF amputation was most common accounting for 68.2% of patients, followed by HX (13.6%), TT amputation (9.1%), and HP (9.1%), respectively.

Table 1. Demographic and clinical characteristics of included children/adolescents with lower-extremity amputation ($n = 22$).

Variable	Subcategory	Total Population ($n = 22$)
	Age (years); mean (SD)	
		12 (5.1)
	Gender; n (%)	
	Male	14 (63.6%)
	Female	8 (36.4%)
	Causes of Amputation; n (%)	
	Tumor	16 (72.7%)
	Infection	1 (4.5%)
	Dysmelia	3 (13.6%)
	Circulation	2 (9.1%)
	Total	22 (100%)
	Level of Amputation; n (%)	
	Transtibial	2 (9.1%)
	Transfemoral	15 (68.2%)
	Hemipelvectomy	2 (9.1%)
	Hip-disarticulation	3 (13.6%)
	Total	22 (100%)
	Complications; n (%)	
		10 (45.45%)
	Revision Surgery due to complications; n (%)	
		10 (45.45%)

n: Number; SD: Standard Deviation.

3.2. Complications following Amputations

Complications occurred in 10 (45.45%) out of 22 amputated patients, all of which were residual limb complications. Based on an intact growth plate, which is present in transmetaphyseal amputations (at femoral and tibial levels) (Figure 2), impaling of the residual limb occurred. This happens mainly due to continuous longitudinal growth of the bone leading to excessive stress on soft tissue. As a result, 9 of 17 patients (52.9%) experienced stump impalement (Figure 3).

In four of the nine recorded patients with limb impalement as a complication, a shorting of the bone and a remolding of the distal end of the stump (deperiosteostomy) was performed during amputation. This procedure was not used in the remaining five patients.

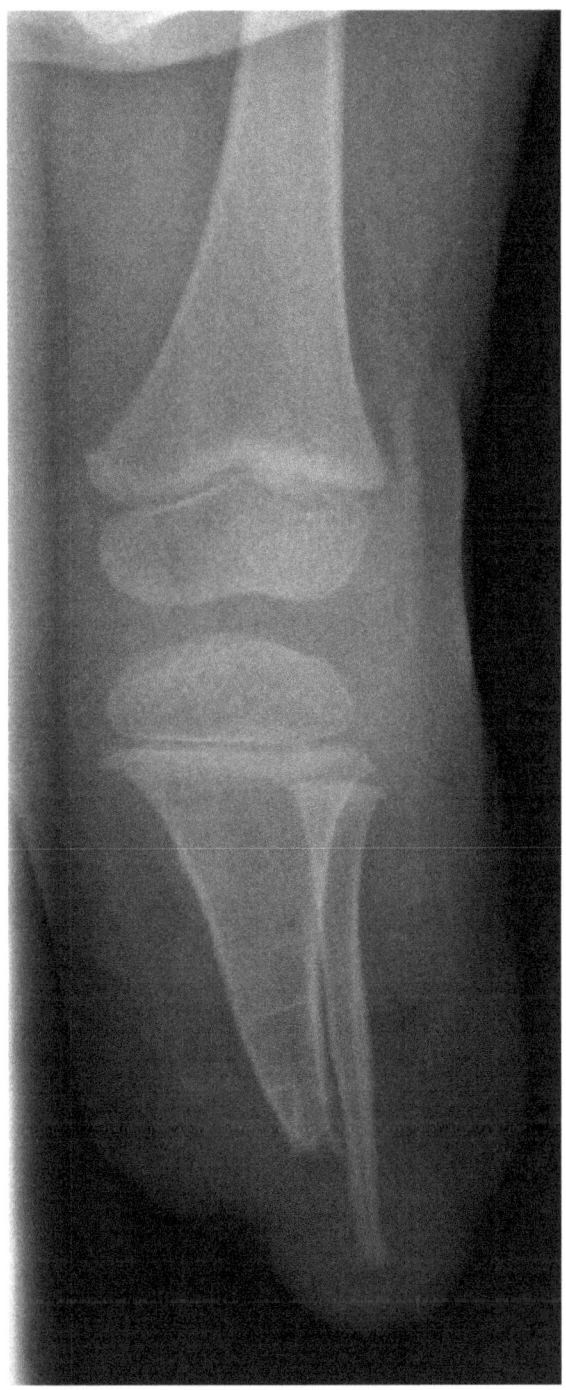

Figure 2. Postoperative X-ray of transtibial amputation.

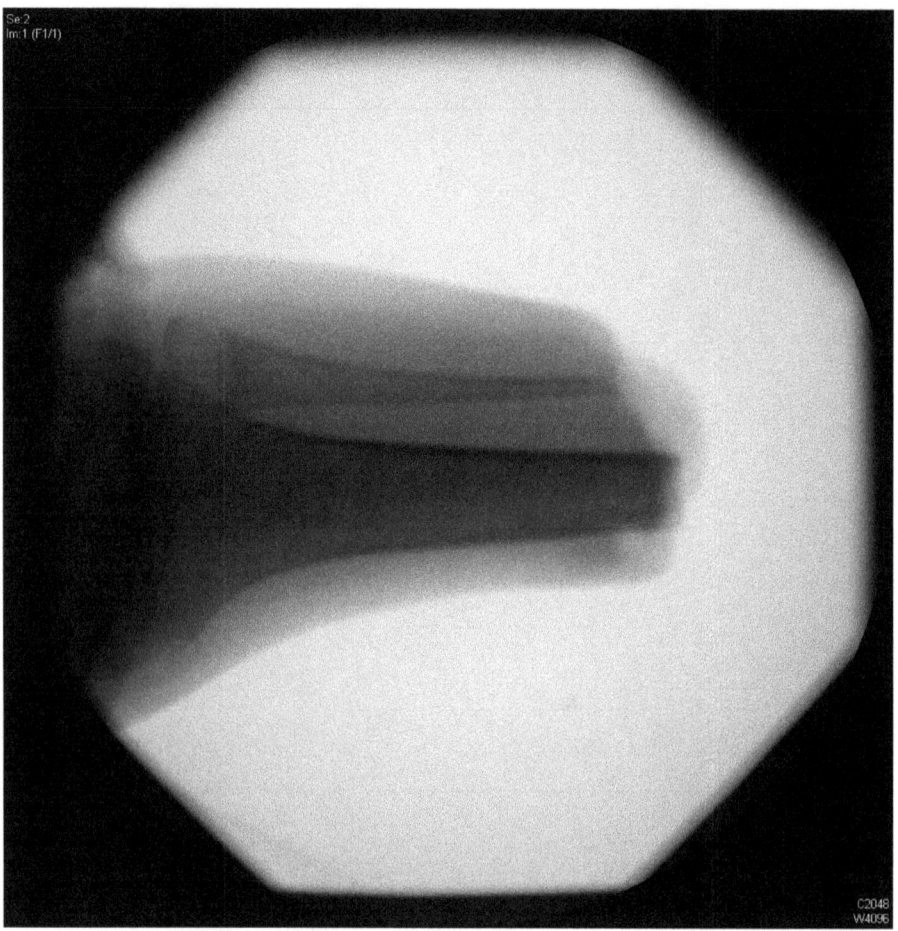

Figure 3. X-ray image of stump spike.

3.3. Revisions Secondary to Complications

Revision surgeries following amputation were performed in 10 patients that experienced postoperative complications, 9 of which received bony revisions accounting for 90% of all revisions, while 1 case had soft tissue revision. A summary of bony revision procedures that were carried out is provided in Table 2. Stump shortening and stump revision was most common in our population, accounting for 33.3% of revisions.

Table 2. Summary of the bony revision procedures that were performed in complicated amputated patients.

Variables	Number (%)
Revision with stump shortening + reconstruction with bone cartilage cap plasty	1 (11.1%)
Stump revision with ablation of bone tips	1 (11.1%)
Stump shortening and stump revision	3 (33.3%)
Stump shortening with periosteoplasty	2 (22.2%)

Table 2. *Cont.*

Variables	Number (%)
Stump cap plasty with bone wedge from iliac crest	1 (11.1%)
Resection of exostosis and bony aspects	1 (11.1%)
Total	9 (100%)

4. Discussion

Major limb amputation has been perceived as a frequent surgical procedure attempted in many orthopedic, general, vascular, and trauma settings, mainly for life-saving purposes. That being said, amputation is commonly associated with a substantial impact on the affected individual's social and psychological status [7,8]. The patterns of amputation indications, frequency, and levels, as well as subsequent complications and need for revision surgeries, are widely variable based on the age of patients, settings, and country in which they are carried out [1,6]. Therefore, we conducted this retrospective analysis of children and adolescent patients who underwent lower-limb amputation at our institution over a 10-year period to report patterns of amputation indications, complications, and revision surgery.

A total of 22 patients were included for descriptive analysis, following the exclusion of 1 case that did not match our eligibility criteria. All of them were children or adolescents with a mean age of 12 years. We observed a male predominance accounting for 63.6% of amputated patients. This observation stands in line with the recent literature [9–13]. Although, most of the available evidence provides data in adult patients, and it therefore seems that male predominance in amputation is a common observation across all age groups. However, this still warrants further investigation to determine the reasons behind this predominance, as the presented sample size is too small for a principal generalization.

Indications for limb amputation, particularly within pediatric population, vary greatly in different settings and countries. For instance, some reports indicate almost 80 to 90% of limb amputations in adults occur as a result of vascular abnormality in developed countries [14–16] while in developing countries, trauma and infections are perceived as the most prevalent indications for limb amputations [3,4]. It is assumed that in developed countries, pediatric amputations are mainly performed to treat tumors, while in developing countries, trauma and infections are the most common indications. In this study, tumors were the leading cause of amputation in children/adolescents, followed by dysmelia. This is somewhat consistent with the study by Chalya et al. [6], where vascular abnormalities were ranked third as a cause of lower-limb amputation; however, diabetic foot and trauma were ranked first and second, respectively. Of note, the authors included individuals of all age groups, while most of them had an age ranging between 41 and 50 years. Similar to the previous study, Jahmani et al. [5] reported diabetic foot (41.9%) and trauma (38.4%) as leading indications for amputation. The authors studied indications for lower-limb amputation in patients with (0–10) and (11–20) years of age, of which primary bone cancer and trauma were reported as the common indication for amputation within each of these age groups, respectively. The differences in indication for amputation between this study and recent literature could be related to this unique and young age group within the analyzed cohort.

Of note, in our population, the decision of which type of amputation was to be carried out was solely dependent on the findings of tumor extension, while putting into consideration an appropriate safety margin. In our study, TF amputation was the most frequent level of lower-limb amputation among children and adolescents. This is consistent with current literature, where above-knee amputation was reported as the most common level of amputation, both in the adult and pediatric population [10,17,18].

We observed many complications in our patients undergoing lower-limb amputation, accounting for 45.5% of the studied population. All observed complications were residual limb complications, with stump impalement or bony overgrowth being most frequent (nine patients). In four of nine patients, deperiosteostomy was performed to tackle this complication. Preservation of the length of limb in this population is of great importance, mainly because the lost distal growth plate accounts for approximately 75% of vertical femoral growth. In these patients, TF amputations lead to a very short stump leading to a complex biomechanical situation regarding prosthetic fitting. On the other hand, TT amputation, although preserving the proximal growth plate, often leads to bony overgrowth at the distal end, which subsequently may continue growing until growth is stationary within amputated individuals [1]. Consistent with our findings, bony overgrowth is reported as the most prevalent complication following lower-limb amputation in adolescents, with rates ranging from 4 to 50% [19–24]. Importantly, age, location, indication for amputation, and level of amputations are perceived as attributable factors for such prevalence, whereas younger individuals are more likely to experience this complication [19,20,25]. This could be the reason for this complication being so frequent in our population, secondary to the young age of included individuals.

It is important to highlight an unfamiliar observation in one of our cases, where the fibula outgrew the tibia following amputation (Figure 4). Although the surgery was performed correctly and no epiphysiodesis was performed, this observation remains unclear.

More so, all amputated individuals in our study who experienced postoperative complications had undergone revision surgery (10 out of 10 patients). Little is reported regarding the value of revision surgery on lower-limb amputation, particularly in the pediatric population due to the scarcity of evidence in this particular field. In a recent analysis of 71 revision surgeries in patients who underwent lower-limb amputation, it was reported that soft-tissue pathology (31.0%) was the most common indication for revision surgery followed by infections (31.0%) and bone pathology (18.3%), respectively [26]. This differs from our observation, since in our series, nine patients underwent bony revision, whilst only one case underwent soft tissue revision surgery. This discrepancy could be related to indication for amputation in the first place, as in our study, tumor (mainly osteosarcoma) was the main indication for amputation, whereas trauma was most common for amputation in the previous study [26]. This highlights an important observation relating to the association between the primary indication for amputation and subsequent complications and revision surgeries. Nevertheless, larger and prospective studies are needed to further investigate this observation. That being said, it is of great importance to mention that this problem of bony impalement begins early in these patients, and due to the bone overgrowth, there is a significant stress on the surrounding soft tissues, leading to unequivocal growth and eventually penetration. This in turn results in a significant impact of affected patients' life in terms of pain and activities of daily living which can also negatively impact the affected child's mental health. In these circumstances, revision surgery is considered a necessary function-improving intervention.

Surgical options for revision surgery in children and adolescents include stump shortening with the option of temporary epiphysiodesis of the proximal growth plates. However, the resulting reduced bone growth can complicate restoration in very short residual limbs and lead to instability in the overlying joint, making length preservation/gain advantageous for prosthetic restoration. Even an operation according to Ertl does not solve the problem of the bone growing further. The orthopedic technical restoration with traction liners and the prosthetic restoration with stretching/tensioning of the soft tissues (i.e., pin system) should be optimized accordingly to reduce revision interventions during growth.

Of note, infantile amputation is a rare occurrence and our study is the first to provide valuable insights into lower-limb amputation patterns and complications in children and adolescents in Germany over a 10-year period. Despite the high revision rate due to bony impalement, there is no alternative to amputation in terms of providing good functional outcome. That being said, our study has several limitations, the biggest of which being the limited sample size; however, because lower-limb amputation in pediatric populations is rare, we could analyze this population's characteristics in a larger dataset, even though a retrospective design limits the conclusions that could be drawn from it, given the lack of important data outlining a better perspective on this patient population. Therefore, future research should include a larger, more widely representative dataset to further investigate, describe and analyze lower-limb amputation patterns in pediatric patients.

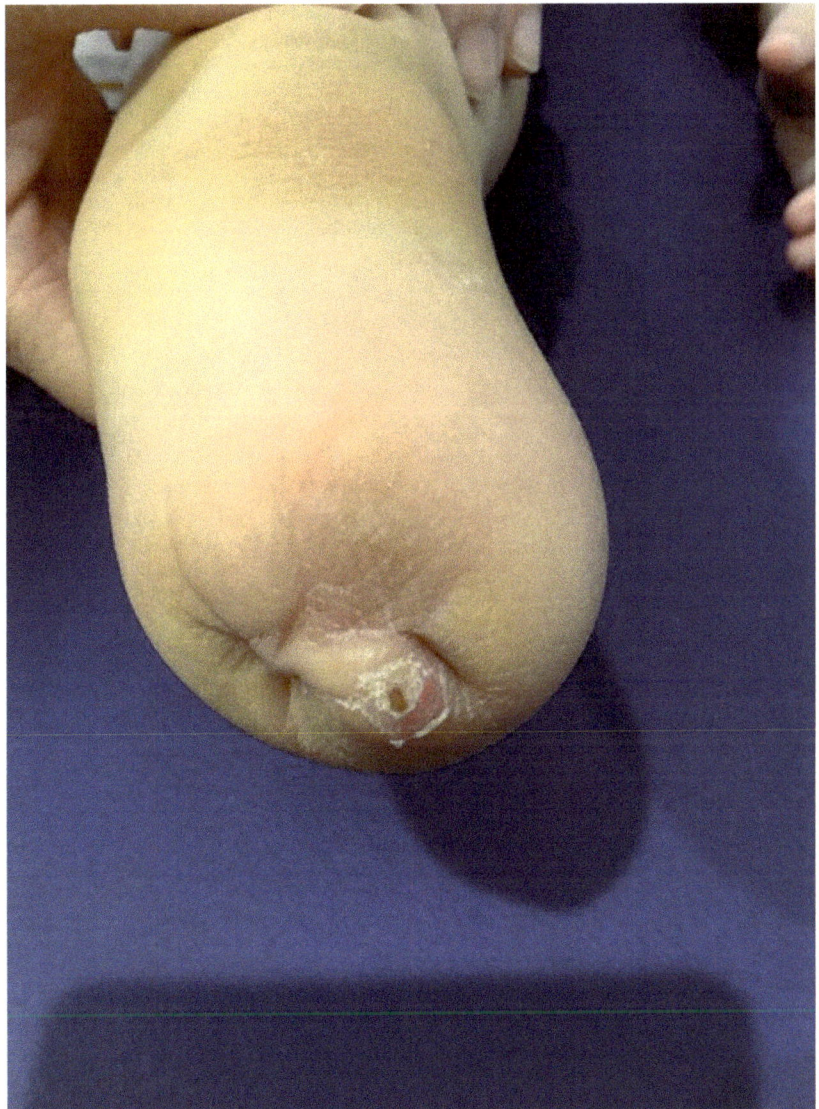

Figure 4. A clinical image showing an unfamiliar observation of the fibula outgrowing the tibia in an amputated case.

5. Conclusions

Lower-limb amputation in children and adolescents is a rare encounter, which is more predominant in males and is commonly indicated due to bone tumors. TF amputation is the most common level of amputation. Postoperative complications are reported in nearly half the amputated population, besides bony overgrowth. Most of these complications indicate and result in revision surgery to correct for the occurring abnormality, of which stump growth is most common. Despite the high revision rate, it must be noted that amputation is without alternative in these cases. In addition, modern prosthesis fitting usually enables patients to have very good everyday function.

Author Contributions: Conceptualization: A.H.; methodology: A.H.; software: A.H. and S.G.; validation: A.H. and S.G.; formal analysis: A.H. and S.G.; investigation: A.H. and S.G.; resources: A.H.; data curation: S.G. and A.H.; writing—original draft preparation: A.H. and M.G.; writing—review and editing: A.H., C.P., J.K., B.L., M.A., and T.R.; visualization: S.G.; supervision: A.H.; project administration: A.H. All authors have read and agreed to the published version of the manuscript.

Funding: The authors have not declared a specific grant for this research from any funding agency in the public, commercial or not-for-profit sectors. For the publication fee we acknowledge financial support by Deutsche Forschungsgemeinschaft within the funding programme "Open Access Publikationskosten" as well as by Heidelberg University.

Institutional Review Board Statement: This research study was conducted in accordance with the Declaration of Helsinki, and was approved on 23 September 2019 by the ethics committee, Medical Faculty of Heidelberg (protocol registration number: S-649/2019).

Informed Consent Statement: Patient consent was waived due to minimal risk.

Data Availability Statement: All the Data analyzed in this manuscript can be provided upon request by contacting the corresponding author.

Acknowledgments: Statistical advice was provided by Thomas Bruckner, Institute for Medical Biometry and Informatics in Heidelberg.

Conflicts of Interest: The authors declare no conflict of interest. Regardless, Tobias Renkawitz has received research support and personal fees from Arbeitsgemeinschaft Endoprothetik (AE), DGOU, DGOOC; BVOU, DePuy International, Otto Bock Foundation, Deutsche Arthrose Hilfe, Aesculap, Zimmer, Stiftung Oskar Helene Heim Berlin, Vielberth Foundation Regensburg, the German Ministry of Education and Research as well as the German Federal Ministry of Economic Cooperation and Development. Axel Horsch received research support from Arthrose Hilfe and Ipsen.

References

1. Griffet, J. Amputation and prosthesis fitting in paediatric patients. *Orthop. Traumatol. Surg. Res.* **2016**, *102* (Suppl. 1), S161–S175. [CrossRef] [PubMed]
2. Masood Jawaid, I.A.; Kaimkhani, G.M. Current indications for major lower limb amputations at Civil Hospital, Karachi. *Pak. J. Surg.* **2008**, *24*, 228–231.
3. Abou-Zamzam, A.M., Jr.; Teruya, T.H.; Killeen, J.D.; Ballard, J.L. Major lower extremity amputation in an academic vascular center. *Ann. Vasc. Surg.* **2003**, *17*, 86–90. [CrossRef]
4. Olasinde, A.A.; Oginni, L.M.; Bankole, J.O.; Oluwadiya, K.S. Indications for amputations in Ile-Ife, Nigeria. *Niger. J. Med. J. Natl. Assoc. Resid. Dr. Niger.* **2002**, *11*, 118–121.
5. Jahmani, R.; Paley, D. *Stump Overgrowth after Limb Amputation in Children, In Limb Amputation*; IntechOpen: London, UK, 2019.
6. Chalya, P.L.; Mabula, J.B.; Dass, R.M.; Ngayomela, I.H.; Chandika, A.B.; Mbelenge, N.; Gilyoma, J.M. Major limb amputations: A tertiary hospital experience in northwestern Tanzania. *J. Orthop. Surg. Res.* **2012**, *7*, 18. [CrossRef]
7. Paudel, B.; Shrestha, B.K.; Banskota, A.K. Two faces of major lower limb amputations. *Kathmandu Univ. Med. J.* **2005**, *3*, 212–216.
8. Van Der Meij, W.K.N. *No Leg to Stand On: Historical Relation between Amputation Surgery and Prostheseology*; University of Groningen: Groningen, The Netherlands, 1995.
9. Jenyo, M.; Diya, K.; Olakulehin, O. Limb amputations in Osogbo, Nigeria. *Afr. J. Trauma* **2004**, *2*, 80–82.
10. Kidmas, A.; Nwadiaro, C.; Igun, G. Lower limb amputation in Jos, Nigeria. *East Afr. Med. J.* **2004**, *81*, 427–429. [CrossRef]
11. Nwankwo, O.; Katchy, A. Surgical limb amputation: A five-year experience at Hilltop Orthopedic Hospital Enugu, Nigeria. *Niger. J. Orthop. Trauma* **2004**, *3*, 139–149. [CrossRef]
12. Sié Essoh, J.B.; Kodo, M.; Djè Bi Djè, V.; Lambin, Y. Limb amputations in adults in an Ivorian teaching hospital. *Niger. J. Clin. Pract.* **2009**, *12*, 245–247.
13. Solagberu, B. The scope of amputations in a Nigerian teaching hospital. *Afr. J. Med. Med. Sci.* **2001**, *30*, 225–227. [PubMed]
14. Greive, A.C.; Lankhorst, G.J. Functional outcome of lower-limb amputees: A prospective descriptive study in a general hospital. *Prosthet. Orthot. Int.* **1996**, *20*, 79–87. [CrossRef] [PubMed]
15. Pernot, H.F.; Winnubst, G.M.; Cluitmans, J.J.; De Witte, L.P. Amputees in Limburg: Incidence, morbidity and mortality, prosthetic supply, care utilisation and functional level after one year. *Prosthet. Orthot. Int.* **2000**, *24*, 90–96. [CrossRef] [PubMed]

16. Rommers, G.M.; Vos, L.D.; Groothoff, J.W.; Schuiling, C.H.; Eisma, W.H. Epidemiology of lower limb amputees in the north of The Netherlands: Aetiology, discharge destination and prosthetic use. *Prosthet. Orthot. Int.* **1997**, *21*, 92–99. [CrossRef]
17. Umaru, R.; Gali, B.; Ali, N. Role of inappropriate traditional splintage in limb amputation in Maiduguri, Nigeria. *Ann. Afr. Med.* **2004**, *3*. Available online: https://tspace.library.utoronto.ca/handle/1807/4100 (accessed on 17 May 2022).
18. Yusof, M.I.; Sulaiman, A.R.; Muslim, D.A. Diabetic foot complications: A two-year review of limb amputation in a Kelantanese population. *Singap. Med. J.* **2007**, *48*, 729–732.
19. Abraham, E.; Pellicore, R.J.; Hamilton, R.C.; Hallman, B.W.; Ghosh, L. Stump overgrowth in juvenile amputees. *J. Pediatric Orthop.* **1986**, *6*, 66–71. [CrossRef]
20. Aitken, G. Overgrowth of the amputation stump. *Interclin Inf. Bull* **1962**, *1*, 66–71.
21. Aitken, G.T. Surgical Amputation in Children. *J. Bone Jt. Surg.* **1963**, *45*, 1735–1741. [CrossRef]
22. Fedorak, G.T.; Watts, H.G.; Cuomo, A.V.; Ballesteros, J.P.; Grant, H.J.; Bowen, R.E.; Scaduto, A.A. Osteocartilaginous transfer of the proximal part of the fibula for osseous overgrowth in children with congenital or acquired tibial amputation: Surgical technique and results. *J. Bone Jt. Surg.* **2015**, *97*, 574–581. [CrossRef]
23. O'Neal, M.L.; Bahner, R.; Ganey, T.M.; Ogden, J.A. Osseous overgrowth after amputation in adolescents and children. *J. Pediatric Orthop.* **1996**, *16*, 78–84. [CrossRef]
24. Tenholder, M.; Davids, J.R.; Gruber, H.E.; Blackhurst, D.W. Surgical management of juvenile amputation overgrowth with a synthetic cap. *J. Pediatric Orthop.* **2004**, *24*, 218–226. [CrossRef]
25. Abraham, E. Operative treatment of bone overgrowth in children who have an aquired or congenital amputation. *J. Bone Jt. Surg.* **1996**, *78*, 1287–1288. [CrossRef]
26. Bourke, H.E.; Yelden, K.C.; Robinson, K.P.; Sooriakumaran, S.; Ward, D.A. Is revision surgery following lower-limb amputation a worthwhile procedure? A retrospective review of 71 cases. *Injury* **2011**, *42*, 660–666. [CrossRef] [PubMed]

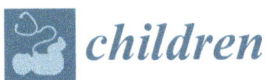

Review

Extraosseous Ewing Sarcoma in Children: A Systematic Review and Meta-Analysis of Clinicodemographic Characteristics

Maher Ghandour [1], Burkhard Lehner [1], Matthias Klotz [2], Andreas Geisbüsch [1], Jakob Bollmann [1], Tobias Renkawitz [1] and Axel Horsch [1,*]

1 Department of Orthopedics, Heidelberg University Hospital, 69129 Heidelberg, Germany
2 Orthopedics and Trauma Surgery, Marienkrankenhaus Soest, 59494 Soest, Germany
* Correspondence: axel.horsch@med.uni-heidelberg.de

Abstract: Background: We conducted this systematic review to provide comprehensive evidence on the prevalence, clinical features and outcomes of young extraosseous Ewing sarcoma (EES) cases. **Methods:** PubMed, Scopus, Web of Science, and Google Scholar were searched for articles reporting the occurrence of EES among children and adolescents (<21 years). The primary outcome included the rate of occurrence of EES among children and adolescents, while the secondary outcomes included the descriptive analyses of the demographic characteristics, tumor characteristics, and clinical outcomes of the affected cases. The data are reported as the effect size (ES) and its corresponding 95% confidence interval (CI). **Results:** A total of 29 studies were included. Twenty-four reported instances of childhood disease among all the EES cases [ES = 30%; 95%CI: 29–31%], while five studies reported extraosseous cases among the pediatric EES cases [ES = 22%; 95%CI: 13–31%]. The thorax is the most common location of childhood EES [33%; 95%CI: 20–46%] followed by the extremities [31%; 95%CI: 22–40%]. Concurrent chemotherapy and radiotherapy [57%; 95%CI: 25–84%] was the most commonly implemented management protocol in the pediatric EES cases. The rate of no evidence of disease and 5-year overall survival was 69% for both outcomes. Mortality occurred in 29% of cases, while recurrence and secondary metastasis occurred in 35% and 16% of cases, respectively. **Conclusions:** Our findings provide insight into the clinical features and outcomes of EES among children and adolescents.

Keywords: Ewing sarcoma; extraosseous; children

1. Introduction

The Ewing sarcoma family of tumors (ESFT) is a collection of small, rounded tumor cells that have similar neural histological and genetic characteristics [1–4]. ESFT is categorized into four types based on the origin of the tumor: Ewing sarcoma of the bone, peripheral primitive neuroectodermal tumor (pPNET), Askin tumor, which originates from the chest wall, and, finally, the extraosseous or extraskeletal Ewing sarcoma (EES). EES, which occurs in around 20% of ES cases, typically originates from the soft tissues of the trunk and extremities [5], and the majority of these cases are reported among patients who are 10–30 years of age [6].

Based on a previous report, the incidence of EES is 0.4 per million individuals, which is lower than that of ES of the bone by 10-fold [7]. Although uncommon, the occurrence of EES seems to have a bimodal distribution, where there is a peak in the occurrence rate among children (<5 years) and adults (>35 years) [8], with an increased likelihood of presenting among older populations compared to ES of the bone. Unlike Ewing sarcoma of the bone, no evidence supports a link between the tumor and race or biological sex [8–10].

The management of EES includes surgery [11] and chemotherapy [10,12,13] in resectable tumors. Under unresectable conditions, radiotherapy is usually considered [14].

According to the National Comprehensive Cancer Network (NCCN), the optimum management of EES remains not clearly defined [15,16], although some studies have highlighted an added value of surgery among EES cases compared to Ewing sarcoma of the bone in terms of better survival rates [17,18]. In general, the prognosis of EES is more favorable than that of the bone [9,10].

To date, there is no clear picture regarding the occurrence rate of EES among children and adolescents (<21 years), as well as their demographic characteristics, tumor characteristics (i.e., location), treatment modalities, and clinical outcomes (i.e., survival, mortality, recurrence). Therefore, we conducted this systematic review and meta-analysis to provide collective evidence regarding the clinical characteristics and outcomes in this patient population.

2. Materials and Methods

2.1. Study Design and Search Strategy

This systematic review was performed in accordance with the Preferred Reporting Items for Systematic Reviews and Meta-Analyses (PRISMA) guidelines [19]. A protocol was not registered, since it is not mandatory, as per several recommendations [20,21]. On 26 July 2022, PubMed, Scopus, Web of Science, and Google Scholar were searched for articles that report the presentation of EES in the pediatric population (children and young adolescents <21 years of age). Of note, only the first 200 records from Google Scholar were retrieved and screened according to recently published guidelines [22]. We updated the database search on 24 August 2022 to ensure that no additional relevant reports had been published prior to the qualitative and quantitative analyses [23].

We used a combination of keywords and terms in our search, which included the following: ("Ewing Sarcoma" OR "Ewing's Sarcoma") AND (adolescen* OR Child* OR Pediatric* OR "young adult") AND ("soft tissue" OR extraskeletal OR extraosseous) AND (clinicopathologic* OR "clinical feautre" OR "clinical characteristic*" OR "clinical outcome*"). The terms of the Medical Subject Headings (MeSH) were also added (particularly in PubMed) to retrieve all the possibly relevant articles. The detailed search criteria used for each database are described in Supplementary Table S1.

Moreover, we conducted a manual search to find any relevant articles that may have potentially been excluded during the screening phase or were not found during the database search [24,25]. This strategy was conducted through three different approaches: (1) screening the titles of the reference list of the final included papers, (2) reading the titles and abstracts of articles similar to final included studies through the "similar articles" function on PubMed, and (3) conducting a random search on Google using keywords similar to those of the original database search, such as: "Ewing sarcoma" + "child". It is noteworthy that no filters were used during the database search regarding the language of the research paper, year in which the paper was published, or the country of the first author.

2.2. Eligibility Criteria

The methodology and design of this review were conducted as per the PICO framework [26,27], including the population (pediatric cases of EES), intervention (none), comparison (none), and outcome (primary outcome: prevalence rate of EES in children and adolescents; secondary outcomes: clinicodemographic characteristics, tumor characteristics, and clinical outcomes in pediatric cases of EES).

For articles to be included, a study had to: (1) report original data, (2) include cases of EES, (3) report cases aged <21 years. On the other hand, studies were excluded if they were compliant with one of the following criteria: (1) non-original research (i.e., review articles, editorials without human data, commentaries, theses, conference abstracts/posters, and books), (2) animal, in vivo, and in vitro studies, (3) case reports and case series of <5 cases, (4) studies reporting EES cases of mixed ages (children, adolescents, adults, and elderly) without stratifying the cases according to their age, (5) studies reporting Ewing sarcomas of mixed origin (extraosseous and skeletal) in children without stratifying the cases according to their origin, and (6) duplicated records.

2.3. Screening and Study Selection

Following the retrieval of records through the database search [28], the references were imported to EndNote (Version 8) for duplicate removal and to organize the screening sheet [29]. The screening sheet included the following: article ID, list of authors' names, year of publication (YOP), research paper's title, DOI, journal name, and abstract. The screening was carried out in three separate stages: title, abstract, and full-text screening. All of these steps were performed by two sets of two reviewers each. Any differences between the reviewers were reviewed and resolved by the senior author [30].

Significantly, upon reviewing the literature, two categories of articles were found to be consistent with our eligibility criteria. The first group of articles included patients with EES, among whom pediatric cases were counted, and the second group of articles included pediatric cases, of whom the origin of Ewing sarcoma was determined (extraosseous or skeletal). Both of these categories were included, extracted, and presented separately in our review.

2.4. Extraction and Quality Assessment

The data extraction process was carried out in a similar manner as the screening stage [31]. The senior author designed a pilot data extraction sheet through the Excel software (version 2021) that was consistent with the study objectives. The sheet included 5 domains. The first domain highlighted the baseline characteristics of the included studies (authors' names, year of publication, country, study design, sample size, and follow-up duration). The second domain included the demographic characteristics of the included participants, such as age and biological sex. The third domain included the location of the EES among the pediatric cases (i.e., cranium, female genital tract, orbit, head and neck, pelvis, extremities, thorax, abdomen). The fourth domain included the tumor's characteristics (i.e., management modalities (i.e., surgery alone, surgery combined with radiotherapy, surgery combined with chemotherapy, etc.). The final domain included the patients' clinical outcomes in terms of the overall survival (OS), progression-free survival (PFS), disease-specific survival (DSS), secondary metastasis, no evidence of disease (NED), mortality, and recurrence. Two reviewers extracted the data from the included studies for further qualitative and quantitative synthesis, as per the recommended guidelines [32,33].

2.5. Data Synthesis

All quantitative analyses were conducted using the STATA software (version 17) with the metaprop command [34]. The exact cimethod [34] was used to pool the effect size (ES)—occurrence rate of EES in the pediatric cases—along with its 95% confidence interval (CI). Importantly, for the purposes of discussing the findings of our review, the term ES will refer to the effect size and not Ewing sarcoma (which will not be abbreviated in this manuscript). The random-effects and fixed-effects models were used according to the presence or absence of heterogeneity, respectively [35,36]. Heterogeneity was measured using the I^2 statistic, where a value of >50% or a p-value of <0.05 indicates significant heterogeneity.

3. Results
3.1. Search Results

A summary of the results of the electronic database search, as well as the screening stage, is provided in Figure 1. The initial database search resulted in 2611 references, out of which 179 duplicated records were found and removed using the EndNote software (version 8). The titles and abstracts of 2432 articles were screened, resulting in 276 articles eligible for full-text screening. The full texts of six studies were not found and, therefore, these were excluded. A total of 241 studies were excluded as follows: adult cases (n = 22), skeletal involvement (n = 23), case reports (n = 73), duplicated records (n = 2), elderly cases (n = 2), in vitro studies (n = 3), mixed-age populations (n = 82), no data on sarcoma origin (n = 5), non-Ewing sarcoma (n = 23), and reviews (n = 6). The updated and manual search yielded no more studies, so that the final number of included studies was equal to 29 reports. Twenty-four articles reported the rate of childhood cases among those with EES (of all ages), while five studies reported the rate of extraosseous involvement in pediatric Ewing sarcoma (of mixed origin—skeletal and extraosseous) cases.

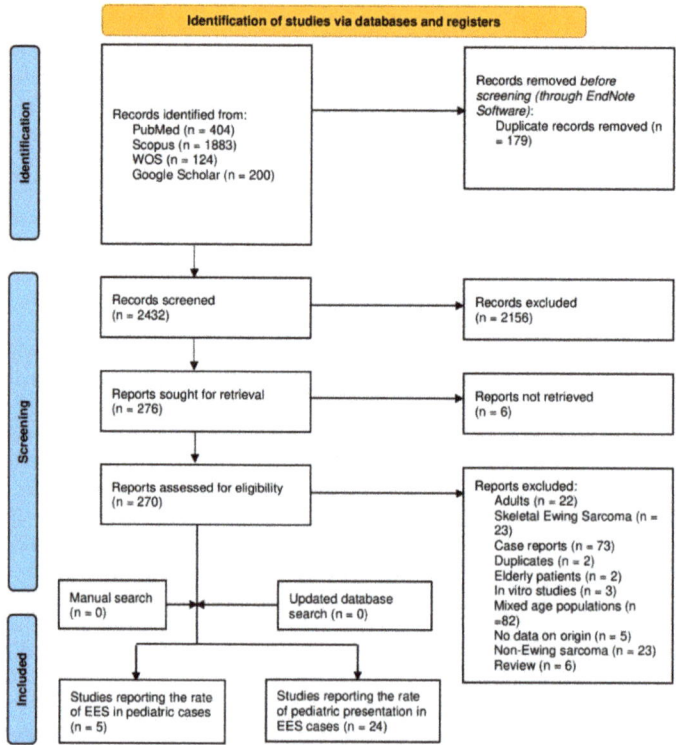

Figure 1. A PRISMA diagram showing the database search and screening results of the review.

3.2. Baseline Characteristics of the Included Studies

The baseline characteristics of the included studies are presented in Table 1. Among the 24 studies that reported the rate of childhood cases among all the EES cases (adults and children), two were conducted in the United Kingdom (UK), two in China, one in Germany, three in India, three in Italy, one in Japan, one in Korea, one in Turkey, and ten in the United States (US). Five studies were case series, fourteen were retrospective chart reviews, one was a registry-based study, three were SEER-based studies, and one was a secondary analysis of three prospective studies. The number of included patients with EES in the individual studies ranged from 8 [37–39] to as high as 3178 [40] patients, with a total sample size of 5752 patients with EES. The follow-up was reported in 16 studies, ranging from as low as 0.9 [41] months to as high as 349 months [42].

Among the five studies that reported the rate of EES among children with ES, one study was conducted in the Netherlands, three in the US, and one in China. Three studies were retrospective chart reviews, one was a multicenter cohort study, and one was a secondary analysis of two clinical trials. The sample size of included pediatric patients with Ewing sarcoma ranged from 18 [43] to 1039 cases [9], with an overall sample size of 1190. The follow-up duration was reported in only two studies ranging from 56.4 [44] to 120 months [45].

Table 1. Baseline characteristics of the included studies.

Author (YOP)	Country	Design	Sample	FU (Months)
Studies reporting the rate of childhood among all EES Cases (adults and children)				
Banerjee (1997) [37]	UK	Case series	8	5–12
Biswas (2014) [46]	India	Chart review	374	25 *
Boyce-Fappiano (2021) [2]	USA	Chart review	60	74 *
Casanova (2007) [47]	Italy	Case series	52	120 *
Chen (2019) [48]	USA	Chart review	31	24.8
Chiang (2017) [49]	USA	Chart review	19	NR
Deshpande (2021) [38]	India	Case series	8	15–43
Gupta (2010) [50]	USA	Chart review	53	46.8 *
Jiang (2018) [40]	China	SEER-based study	3178	NR
Koka (2021) [39]	USA	Case series	8	52.63
Koscielniak (2021) [4]	Germany	Secondary analysis of three prospective studies	243	84 *
Lee (2010) [51]	Korea	Chart review	94	24.9
Livellara (2022) [42]	Italy	Chart review	57	5–349
Muratori (2020) [52]	Italy	Chart review	29	37 *
Murugan (2018) [53]	USA	Chart review	23	5–156
Pradhan (2011) [54]	UK	Chart review	253	87
Qureshi (2013) [55]	India	Chart review	32	NR
Raney (1997) [56]	USA	Registry-based study	130	NR
Neriman (2009) [57]	Turkey	Case series	13	NR
Takenaka (2016) [58]	Japan	Chart review	74	44 *
Tarek (2020) [41]	USA	Chart review	30	0.9
Verma (2017) [59]	USA	SEER-based study	415	NR
Wong (2015) [60]	USA	SEER-based study	550	NR
Xie (2010) [61]	China	Chart review	18	NR
Studies reporting the rate of EES among cases of childhood Ewing sarcoma				
Bosma (2022) [45]	The Netherlands	Multicenter cohort	60	120
Cash (2015) [9]	USA	Secondary analysis of 2 clinical trials	1039	NR
Huh (2017) [44]	USA	Chart review	42	56.4 *
Majeed (2019) [62]	USA	Chart review	31	NR
Xiao (2016) [43]	China	Chart review	18	NR

* Data are reported as the median and not the mean. YOP: year of publication; USA: United States of America; NR: not reported; UK: United Kingdom; FU: follow-up; EES: extraosseous Ewing sarcoma.

3.3. Demographic Characteristics of the Included Participants

The demographic characteristics of the included patients are illustrated in Table 2. Among the studies that included patients with EES regardless of their age, the rate of affected children ranged from as low as 5.63% (31 out of 550 cases) [60] to as high as 100% [55,56]. The pooled rate of childhood EES among the patients with EES was 30% [3001 patients, 95%CI: 29–31%; I^2 = 99.01%]. Out of the pediatric cases diagnosed with EES, 52.45% were males (224 out of 427 patients).

Table 2. The demographic characteristics of the included participants in each study with an overall estimation of the rate of the presentation with EES in childhood.

Author (YOP)	Rate of Pediatric Cases in EES				Biological Sex (Male)		
	N	T	%	Definition	N	T	%
Studies reporting the rate of childhood among all EES cases (adults and children)							
Banerjee (1997) [37]	6	8	75.00%	9–17	3	6	50%
Biswas (2014) [46]	29	60	48.33%	≤15	-	-	-
Boyce-Fappiano (2021) [2]	14	60	23.33%	≤20	-	-	-
Casanova (2007) [47]	9	9	100.00%	1–18	-	-	-
Chen (2019) [48]	17	31	54.83%	<20	-	-	-
Chiang (2017) [49]	4	19	21.05%	12–16	0	4	0%
Deshpande (2021) [38]	6	8	75.00%	1–13	2	6	33.33%
Gupta (2010) [50]	2	29	6.89%	0.3–16.2	-	-	-
Jiang (2018) [40]	413	981	42.09%	0–19	-	-	-
Koka (2021) [39]	4	8	50.00%	2–8	4	4	100%
Koscielniak (2021) [4]	221	243	90.94%	1–21	118	221	53.39%
Lee (2010) [51]	21	94	22.34%	≤12	-	-	-
Livellara (2022) [42]	18	57	31.57%	≤12	-	-	-
Muratori (2020) [52]	20	29	68.96%	<20	-	-	-
Murugan (2018) [53]	4	23	17.39%	8–19	2	4	50%
Pradhan (2011) [54]	70	129	54.26%	<16	-	-	-
Qureshi (2013) [55]	32	32	100.00%	1–19	23	32	71.87%
Raney (1997) [56]	130	130	100.00%	1–20	61	130	46.92%
Neriman (2009) [57]	13	13	100.00%	-	7	13	53.84%
Takenaka (2016) [58]	3	25	12.00%	-	-	-	-
Tarek (2020) [41]	7	30	23.33%	1–19	4	7	57.14%
Verma (2017) [59]	164	415	39.51%	0–18	-	-	-
Wong (2015) [60]	31	550	5.63%	<12 months	-	-	-
Xie (2010) [61]	9	18	50.00%	<18	-	-	-
Total	1247	3001	ES = 0.30 [95%CI: 0.29–0.31]		224	427	52.45%

Author (YOP)	Rate of EES in Pediatric Cases				Biological sex (Male)		
	N	T	%		N	T	%
Studies reporting the rate of EES among cases of childhood Ewing sarcoma							
Bosma (2022) [45]	6	60	10.00%	-	-	-	-
Cash (2015) [9]	213	1039	20.50%	-	116	213	54.46%
Huh (2017) [44]	6	42	14.28%	-	-	-	-
Majeed (2019) [62]	10	31	32.25%	-	-	-	-
Xiao (2016) [43]	10	18	55.55%	-	6	10	60.00%
Total	245	1190	ES = 0.22 [95%CI: 0.13–0.31]		122	223	54.70%

YOP: year of publication, N: number, T: total sample size, EES: extraosseous Ewing sarcoma.

Among the studies that included pediatric cases of Ewing sarcoma regardless of its origin, the rate of presentation with a disease of extraosseous origin ranged from 10% (6 out of 60 cases) [45] to 55.55% (10 out of 18 cases) [42], with an overall pooled rate of 22%

[1190 patients, 95%CI: 13–31%; I^2 = 19.28%]. Out of the pediatric cases diagnosed with EES, 54.70% (122 out of 223) were males.

3.4. The Location of EES in the Pediatric Cases

Among the included studies, only 13 reported data regarding the location of EES among the pediatric cases (Table 3). The pooled meta-analysis revealed that the thorax was the predominant site where EES occurred [33%; 95%CI: 20–46%] followed by the extremities [31%; 95%CI: 22–40%], the head and neck [14%; 95%CI: 7–21%], the pelvis [13%; 95%CI: 9–16%], the abdomen [10%; 95%CI: 4–16%], the spine [8%; 95%CI: 6–11%], the intracranial space [8%; 95%CI: 1–33%], and finally the orbit [2%; 95%CI: 0–4%]. Of note, among the pediatric cases, the occurrence of EES in the skin, the kidney, and the female genital tract was scarcely reported, and the performance of a meta-analysis was not feasible due to the lack of sufficient data.

Table 3. The location of extraosseous Ewing sarcoma in the pediatric cases.

Author (YOP)	Total	Skin—Subcutaneous Tissue (N)	Kidney (N)	Intra-cranial (N)	Female Genital Tract (N)	Orbit (N)	H&N (N)	Pelvis (N)	Spine (N)	Thorax (N)	Abdomen (N)	Extremity (N)
Banerjee (1997) [37]	6	6	-	-	-	-	-	-	-	-	-	-
Biswas (2014) [46]	-	-	-	-	-	-	-	-	-	-	-	-
Boyce-Fappiano (2021) [2]	-	-	-	-	-	-	-	-	-	-	-	-
Casanova (2007) [47]	-	-	-	-	-	-	-	-	-	-	-	-
Chen (2019) [48]	17	-	-	17	-	-	-	-	-	-	-	-
Chiang (2017) [49]	4	-	-	-	4	-	-	-	-	-	-	-
Deshpande (2021) [38]	6	-	-	6	-	-	-	-	-	-	-	-
Gupta (2010) [50]	-	-	-	-	-	-	-	-	-	-	-	-
Jiang (2018) [40]	-	-	-	-	-	-	-	-	-	-	-	-
Koka (2021) [39]	4	-	-	-	-	4	-	-	-	-	-	-
Koscielniak (2021) [4]	221	-	-	-	-	-	40	26	23	48	24	65
Lee (2010) [51]	-	-	-	-	-	-	-	-	-	-	-	-
Livellara (2022) [42]	-	-	-	-	-	-	-	-	-	-	-	-
Muratori (2020) [52]	-	-	-	-	-	-	-	-	-	-	-	-
Murugan (2018) [53]	4	-	4	-	-	-	-	-	-	-	-	-
Pradhan (2011) [54]	-	-	-	-	-	-	-	-	-	-	-	-
Qureshi (2013) [55]	32	-	-	-	-	-	-	11	-	-	1	19
Raney (1997) [56]	130	-	-	-	-	2	8	-	-	32	20	26
Neriman (2009) [57]	13	-	-	1	-	3	-	-	-	-	-	5
Takenaka (2016) [58]	-	-	-	-	-	-	-	-	-	-	-	-
Tarek (2020) [41]	7	-	7	-	-	-	-	-	-	-	-	-
Verma (2017) [59]	-	-	-	-	-	-	-	-	-	-	-	-
Wong (2015) [60]	-	-	-	-	-	-	-	-	-	-	-	-
Xie (2010) [61]	-	-	-	-	-	-	-	-	-	-	-	-
Bosma (2022) [45]	-	-	-	-	-	-	-	-	-	-	-	-
Cash (2015) [9]	213	-	-	-	-	-	17	29	15	92	-	56
Huh (2017) [44]	-	-	-	-	-	-	-	-	-	-	-	-
Majeed (2019) [62]	-	-	-	-	-	-	-	-	-	-	-	-
Xiao (2016) [43]	10	-	-	-	-	-	2	1	0	6	-	0
Total	N/T	6/6	11/11	24/36	4/4	9/147	78/606	56/444	38/444	178/574	45/383	171/619
	%	100	100	66.66	100	6.12	12.87	12.61	8.55	31.01	11.75	27.62
ES [95%CI]		N/A	N/A	0.08 [0.01–0.33]	N/A	0.02 [0.0–0.04]	0.14 [0.07–0.21]	0.13 [0.09–0.16]	0.08 [0.06–0.11]	0.33 [0.20–0.46]	0.10 [0.04–0.16]	0.31 [0.22–0.40]

YOP: year of publication; N: number of cases; T: total number of pediatric cases of EES; EES: extraosseous Ewing sarcoma; H&N: head and neck; ES: effect size; CI: confidence interval.

3.5. The Characteristics of EES among the Pediatric Cases

Among the included studies, the management modalities in childhood EES were described and reported in ten studies (Table 4), among which concurrent chemotherapy and radiotherapy [13 patients, 57%; 95%CI: 25–84%] was the most frequently employed treatment protocol, followed by surgery combined with radiotherapy [236 patients, 55%; 95%CI: 28–82%], surgery alone [223 patients, 53%; 95%CI: 37–68%], surgery combined with chemotherapy [36 patients, 29%; 95%CI: 5–52%], and finally radiotherapy alone [219 patients, 16%; 95%CI: 11–21%].

Table 4. Trends in the management modalities of pediatric cases of extraosseous Ewing sarcoma reported in the literature.

Author (YOP)	Surgery Alone		RT Alone		Surgery + RT		Surgery + CT		Concurrent CT with RT	
	N	T	N	T	N	T	N	T	N	T
Banerjee (1997) [37]	-	-	-	-	-	-	3	6	-	-
Biswas (2014) [46]	-	-	-	-	-	-	-	-	-	-
Boyce-Fappiano (2021) [2]	-	-	-	-	-	-	-	-	-	-
Casanova (2007) [47]	-	-	-	-	6	9	-	-	6	6
Chen (2019) [48]	-	-	-	-	-	-	-	-	-	-
Chiang (2017) [49]	3	4	-	-	1	4	0	4	-	-
Deshpande (2021) [38]	-	-	-	-	5	6	1	6	-	-
Gupta (2010) [50]	-	-	-	-	-	-	-	-	-	-
Jiang (2018) [40]	-	-	-	-	-	-	-	-	-	-
Koka (2021) [39]	-	-	-	-	3	4	-	-	-	-
Koscielniak (2021) [4]	-	-	-	-	-	-	-	-	-	-
Lee (2010) [51]	-	-	-	-	-	-	-	-	-	-
Livellara (2022) [42]	-	-	-	-	-	-	-	-	-	-
Muratori (2020) [52]	-	-	-	-	-	-	-	-	-	-
Murugan (2018) [53]	-	-	-	-	-	-	-	-	-	-
Pradhan (2011) [54]	-	-	-	-	-	-	-	-	-	-
Qureshi (2013) [55]	-	-	-	-	-	-	-	-	-	-
Raney (1997) [56]	-	-	-	-	-	-	-	-	-	-
Neriman (2009) [57]	-	-	-	-	-	-	13	13	-	-
Takenaka (2016) [58]	-	-	-	-	-	-	-	-	-	-
Tarek (2020) [41]	-	-	-	-	-	-	7	7	4	7
Verma (2017) [59]	-	-	-	-	-	-	-	-	-	-
Wong (2015) [60]	-	-	-	-	-	-	-	-	-	-
Xie (2010) [61]	-	-	-	-	-	-	-	-	-	-
Bosma (2022) [45]	4	6	1	6	-	-	-	-	-	-
Cash (2015) [9]	99	213	34	213	63	213	-	-	-	-
Huh (2017) [44]	-	-	-	-	-	-	-	-	-	-
Majeed (2019) [62]	-	-	-	-	-	-	-	-	-	-
Xiao (2016) [43]	-	-	-	-	-	-	-	-	-	-
Total	106	223	35	219	78	236	24	36	10	13
%	47.53%		15.98%		33.05%		66.67%		76.92%	
ES [95%CI]	0.53 [0.37–0.68]		0.16 [0.11–0.21]		0.55 [0.28–0.82]		0.29 [0.05–0.52]		0.57 [0.25–0.84]	

YOP: year of publication; CT: chemotherapy; RT: radiotherapy; ES: effect size; CI: confidence interval; N: number of cases; T: total sample of pediatric cases of EES; EES: extraosseous Ewing sarcoma.

3.6. The Clinical Outcomes of EES among the Pediatric Cases

The clinical outcomes associated with childhood EES are presented in Table 5. The 5-year OS was reported in 11 studies, out of which 664/1066 pediatric EES cases survived. The pooled 5-year OS rate was 69% [95%CI: 56–81%]. The 5-year PFS, DSS, and DMFS were reported in only a single study, which was not enough to derive conclusions or be for the data to be included in a meta-analysis. Seven studies reported no evidence of disease among 257 out of the 288 cases, with a pooled rate of 69% [95%CI: 51–87%]. Morality was reported in ten studies, where 120 deaths occurred among 404 pediatric cases of EES, with a pooled mortality rate of 29% [95%CI: 25–33%]. Meanwhile, recurrence was reported in five studies (19 cases out of 60 pediatric EES cases), with a pooled recurrence rate of 35% [95%CI: 16–54%]. Finally, secondary metastasis was reported in three studies, occurring in 38 cases out of 236 pediatric EES patients, with a pooled rate of 16% [95%CI: 11–21%].

Table 5. The clinical outcomes of pediatric patients with extraosseous Ewing sarcoma.

Author (YOP)	5-Year OS		5-Year PFS		5-Year DSS		5-Year DMFS		Mortality		NED		Recurrence		Secondary Metastasis	
	N	T	N	T	N	T	N	T	N	T	N	T	N	T	N	T
Banerjee (1997) [37]	-	-	-	-	-	-	-	-	1	6	-	-	-	-	1	6
Biswas (2014) [46]	16	29	11	29	-	-	-	-	-	-	-	-	-	-	-	-
Boyce-Fappiano (2021) [2]	-	-	-	-	12	14	9	14	-	-	9	14	-	-	-	-
Casanova (2007) [47]	9	9	-	-	-	-	-	-	1	9	-	-	-	-	1	9
Chen (2019) [48]	-	-	-	-	-	-	-	-	-	-	-	-	-	-	-	-
Chiang (2017) [49]	-	-	-	-	-	-	-	-	1	4	2	4	-	-	-	-
Deshpande (2021) [38]	-	-	-	-	-	-	-	-	1	6	4	6	2	6	-	-
Gupta (2010) [50]	-	-	-	-	-	-	-	-	-	-	-	-	-	-	-	-
Jiang (2018) [40]	268	413	-	-	-	-	-	-	-	-	-	-	-	-	-	-
Koka (2021) [39]	-	-	-	-	-	-	-	-	1	4	3	4	-	-	-	-
Koscielniak (2021) [4]	73	221	-	-	-	-	-	-	65	221	209	221	-	-	36	221
Lee (2010) [51]	16	21	-	-	-	-	-	-	-	-	-	-	-	-	-	-
Livellara (2022) [42]	17	18	-	-	-	-	-	-	-	-	-	-	-	-	-	-
Muratori (2020) [52]	14	20	-	-	-	-	-	-	-	-	-	-	-	-	-	-
Murugan (2018) [53]	-	-	-	-	-	-	-	-	1	4	-	-	1	4	-	-
Pradhan (2011) [54]	-	-	-	-	-	-	-	-	-	-	-	-	-	-	-	-
Qureshi (2013) [55]	26	32	-	-	-	-	-	-	-	-	29	32	6	32	-	-
Raney (1997) [56]	61	87	-	-	-	-	-	-	42	130	-	-	-	-	-	-
Neriman (2009) [57]	-	-	-	-	-	-	-	-	4	13	-	-	7	11	-	-
Takenaka (2016) [58]	2	3	-	-	-	-	-	-	-	-	-	-	-	-	-	-
Tarek (2020) [41]	-	-	-	-	-	-	-	-	3	7	1	7	3	7	-	-
Verma (2017) [59]	-	-	-	-	-	-	-	-	-	-	-	-	-	-	-	-
Wong (2015) [60]	-	-	-	-	-	-	-	-	-	-	-	-	-	-	-	-
Xie (2010) [61]	-	-	-	-	-	-	-	-	-	-	-	-	-	-	-	-
Bosma (2022) [45]	-	-	-	-	-	-	-	-	-	-	-	-	-	-	-	-
Cash (2015) [9]	162	213	-	-	-	-	-	-	-	-	-	-	-	-	-	-
Huh (2017) [44]	-	-	-	-	-	-	-	-	-	-	-	-	-	-	-	-
Majeed (2019) [62]	-	-	-	-	-	-	-	-	-	-	-	-	-	-	-	-
Xiao (2016) [43]	-	-	-	-	-	-	-	-	-	-	-	-	-	-	-	-
Total	664	1066	11	29	12	14	9	14	120	404	257	288	19	60	38	236
%	62.28%		37.93%		85.71%		64.28%		29.70%		89.23%		31.66%		16.10%	
ES [95%CI]	0.69 [0.56–0.81]		N/A		N/A		N/A		0.29 [0.25–0.33]		0.69 [0.51–0.87]		0.35 [0.16–0.54]		0.16 [0.11–0.21]	

YOP: year of publication; N: number of cases of the outcome; T: total number of pediatric cases of EES; EES: extraosseous Ewing sarcoma; ES: effect size; CI: confidence interval; OS: overall survival; PFS: progression-free survival; DSS: disease-specific survival; NED: no evidence of disease; DMFS: distant-metastatic free survival; N/A: not applicable for meta-analysis

4. Discussion

There is limited evidence regarding the occurrence rate and clinical characteristics of EES in children. Our systematic review is the first to comprehensively discuss the prevalence, clinical features, and outcomes of EES patients of pediatric age (less than 21 years). A summary of our key findings can be found in Table 6. Overall, a total of

29 studies reporting on 5752 patients were analyzed. In our study, we found that the rate of affected children and adolescents with EES in a population with EES (mixed age) varied substantially between the studies, ranging from 5.63% [60] to as high as 100% [55]. This discrepancy could be related to the design and methodology of the included studies, since some studies included patients with EES regardless of the age group at baseline, while a few studies included pediatric cases of EES at baseline [55,56]. Overall, our meta-analysis revealed that 30% of the EES cases occurred among children and adolescents. Consistent with previous observations [8,9], no link was noted between EES presentation in children and biological sex. The pooled rate of male pediatric patients with EES was 52.45%, which is relatively similar to that of female cases (47.55%).

Table 6. Summary of the key findings on the pediatric EES cases in our review.

Outcome	Category	The Rate of Children among Patients with EES	The Rate of Extraosseous Origin in Pediatric Cases of ES
Prevalence			
	N/T	1247/3001	245/1190
	% [95%CI]	30% [29–31%]	22% [13–31%]
Biological sex			
	N/T	224/427	122/223
	%	52.45%	54.70%
Location of EES in pediatric cases			
Most common	Thorax	33% [20–46%]	
	Extremity	31% [22–40%]	
Least common	Orbit	2% [0–4%]	
Clinical outcomes			
	5-year OS	69% [56–81%]	
	Mortality	29% [25–33%]	
	NED	69% [51–87%]	
	Recurrence	35% [16–54%]	
	2ry metastasis	16% [11–21%]	

In addition, five studies included children affected with ES at baseline, and then the origin of the tumor was analyzed in these cases. The rate of EES out of all the ES types ranged from 10% to 55.55% among the individual studies. Again, the difference in reported rates could be related to the design and methodology implemented in each study. That being said, in our meta-analysis, the rate of EES occurrence among the pediatric ES cases was 22%, of whom 54.70% were males.

Data on the location of EES among pediatric cases is scarce, since the majority of the available studies in the literature include patients with mixed ages and tend to stratify the outcomes (i.e., survival) based on age (children vs. adults or the elderly), without stratifying the clinical characteristics or tumor characteristics based on the age of the examined patients. Therefore, the data reported in our review regarding the EES location in the pediatric cases rely mainly on case series with a case-by-case description of the tumor characteristics. Thirteen studies reported relevant data on the location of EES, and our pooled meta-analysis revealed that the thorax is the most predominant origin for EES in children and adolescents, followed by the extremities, the head and neck, the pelvis, the abdomen, the spine, and the intracranial space, respectively. In certain cases, the EES originated in the orbit among the pediatric cases; however, the occurrence rate did not surpass the rare event assumption (>5%). Additionally, other sites, such as the great toe [63], the mesocolon [64], the frontal sinus [65], and the penis [66], have been described as rare cases. Moreover, the kidneys [41,53], the skin [37], and the female genital tract [49] have been reported as sites of origin of EES in pediatric cases in several case series; however, not enough data were present to perform a meta-analysis of the prevalence in this case.

There is a debate on the best management approach for EES cases occurring in children, and this uncertainty is related to the rarity of EES, the discrepancy in its clinical presentation, and the differences in the patients' characteristics [67]. In addition, this patient population is underrepresented in clinical trials directed towards the investigation of the efficacy and safety of various treatment modalities among pediatric cases of EES. In our review, only ten studies reported the treatment modalities according to different age groups, and the majority of the data were pooled from case series. Overall, the majority of cases were treated with concurrent chemotherapy and radiotherapy (57% of cases), followed by surgery and radiotherapy (55%), surgery alone (53%), surgery and chemotherapy (29%), and radiotherapy alone in cases of unresectable tumors (16%). It is important to mention that the confidence interval of these reported rates is wide, reflecting the imprecision of the reported effect estimates. Therefore, these data should be interpreted with caution and should not be perceived as representative of the EES pediatric population. More data from properly designed research studies are still needed to confirm this observation. Additionally, the available data did not present survival outcomes stratified by these treatment modalities in the pediatric cases separately. Therefore, future studies should carefully consider stratifying data (clinical characteristics and outcomes) based on the origin of the tumor (skeletal vs. extraskeletal) and age of the included patients (children vs. adults vs. the elderly).

In our study, we found that a great proportion of pediatric EES patients have a preferable prognosis in terms of their 5-year overall survival (with an overall rate of 69%), which is consistent with that of cases with no evidence of disease following treatment (an overall rate of 69%). However, mortality was documented in almost one-third of the pediatric EES population (120 deaths out of 404 cases, an overall rate of 29%). Additionally, recurrence was reported in 35% of cases, while secondary metastasis was reported in 16%. That being said, these rates should be based on the available data of 11 studies out of the 29 studies included in our review. Therefore, the presented data are not generalizable to the whole EES pediatric population.

Meanwhile, our review has several limitations. The most important is the fact that our estimates regarding the prevalence of childhood EES among EES cases (of all ages) or the prevalence of cases of extraosseous origin among the pediatric Ewing sarcoma cases could be overestimated, since the majority of the included studies investigated EES cases and not the Ewing sarcoma population as a whole. In addition, most of these studies are based on retrospective analyses and not cross-sectional in design, which further limits the generalizability of our findings.

5. Conclusions

Although it is difficult to draw solid conclusions, our results highlight the proportion of children affected by extraosseous Ewing sarcoma, with a special focus on the demographic characteristics, tumor characteristics, and clinical outcomes of the affected patients.

Supplementary Materials: The following supporting information can be downloaded at: https://www.mdpi.com/article/10.3390/children9121859/s1, Table S1: The detailed search strategy employed in each electronic database.

Author Contributions: Conceptualization: M.G. and A.H.; methodology: M.G. and A.H.; software: M.G., A.H. and M.K.; validation: M.G., A.H. and M.K.; investigation: M.G., A.H. and M.K.; writing—original draft preparation: A.H. and M.G.; writing—review and editing: A.H., M.G., B.L., M.K., J.B., A.G. and T.R.; visualization: M.G. All authors have read and agreed to the published version of the manuscript.

Funding: This research received no external funding.

Institutional Review Board Statement: Not applicable.

Informed Consent Statement: Not applicable.

Data Availability Statement: The data presented in this manuscript can be provided by the corresponding author upon reasonable request.

Conflicts of Interest: The authors declare no conflict of interest. Regardless, Tobias Renkawitz has received research support and personal fees from Arbeitsgemeinschaft Endoprothetik (AE), DGOU, DGOOC, BVOU, DePuy International, the Otto Bock Foundation, Deutsche Arthrose Hilfe, Aesculap, Zimmer, Stiftung Oskar Helene Heim Berlin, Vielberth Foundation Regensburg, the German Ministry of Education and Research, as well as the German Federal Ministry of Economic Cooperation and Development. Axel Horsch received research support from Arthrose Hilfe and Ipsen.

References

1. Abboud, A.; Masrouha, K.; Saliba, M.; Haidar, R.; Saab, R.; Khoury, N.; Tawil, A.; Saghieh, S. Extraskeletal Ewing sarcoma: Diagnosis, management and prognosis. *Oncol. Lett.* **2021**, *21*, 354. [CrossRef]
2. Boyce-Fappiano, D.; Guadagnolo, B.A.; Ratan, R.; Wang, W.L.; Wagner, M.J.; Patel, S.; Livingston, J.A.; Lin, P.P.; Diao, K.; Mitra, D. Evaluating the soft tissue sarcoma paradigm for the local management of extraskeletal Ewing sarcoma. *Oncologist* **2021**, *26*, 250–260. [CrossRef]
3. Bradford, K.; Nobori, A.; Johnson, B.; Allen-Rhoades, W.; Naik-Mathuria, B.; Panosyan, E.H.; Gotesman, M.; Lasky, J.; Cheng, J.; Ikeda, A. Primary renal Ewing sarcoma in children and young adults. *J. Pediatr. Hematol. Oncol.* **2020**, *42*, 474. [CrossRef]
4. Koscielniak, E.; Sparber-Sauer, M.; Scheer, M.; Vokuhl, C.; Kazanowska, B.; Ladenstein, R.; Niggli, F.; Ljungman, G.; Paulussen, M.; Bielack, S.S. Extraskeletal Ewing sarcoma in children, adolescents, and young adults. An analysis of three prospective studies of the Cooperative Weichteilsarkomstudiengruppe (CWS). *Pediatr. Blood Cancer* **2021**, *68*, e29145. [CrossRef]
5. Balamuth, N.J.; Womer, R.B. Ewing's sarcoma. *Lancet. Oncol.* **2010**, *11*, 184–192. [CrossRef]
6. Iwamoto, Y. Diagnosis and treatment of Ewing's sarcoma. *Jpn. J. Clin. Oncol.* **2007**, *37*, 79–89. [CrossRef]
7. Van den Berg, H.; Heinen, R.C.; van der Pal, H.J.; Merks, J.H. Extra-osseous Ewing sarcoma. *Pediatr. Hematol. Oncol.* **2009**, *26*, 175–185. [CrossRef]
8. Applebaum, M.A.; Worch, J.; Matthay, K.K.; Goldsby, R.; Neuhaus, J.; West, D.C.; Dubois, S.G. Clinical features and outcomes in patients with extraskeletal Ewing sarcoma. *Cancer* **2011**, *117*, 3027–3032. [CrossRef]
9. Cash, T.; McIlvaine, E.; Krailo, M.D.; Lessnick, S.L.; Lawlor, E.R.; Laack, N.; Sorger, J.; Marina, N.; Grier, H.E.; Granowetter, L.; et al. Comparison of clinical features and outcomes in patients with extraskeletal versus skeletal localized Ewing sarcoma: A report from the Children's Oncology Group. *Pediatr. Blood Cancer* **2016**, *63*, 1771–1779. [CrossRef]
10. Lynch, A.D.; Gani, F.; Meyer, C.F.; Morris, C.D.; Ahuja, N.; Johnston, F.M. Extraskeletal versus Skeletal Ewing Sarcoma in the adult population: Controversies in care. *Surg. Oncol.* **2018**, *27*, 373–379. [CrossRef]
11. Bailey, K.; Cost, C.; Davis, I.; Glade-Bender, J.; Grohar, P.; Houghton, P.; Isakoff, M.; Stewart, E.; Laack, N.; Yustein, J. Emerging novel agents for patients with advanced Ewing sarcoma: A report from the Children's Oncology Group (COG) New Agents for Ewing Sarcoma Task Force. *F1000Research* **2019**, *8*, 493. [CrossRef]
12. Mori, Y.; Kinoshita, S.; Kanamori, T.; Kataoka, H.; Joh, T.; Iida, S.; Takemoto, M.; Kondo, M.; Kuroda, J.; Komatsu, H. The successful treatment of metastatic extraosseous Ewing sarcoma with pazopanib. *Intern. Med.* **2018**, *57*, 2753–2757. [CrossRef]
13. Saiz, A.M.; Gingrich, A.A.; Canter, R.J.; Kirane, A.R.; Monjazeb, A.M.; Randall, R.L.; Thorpe, S.W. Role of radiation therapy in adult extraskeletal Ewing's sarcoma patients treated with chemotherapy and surgery. *Sarcoma* **2019**, *2019*, 5413527. [CrossRef]
14. Dunst, J.; Schuck, A. Role of radiotherapy in Ewing tumors. *Pediatr. Blood Cancer* **2004**, *42*, 465–470. [CrossRef]
15. Biermann, J.S. Updates in the treatment of bone cancer. *J. Natl. Compr. Cancer Netw.* **2013**, *11*, 681–683. [CrossRef]
16. Casali, P.G.; Bielack, S.; Abecassis, N.; Aro, H.T.; Bauer, S.; Biagini, R.; Bonvalot, S.; Boukovinas, I.; Bovee, J.; Brennan, B.; et al. Bone sarcomas: ESMO-PaedCan-EURACAN Clinical Practice Guidelines for diagnosis, treatment and follow-up. *Ann. Oncol. Off. J. Eur. Soc. Med. Oncol.* **2018**, *29*, iv79–iv95. [CrossRef]
17. Covelli, H.D.; Beekman, J.F.; Kingry, R.L. Extraskeletal Ewing's sarcoma: Prolonged survival with recurrence after operation. *South. Med. J.* **1980**, *73*, 1294–1295. [CrossRef]
18. Rud, N.P.; Reiman, H.M.; Pritchard, D.J.; Frassica, F.J.; Smithson, W.A. Extraosseous Ewing's sarcoma. A study of 42 cases. *Cancer* **1989**, *64*, 1548–1553. [CrossRef]
19. Page, M.J.; McKenzie, J.E.; Bossuyt, P.M.; Boutron, I.; Hoffmann, T.C.; Mulrow, C.D.; Shamseer, L.; Tetzlaff, J.M.; Akl, E.A.; Brennan, S.E. The PRISMA 2020 statement: An updated guideline for reporting systematic reviews. *Syst. Rev.* **2021**, *10*, 89. [CrossRef]
20. Booth, A.; Sutton, A.; Clowes, M.; Martyn-St James, M. *Systematic Approaches to a Successful Literature Review*; SAGE: Thousand Oaks, CA, USA, 2021.
21. Liang, L.; Hou, X.; Bailey, K.R.; Zhang, Y.; Tymchak, W.; Qi, Z.; Li, W.; Banh, H.L. The association between hyperuricemia and coronary artery calcification development: A systematic review and meta-analysis. *Clin. Cardiol.* **2019**, *42*, 1079–1086. [CrossRef]

22. Muka, T.; Glisic, M.; Milic, J.; Verhoog, S.; Bohlius, J.; Bramer, W.; Chowdhury, R.; Franco, O.H. A 24-step guide on how to design, conduct, and successfully publish a systematic review and meta-analysis in medical research. *Eur. J. Epidemiol.* **2020**, *35*, 49–60. [CrossRef] [PubMed]
23. Atkinson, L.Z.; Cipriani, A. How to carry out a literature search for a systematic review: A practical guide. *BJPsych Adv.* **2018**, *24*, 74–82. [CrossRef]
24. Delgado-Rodríguez, M.; Sillero-Arenas, M. Systematic review and meta-analysis. *Med. Intensiv. (Engl. Ed.)* **2018**, *42*, 444–453. [CrossRef]
25. Tawfik, G.M.; Dila, K.A.S.; Mohamed, M.Y.F.; Tam, D.N.H.; Kien, N.D.; Ahmed, A.M.; Huy, N.T. A step by step guide for conducting a systematic review and meta-analysis with simulation data. *Trop. Med. Health* **2019**, *47*, 46. [CrossRef]
26. Eriksen, M.B.; Frandsen, T.F. The impact of patient, intervention, comparison, outcome (PICO) as a search strategy tool on literature search quality: A systematic review. *J. Med. Libr. Assoc. JMLA* **2018**, *106*, 420. [CrossRef] [PubMed]
27. Santos, C.M.d.C.; Pimenta, C.A.d.M.; Nobre, M.R.C. The PICO strategy for the research question construction and evidence search. *Rev. Lat. Am. Enferm.* **2007**, *15*, 508–511. [CrossRef]
28. Bethel, A.C.; Rogers, M.; Abbott, R. Use of a search summary table to improve systematic review search methods, results, and efficiency. *J. Med. Libr. Assoc. JMLA* **2021**, *109*, 97. [CrossRef]
29. Bramer, W.M.; Giustini, D.; de Jonge, G.B.; Holland, L.; Bekhuis, T. De-duplication of database search results for systematic reviews in EndNote. *J. Med. Libr. Assoc. JMLA* **2016**, *104*, 240. [CrossRef]
30. Ghogomu, E.A.; Maxwell, L.J.; Buchbinder, R.; Rader, T.; Pardo, J.P.; Johnston, R.V.; Christensen, R.D.; Rutjes, A.W.; Winzenberg, T.M.; Singh, J.A. Updated method guidelines for cochrane musculoskeletal group systematic reviews and metaanalyses. *J. Rheumatol.* **2014**, *41*, 194–205. [CrossRef]
31. Sargeant, J.; O'Connor, A. Conducting systematic reviews of intervention questions II: Relevance screening, data extraction, assessing risk of bias, presenting the results and interpreting the findings. *Zoonoses Public Health* **2014**, *61*, 39–51. [CrossRef]
32. Büchter, R.B.; Weise, A.; Pieper, D. Development, testing and use of data extraction forms in systematic reviews: A review of methodological guidance. *BMC Med. Res. Methodol.* **2020**, *20*, 259. [CrossRef] [PubMed]
33. Rao, S.; Moon, K. Literature search for systematic reviews. In *Principles and Practice of Systematic Reviews and Meta-Analysis*; Springer: Berlin/Heidelberg, Germany, 2021; pp. 11–31.
34. Nyaga, V.N.; Arbyn, M.; Aerts, M. Metaprop: A Stata command to perform meta-analysis of binomial data. *Arch. Public Health* **2014**, *72*, 39. [CrossRef] [PubMed]
35. Higgins, J.P.; Thompson, S.G. Quantifying heterogeneity in a meta-analysis. *Stat. Med.* **2002**, *21*, 1539–1558. [CrossRef] [PubMed]
36. Petitti, D.B. Approaches to heterogeneity in meta-analysis. *Stat. Med.* **2001**, *20*, 3625–3633. [CrossRef]
37. Banerjee, S.S.; Agbamu, D.; Eyden, B.P.; Harris, M. Clinicopathological characteristics of peripheral primitive neuroectodermal tumour of skin and subcutaneous tissue. *Histopathology* **1997**, *31*, 355–366. [CrossRef]
38. Deshpande, G.; Epari, S.; Gupta, C.; Shetty, O.; Gurav, M.; Chinnaswamy, G.; Moiyadi, A.; Gupta, T. Primary intracranial Ewing sarcoma/peripheral primitive neuroectodermal tumor, an entity of unacquaintance: A series of 8 cases. *Child's Nerv. Syst.* **2021**, *37*, 839–849. [CrossRef]
39. Koka, K.; Rahim, F.E.; El-Hadad, C.; Bell, D.; Debnam, J.M.; Guo, Y.; Esmaeli, B. Primary Ewing's sarcoma with orbit involvement: Survival and visual outcomes after eye-sparing multidisciplinary management in eight patients. *Head Neck* **2021**, *43*, 3857–3865. [CrossRef]
40. Jiang, S.; Wang, G.; Chen, J.; Dong, Y. Comparison of clinical features and outcomes in patients with extraskeletal vs skeletal Ewing sarcoma: An SEER database analysis of 3,178 cases. *Cancer Manag. Res.* **2018**, *10*, 6227. [CrossRef]
41. Tarek, N.; Said, R.; Andersen, C.R.; Suki, T.S.; Foglesong, J.; Herzog, C.E.; Tannir, N.M.; Patel, S.; Ratan, R.; Ludwig, J.A. Primary ewing sarcoma/primitive neuroectodermal tumor of the kidney: The md anderson cancer center experience. *Cancers* **2020**, *12*, 2927. [CrossRef]
42. Livellara, V.; Bergamaschi, L.; Puma, N.; Chiaravalli, S.; Podda, M.; Casanova, M.; Gasparini, P.; Pecori, E.; Alessandro, O.; Nigro, O. Extraosseous Ewing sarcoma in children and adolescents: A retrospective series from a referral pediatric oncology center. *Pediatr. Blood Cancer* **2022**, *69*, e29512. [CrossRef]
43. Xiao, H.; Bao, F.; Tan, H.; Wang, B.; Liu, W.; Gao, J.; Gao, X. CT and clinical findings of peripheral primitive neuroectodermal tumour in children. *Br. J. Radiol.* **2016**, *89*, 20140450. [CrossRef]
44. Huh, W.W.; Daw, N.C.; Herzog, C.E.; Munsell, M.F.; McAleer, M.F.; Lewis, V.O. Ewing sarcoma family of tumors in children younger than 10 years of age. *Pediatr. Blood Cancer* **2017**, *64*, e26275. [CrossRef]
45. Bosma, S.E.; van der Heijden, L.; Sierrasesúmaga, L.; Merks, H.J.; Haveman, L.M.; van de Sande, M.A.; San-Julián, M. What Do We Know about Survival in Skeletally Premature Children Aged 0 to 10 Years with Ewing Sarcoma? A Multicenter 10-Year Follow-Up Study in 60 Patients. *Cancers* **2022**, *14*, 1456. [CrossRef]
46. Biswas, B.; Shukla, N.; Deo, S.; Agarwala, S.; Sharma, D.; Vishnubhatla, S.; Bakhshi, S. Evaluation of outcome and prognostic factors in extraosseous Ewing sarcoma. *Pediatr. Blood Cancer* **2014**, *61*, 1925–1931. [CrossRef]
47. Casanova, M.; Meazza, C.; Gronchi, A.; Fiore, M.; Zaffignani, E.; Podda, M.; Collini, P.; Gandola, L.; Ferrari, A. Soft-tissue sarcomas of the extremities in patients of pediatric age. *J. Child. Orthop.* **2007**, *1*, 195–203. [CrossRef]
48. Chen, J.; Cheng, R.; Fan, F.; Zheng, Y.; Li, Y.; Chen, Y.; Wang, Y. Cranial Ewing sarcoma/peripheral primitive neuroectodermal tumors: A retrospective study focused on prognostic factors and long-term outcomes. *Front. Oncol.* **2019**, *9*, 1023. [CrossRef]

49. Chiang, S.; Snuderl, M.; Kojiro-Sanada, S.; Pi-Sunyer, A.Q.; Daya, D.; Hayashi, T.; Bosincu, L.; Ogawa, F.; Rosenberg, A.E.; Horn, L.-C. Primitive Neuroectodermal Tumors of the Female Genital Tract: A Morphologic, Immunohistochemical and Molecular Study of 19 Cases. *Am. J. Surg. Pathol.* **2017**, *41*, 761. [CrossRef]
50. Gupta, A.A.; Pappo, A.; Saunders, N.; Hopyan, S.; Ferguson, P.; Wunder, J.; O'Sullivan, B.; Catton, C.; Greenberg, M.; Blackstein, M. Clinical outcome of children and adults with localized Ewing sarcoma: Impact of chemotherapy dose and timing of local therapy. *Cancer* **2010**, *116*, 3189–3194. [CrossRef]
51. Lee, J.A.; Kim, D.H.; Lim, J.S.; Koh, J.-S.; Kim, M.S.; Kong, C.-B.; Song, W.S.; Cho, W.H.; Lee, S.-Y.; Jeon, D.-G. Soft-tissue Ewing sarcoma in a low-incidence population: Comparison to skeletal Ewing sarcoma for clinical characteristics and treatment outcome. *Jpn. J. Clin. Oncol.* **2010**, *40*, 1060–1067. [CrossRef]
52. Muratori, F.; Mondanelli, N.; Pelagatti, L.; Frenos, F.; Matera, D.; Beltrami, G.; Innocenti, M.; Capanna, R.; Roselli, G.; Scoccianti, G. Clinical features, prognostic factors and outcome in a series of 29 extra-skeletal Ewing Sarcoma. Adequate margins and surgery-radiotherapy association improve overall survival. *J. Orthop.* **2020**, *21*, 236–239. [CrossRef]
53. Murugan, P.; Rao, P.; Tamboli, P.; Czerniak, B.; Guo, C.C. Primary Ewing sarcoma/primitive neuroectodermal tumor of the kidney: A clinicopathologic study of 23 cases. *Pathol. Oncol. Res.* **2018**, *24*, 153–159. [CrossRef] [PubMed]
54. Pradhan, A.; Grimer, R.; Spooner, D.; Peake, D.; Carter, S.; Tillman, R.; Abudu, A.; Jeys, L. Oncological outcomes of patients with Ewing's sarcoma: Is there a difference between skeletal and extra-skeletal Ewing's sarcoma? *J. Bone Jt. Surg. Br. Vol.* **2011**, *93*, 531–536. [CrossRef] [PubMed]
55. Qureshi, S.S.; Laskar, S.; Kembhavi, S.; Talole, S.; Chinnaswamy, G.; Vora, T.; Ramadwar, M.; Desai, S.; Khanna, N.; Muckaden, M.A. Extraskeletal Ewing sarcoma in children and adolescents: Impact of narrow but negative surgical margin. *Pediatr. Surg. Int.* **2013**, *29*, 1303–1309. [CrossRef] [PubMed]
56. Raney, R.B.; Asmar, L.; Newton, W.A., Jr.; Bagwell, C.; Breneman, J.C.; Crist, W.; Gehan, E.A.; Webber, B.; Wharam, M.; Wiener, E.S.; et al. Ewing's sarcoma of soft tissues in childhood: A report from the Intergroup Rhabdomyosarcoma Study, 1972 to 1991. *J. Clin. Oncol. Off. J. Am. Soc. Clin. Oncol.* **1997**, *15*, 574–582. [CrossRef]
57. Neriman, S.; Cetindag, M.F.; Ilhan, I.E. Treatment of Extraosseous Ewing Sarcoma in Children: Single Center Experience. *Int. J. Hematol. Oncol.* **2009**, *32*, 147–152.
58. Takenaka, S.; Naka, N.; Obata, H.; Joyama, S.; Hamada, K.-I.; Imura, Y.; Kakunaga, S.; Aoki, Y.; Ueda, T.; Araki, N. Treatment outcomes of Japanese patients with Ewing sarcoma: Differences between skeletal and extraskeletal Ewing sarcoma. *Jpn. J. Clin. Oncol.* **2016**, *46*, 522–528. [CrossRef]
59. Verma, V.; Denniston, K.A.; Lin, C.J.; Lin, C. A comparison of pediatric vs. adult patients with the Ewing sarcoma family of tumors. *Front. Oncol.* **2017**, *7*, 82. [CrossRef]
60. Wong, T.; Goldsby, R.E.; Wustrack, R.; Cash, T.; Isakoff, M.S.; DuBois, S.G. Clinical features and outcomes of infants with Ewing sarcoma under 12 months of age. *Pediatr. Blood Cancer* **2015**, *62*, 1947–1951. [CrossRef]
61. Xie, C.-F.; Liu, M.-Z.; Xi, M. Extraskeletal Ewing's sarcoma: A report of 18 cases and literature review. *Chin. J. Cancer* **2010**, *29*, 420–424. [CrossRef]
62. Majeed, S.S.; Muhammad, H.A.; Ali, J.S.; Khudhair, H.H.; Said, A.; Arif, S.O.; Murad, K.M.; Gendari, A.H.; Muhsin, B.M.; Mohammed, S.A. Treatment outcomes of pediatric patients with ewing sarcoma in a war-torn nation: A single-institute experience from Iraq. *J. Glob. Oncol.* **2019**, *4*, 1–9. [CrossRef]
63. Cypel, T.K.S.; Meilik, B.; Zuker, R.M. Extraskeletal Ewing's sarcoma in a great toe of a young boy. *Can. J. Plast. Surg.* **2007**, *15*, 165–168. [CrossRef] [PubMed]
64. Turkyilmaz, Z.; Sonmez, K.; Karabulut, R.; Sen, M.C.; Poyraz, A.; Oguz, A.; Basaklar, A.C. Extraskeletal Ewing sarcoma of the mesocolon in a child. *J. Pediatr. Surg.* **2012**, *47*, e1–e3. [CrossRef] [PubMed]
65. Costa, I.E.; Menezes, A.S.; Lima, A.F.; Rodrigues, B. Extra-skeletal Ewing's sarcoma of the frontal sinus: A rare disorder in pediatric age. *BMJ Case Rep. CP* **2020**, *13*, e232460. [CrossRef]
66. Krakorova, D.A.; Halamkova, J.; Tucek, S.; Bilek, O.; Kristek, J.; Kazda, T.; Zambo, I.S.; Demlova, R.; Kiss, I. Penis as a primary site of an extraskeletal Ewing sarcoma: A case report. *Medicine* **2021**, *100*, e25074. [CrossRef]
67. Salah, S.; Abuhijla, F.; Ismail, T.; Yaser, S.; Sultan, I.; Halalsheh, H.; Shehadeh, A.; Abdelal, S.; Almousa, A.; Jaber, O. Outcomes of extraskeletal vs. skeletal Ewing sarcoma patients treated with standard chemotherapy protocol. *Clin. Transl. Oncol.* **2020**, *22*, 878–883. [CrossRef] [PubMed]

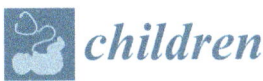

Article
Defining Equinus Foot in Cerebral Palsy

Axel Horsch, Lara Petzinger, Maher Ghandour, Cornelia Putz, Tobias Renkawitz and Marco Götze *

Department of Orthopedics, Heidelberg University Hospital, 69118 Heidelberg, Germany; axel.horsch@med.uni-heidelberg.de (A.H.); lara.petzinger@med.uni-heidelberg.de (L.P.); mghandourmd@gmail.com (M.G.); cornelia.putz@med.uni-heidelberg.de (C.P.); tobias.renkawitz@med.uni-heidelberg.de (T.R.)
* Correspondence: marco.goetze@med.uni-heidelberg.de

Abstract: Background: Equinus foot is the deformity most frequently observed in patients with cerebral palsy (CP). While there is widespread agreement on the treatment of equinus foot, a clear clinical definition has been lacking. Therefore, we conducted this study to evaluate functional changes in gait analysis in relation to maximum possible dorsiflexion (0°, 5°, 10° and 15°) and in two subgroups of CP patients (unilateral and bilateral). Methods: In this retrospective study, CP patients with different degrees of clinically measured maximum dorsiflexion were included. We further subdivided patients into unilaterally and bilaterally affected individuals and also included a healthy control group. All participants underwent a 3D gait analysis. Our goal was to determine the degree of maximum clinical dorsiflexion where the functional changes in range of motion (ROM) and ankle moment and power during gait were most evident. Then, a subgroup analysis was performed according to the affected side. Results: In all, 71 and 84 limbs were analyzed in unilaterally and bilaterally affected subgroups. The clinically 0° dorsiflexion group barely reached a plantigrade position in the 3D gait analysis. Differences in ROM were observed between subgroups. Ankle moment was quite similar between different subgroups but to a lower extent in the unilateral group. All CP patients had reduced ankle power compared to controls. Conclusions: A cutoff value of clinical $\leq 5°$ dorsiflexion is the recommended value for defining a functionally relevant equinus foot in CP patients.

Keywords: cerebral palsy; equinus; dorsiflexion; plantarflexion; definition

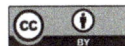

1. Introduction

Equinus foot is the deformity most frequently reported in patients with cerebral palsy (CP) [1]. There are two main types of equinus deformities, and the management approach differs for each type. The first type is known as dynamic equinus, which occurs when the calf muscles become spastic and, in most cases, there is no actual shortening of the gastrosoleus muscle structure yet. Therefore, it is not managed surgically but rather by physical therapy, foot orthosis, casting or botulinum toxin injection i.a. [2]. The second type is referred to as fixed or static equinus with evident contract shortening of the gastrosoleus muscle [3]. In this case, the condition is usually treated surgically by lengthening the affected muscle or its tendon. A wide variety of surgical interventions have been reported in the literature for this type of equinus, and international consensus for treatment has been reached [4,5].

Importantly, proper identification and diagnosis of equinus foot are considered the first step in implementing an appropriate intervention and in reaching a successful outcome [3]. However, there is a clear lack of consensus in the literature on how to properly identify and diagnose equinus foot in CP. A recent survey among 223 orthopedic surgeons highlighted that most of them regularly perform a clinical gait assessment in CP patients they encounter, not specifying if visual or instrumented [6]. However, when it comes to diagnosing equinus foot, their practices differed: 14% rely solely on foot dorsiflexion above plantigrade with an extended knee and neutral hindfoot, and 86% use the "Silfverskjöld test" in addition to the previous approach [6].

In the same context, orthopedic surgeons depend mainly on ankle dorsiflexion to assess equinus; however, there is no clear cutoff value of ankle dorsiflexion to define equinus foot. It is of course difficult to determine such a value, as in CP, equinus must never be considered in isolation; this applies especially for bilateral but also for unilateral CP. The sagittal gait pattern should be identified and described, as the ankle and knee levels are linked by coupling (e.g., the plantar flexion knee extension couple), and treatment should therefore be indicated with caution. Rang's aphorism that "a little equinus is better than calcaneus" can usually be agreed on, and individual decisions have to made with each patient [7].

Surprisingly, only a minority of studies report a cutoff value used to define equinus. For example, Horsch et al. [8] defined equinus foot as $\leq 5°$ of clinical ankle dorsiflexion in the extended knee. However, most reports assessing the efficacy of different surgical interventions for equinus foot did not report a clear diagnostic criterion [9–13]. This lack of a standard diagnostic criterion further demonstrates why the actual prevalence rate of equinus foot in CP patients has been called into question [14]. In addition, most surgeons rely mainly on the change in the degree of ankle dorsiflexion (pre- vs. postintervention) in defining successful surgery or improved clinical outcomes in CP patients with equinus foot [15–19].

Based on the aforementioned observations, a standard clinical criterion needs to be established to define the basis for managing equinus foot in CP patients surgically or conservatively. Such clinical criteria would be of great importance in determining how patients are selected for treatment based on their functional impairment, and this might change the way we look at this condition entirely - from the real prevalence of equinus, to the choice of the proper intervention to the reliable definition of a successful outcome. Therefore, we conducted this current research, using a gait analysis, in an attempt to reach a clinically relevant criterion to define CP patients with equinus foot who are eligible for surgery from those who can be managed otherwise. We also aimed to investigate whether this criterion would be applicable to different subtypes of patients (those unilaterally and bilaterally affected).

2. Materials and Methods

2.1. Study Design and Eligibility Criteria

For this study, data from 173 patients diagnosed with CP were retrospectively reviewed. The data in this work were collected in our motion lab in the time period from 2002 to 2021. Only patients with gross motor function system (GMFCS) I-II were included [20]. Other inclusion criteria were fully available clinical examinations and an instrumented 3D gait analysis, including measurements of the kinetic and kinematic parameters. We searched for patients with a limited range of motion (ROM) in the left leg measured in the clinical examination. More specifically, we included patients with a 0°, 5°, 10° or 15° maximum clinical dorsiflexion in the affected ankle joint. It is common to use 5° steps in stating a joint position, as smaller steps are usually not feasible to determine. The ROM was measured in the knee extension. Therefore, we grouped the patients according to their structural shortening of the calf muscles and did not take the additionally underlying amount of spasticity into account. We excluded patients with a GMFCS level III-IV and ankle dorsiflexion >15°; patients with prior soft tissue surgeries (calf, ischios, psoas, etc.) or botox within the past 6 months before gait analysis; patients that had botulinum toxin injections within 6 months prior to gait analysis; and patients that underwent soft tissue lengthening procedures of the lower limbs in general. We also excluded patients with a maximum clinical dorsiflexion of less than 0°, as this is unanimously seen as a functionally impairing equinus foot, and we tried to establish a value of dorsiflexion that marks the functional shift from good to impaired gait.

2.2. Study Participants and Measurements

We divided the subjects in two groups depending on the characteristics of CP. One group contained patients diagnosed with unilateral, and another group with bilateral, CP. The instrumented 3D gait analysis (IGA) and the clinical examination were performed by a specialized study nurse and a physiotherapist with years of neuro-orthopedic experience, and angles were assessed by a single examiner using a standard goniometer and the neutral zero method. Markers were applied on the skin according to a standard protocol (Plug in Gait Model) [21]. Three markers were used on each foot to measure the ankle movements. One of them was placed on the lateral malleolus, another one on the calcaneus and a third one being the toe marker, which is attached to the second metatarsal bone. Gait patterns were captured by 16 cameras from a Vicon System (Oxford Metrics, Oxford, UK). The data were captured with a 120 Hz frequency. A Woltring filter was used. Additionally, three force plates (Kistler Instruments, Winterthur, Switzerland) measured the kinetic parameters of the patients. All participants were asked to walk a distance of 7 m several times at their own walking speed. This examination was performed barefoot and without any walking aids. All data captured in the gait analysis were visualized as different diagrams for every joint in the sagittal, frontal and transverse plane.

2.3. Statistical Analysis

Study subjects were recruited from a patient cohort of the neuro-orthopedic department of our University Hospital and our established CP patient register. Data were documented in Microsoft Excel. Additionally, we used MatlabR for a graphic representation of the gait analysis data. Normal values were obtained from a group of 50 age-matched healthy patients without any form of gait pathology. The baseline characteristics of participants were presented as numbers and percentages for categorical/dichotomous variables, and as means and standard deviations (SDs) for continuous variables.

3. Results
3.1. Baseline Characteristics of Included Participants

Overall, a total of 155 limbs were analyzed: 71 in the unilateral and 84 in the bilateral group. Meanwhile, 5 patients were excluded from the unilateral groups [GMFC score > 2 ($n = 2$), data gaps in clinical examinations ($n = 2$) and ankle dorsiflexion > 15° ($n = 1$)] and 13 patients were excluded from the bilateral group [GMFCS > 2 ($n = 6$), data gaps in clinical examinations ($n = 4$) and dorsiflexion > 15° ($n = 3$)]. In the unilateral group, 54.9% of the patients were male, 77.5% were GMFCS level I, mean age at the time of IGA was 16.97 (12.13) years, mean weight was 47.16 (21.6) kg and mean height was 151.03 (22.5) cm. Most patients in the bilateral group were also males (56.0%), with GMFCS level II of 72.6% in this group, a mean age of 16 (10.11) years, mean weight of 43.98 (17.12) kg and a mean height of 147.73 (20.64) cm.

3.2. Measured Outcomes in the Bilateral CP Group

The results are demonstrated in three different graphs for every group, divided into ROM, ankle moment and ankle power. Each graph shows a different gait pattern according to the clinically measured dorsiflexion. The norm data are visualized with a gray band in all diagrams for better comparison.

In the bilateral group, 27 patients had a limited maximum dorsiflexion with 0° in the clinical exam and 27 patients could reach 5° dorsiflexion. In 22 patients, 10° dorsiflexion was measured and in 8 patients 15° (Figure 1). The graph shows different curves describing the gait pattern during the gait cycle. The curve representing patients with 0° dorsiflexion in the clinical examination did not reach a plantigrade position of the ankle joint in the gait analysis either. These patients walked in plantarflexion without any heel contact during the whole gait cycle. The gaits corresponding to the patients with 5° and 10° dorsiflexion were similar. In comparison to the 0° patients, they could reach a dorsiflexion in the first 15–50% of the gait cycle. Contemplating the plantarflexion in patients with 5°, 10° and 15° after toe-off (60%), the ROM was approximately comparable to a normal gait. Additionally, the curve for the 15° patients followed a nearly normal course with a slight vaulting pattern in the early stance phase.

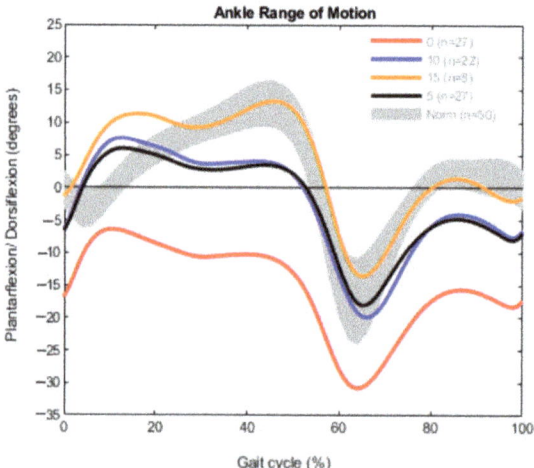

Figure 1. Range of motion measurement in the bilateral group (n = 84).

The moments of dorsiflexion and plantarflexion show a typical M-Shape with two maxima in every curve (Figure 2). All the curves, regardless of the dorsiflexion measured, were comparable. The first maxima were between 0 and 20% of the gait cycle, which represented the loading response and early midstance [22]. After that, the plantarflexion moment was pathologically reduced, followed by the physiological maxima in 40–60% of the gait cycle. In comparison with the norm data, the second peaks were lower than the peak seen in the gait of the norm group. The plantarflexion moment of the patients with 0° dorsiflexion in the clinical exam was the lowest.

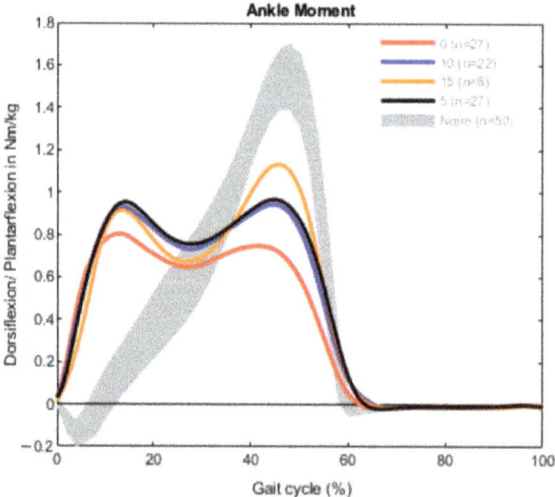

Figure 2. Ankle moment measurement in the bilateral group (n = 84).

The generation of power was reduced in all patients in comparison to the norm data (Figure 3). The power generated in the terminal stance to toe-off was lower than usual in every curve, especially in the group consisting of patients with 0° dorsiflexion. In the beginning of the gait cycle, all graphs show an increased absorption of power, followed by increased power during midstance (10–30% of gait cycle) and a reduced power generation before toe-off (40–60% of gait cycle).

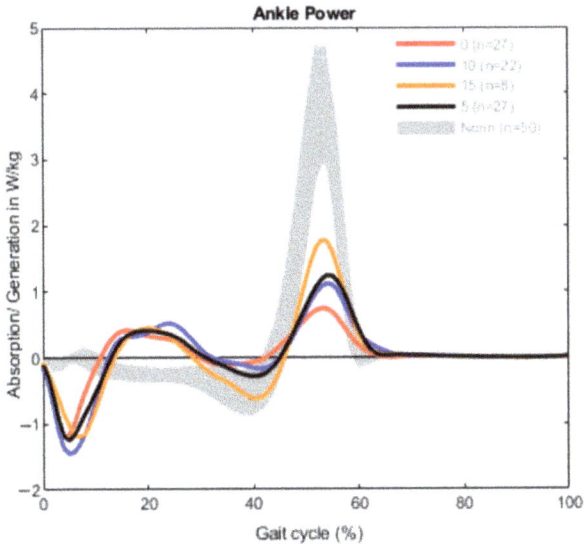

Figure 3. Ankle power measurement in the bilateral group (n = 84).

3.3. Measured Outcomes in the Unilateral Group

In the unilateral group, the subjects were separated into 35 patients with a 0° dorsiflexion at the clinical examination and 15 patients with 5°. Ten subjects could reach a 10° dorsiflexion and 11 patients showed a 15° dorsiflexion. In patients with unilateral CP, the ROM was quite similar to that in the bilaterally affected group (Figure 4). The limbs from the 0° group barely attained dorsiflexion in the gait analysis; instead, the ankle remained in plantarflexion during most of the gait cycle. The other curves (orange, blue and black) stay in the area of the norm data until the swing phase, where all the legs showed an increased plantarflexion.

Referring to the ankle moment, the plantarflexion moment in the loading response was also higher in every curve, but in comparison to the bilaterally affected patients to a lower extent (Figure 5). Additionally, the maximum of the plantarflexion moment during 40–60% of the gait cycle was decreased in every group. The highest moment of plantarflexion appeared in patients with 5° dorsiflexion at the clinical examination.

In patients with unilateral CP, the ankle power was also decreased in all groups during the terminal stance phase to toe-off (Figure 6). Other than in the bilateral group, the absorption-generation pattern of power in the early and midstance was less prominent. Only the 0° patients showed slightly increased power generation in midstance.

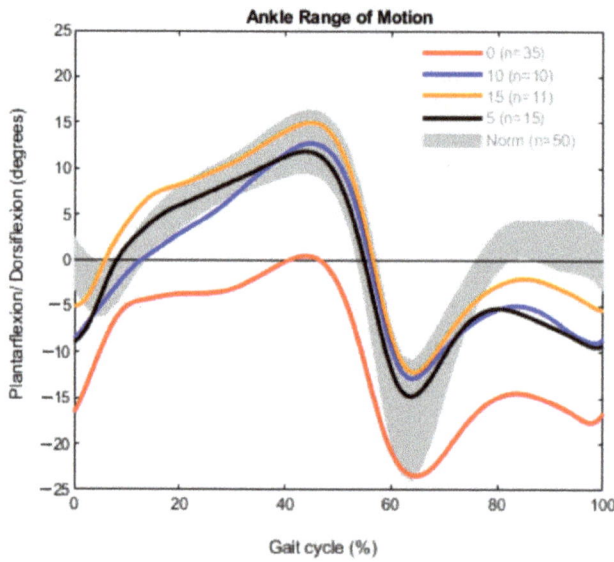

Figure 4. Range of motion measurement in the unilateral group (*n* = 71).

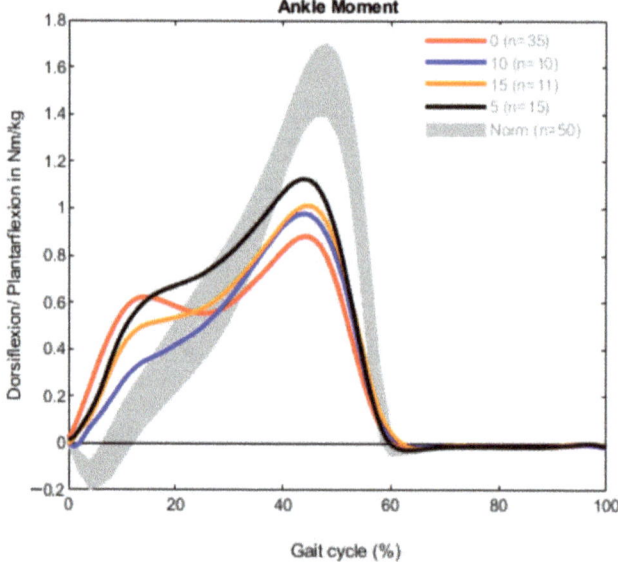

Figure 5. Ankle moment measurement in the unilateral group (*n* = 71).

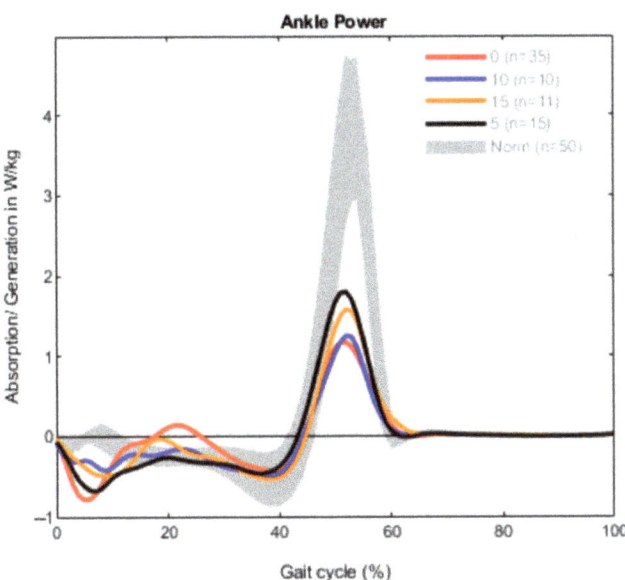

Figure 6. Ankle power measurement in the unilateral group ($n = 71$).

4. Discussion

Normally, during the stance phase (0–60% of the gait cycle), the greatest degree of dorsiflexion is needed just before lifting the heel in a fully extended knee, in which case the ankle has to be in a dorsiflexed, but perpendicular position for smooth ambulation [23,24]. Yet, there is still controversy related to the proper degree of dorsiflexion that is truly required for this to happen. Consequently, it would seem reasonable to use a normal range of values for defining the physiological gait, rather than to apply a definitive value. Based on the literature, this accepted range of normal ankle dorsiflexion lies between 3° and 15° beyond the perpendicular plane when the knee is fully extended [23–25].

Equinus foot is described as decreased ankle joint dorsiflexion; although, there is a lack of consensus on the exact definition and diagnostic criteria. While studies widely agree that static ankle joint equinus represents a reduced range of dorsiflexion at the ankle joint, there is no agreement concerning the degree of dorsiflexion reduction needed for this condition to manifest. Of course, different amounts of spasticity can lead to functionally different patterns. In the present work, we examined the differences in ROM, ankle moment and ankle power in different groups of patients based on the degree of maximum clinical ankle dorsiflexion. Here, among patients in the 0° dorsiflexion group, the subgroup of patients with bilateral CP could not reach plantigrade, and the unilateral subgroup barely reached plantigrade in midstance (40%). Thus, we hypothesize that this value would not be the best cutoff value to define a functionally relevant equinus foot in children with CP.

Owing to this lack of consensus, physicians have used a wide variety of restrictions on dorsiflexion for diagnosis [26]. Sobel et al. [27] proposed that patients have less than 0° of dorsiflexion in order to be diagnosed with equinus (i.e., no step beyond plantigrade), while Orendurff et al. [28] recommended a cutoff value of 5°. On the other hand, Di-Giovanni et al. [29] proposed a minimum value of less than 10° of dorsiflexion, which is consistent with the need for at least 10° of dorsiflexion to maintain a normal gait and avoid possibly increased forefoot loading throughout locomotion [28,30]. The aforementioned recommendations are consistent with Meyer's more recent proposal that, instead of basing an equinus diagnosis on a specific range of dorsiflexion motion, a diagnosis should be verified when the reduction in dorsiflexion reaches a magnitude that increases stress on the Achilles tendon and loading on the forefoot [31]. While it would be expected that forefoot pressure rises during locomotion in order to base an equinus diagnosis on a limit of 10° of dorsiflexion, there is no evidence that this would contribute to the development of defects in the foot or lower leg.

Our results indicate that ankle ROM in children with CP in the unilateral subgroup with 5°, 10° and 15° dorsiflexion was functionally quite similar to that in healthy controls from the beginning of the gait cycle and up to the mid-swing phase (0–75%), typically with more plantarflexion during the end of the cycle as compared to controls. On the other hand, ROM in the bilateral subgroup with 15° dorsiflexion was also similar to that in controls; however, both the 5° and 10° dorsiflexion groups showed reduced dorsiflexion compared to controls during the period from midstance to toe-off (40–60%).

Notably, the ankle joint moment was quite similar in both the uni- and bilateral CP subgroups during the gait cycle; however, the extent of plantarflexion in the bilateral group was higher. In all dorsiflexion groups (0°, 5°, 10° and 15°), the ankle moment throughout the gait cycle was quite comparable. When compared to healthy controls, all of the dorsiflexion groups revealed a higher plantarflexion moment during the loading response that lowered during midstance and never reached a physiological peak in terminal stance. This was consistent in both uni- and bilateral CP groups. This clearly shows that during gait, function as seen in kinetics is often worse than clinical examination and kinematics would suggest. This might be due to differences in the amount of spasticity of the calf muscles and weakness of the foot levers.

So far, equinus deformity itself has not been considered separately for uni- or bilateral involvement in most of the studies published; although, studies often present one group or the other. In our experience, the two groups present differently, with the amount of foot lever weakness being greater in unilaterally affected patients. Recent studies suggest that a functionally separate approach is beneficial, which is also in line with our experience and this assessment [32]. In terms of ankle power, both groups (uni- and bilateral) in our study had reduced power when compared to healthy controls. Similarly, the gait analysis of both groups revealed that reduced ankle power was evident in the period from terminal stance to toe-off (40–60%) as compared to controls. However, both groups had increased power during the loading phase in early stance as compared to healthy controls. The only difference between the two groups was found in the midstance (10–30%): the bilateral group revealed higher power than controls; while in the unilateral group, power was similar to that of the healthy or typically developing (TD) controls.

In addition, although a cutoff point of 10° may increase forefoot loading during locomotion, Orendurff et al. [28] proposed that a dorsiflexion ≤5° should be used for the diagnosis of equinus foot as they found that forefoot pressure was higher in patients with ≤5° dorsiflexion than in patients with more than 5° dorsiflexion ($p < 0.05$). This is consistent with our findings, as we noted that the lowest extent of dorsiflexion was observed in the ≤5° dorsiflexion group as compared to all other groups (0°, 10°, 15° and healthy controls), especially at the loading and midstance phases of the gait cycle where the ankle is at a perpendicular plane and the knee is normally fully extended. In the same context, ankle moment and power in the ≤5° dorsiflexion group were similar to that in other dorsiflexion groups (0°, 10° and 15°) during the whole gait cycle.

Therefore, we recommend taking ≤5° dorsiflexion value as a cutoff point for defining equinus foot deformity at the early phases of gait (loading and midstance) when the knee is normally fully extended and the ankle is in a perpendicular position, especially in bilaterally affected CP patients.

Our study provides a clinically relevant criterion for distinguishing CP patients with impaired function due to equinus from those in whom function is not impaired. This criterion is applicable and easy to use in a clinical setting to identify patients who are in need of treatment and those who possibly are not. That being said, this is a simplistic approach to define a functional relevant equinus, and sagittal gait patterns should always be considered before treatment suggestions are made. Surgeons have to be careful not to contribute to, e.g., crouch gait and impairment of global gait function by trying to improve ankle kinematics solely based on the presence of functionally relevant equinus foot.

The main aim of this study was to estimate a clinically relevant criterion to define CP patients with equinus foot, by reaching a cutoff point of dorsiflexion that can help discriminate CP patients with functional impairment who might be in need of surgical management. In the case of instability in the talonavicular joint, the joint was held during the clinical examination, and then the extent of movement was examined. Since it is not possible to avoid the occurrence of a midfoot break during a gait analysis, this should be considered a clear limitation. However, the purpose of this study was to find a clinical definition for equinus foot with the help of a gait analysis. Our patients were first clinically examined, which ensured that no midfoot break was present. It would also be worth discussing the integration of a foot model in future studies in order to investigate this question more closely.

Our study has several limitations. The most important limitation is the small number of participants within each subgroup (0°, 5°, 10° and 15°) included in our analysis, which further limits the implications drawn from our study and renders it difficult to apply our findings more generally. Additionally, the retrospective nature of our study limits the interpretation of our results. Moreover, we describe the differences observed between the groups studied clinically; thus, more work is required to determine whether these minimal clinical differences also reach statistical significance. Therefore, and based on the aforementioned limitations, future research in this area is still warranted by larger studies with more diverse populations and consideration of sagittal gait patterns to be able to determine whether such definition criteria are applicable for all CP patients, regardless of their clinical and demographic characteristics.

5. Conclusions

In conclusion, a cutoff value $\leq 5°$ maximum clinical dorsiflexion should be used to distinguish between patients who might need treatment from those who do not among CP patients with equinus foot. However, the applicability of this criterion among patients who are unilaterally and bilaterally affected is slightly different; therefore, we recommend considering the laterality of CP when diagnosing patients with equinus foot and when choosing the appropriate management approach for these individuals. This simplistic approach should not leave the sagittal gait pattern unconsidered, as this might lead to impairment of the global gait function.

Author Contributions: Conceptualization: A.H.; methodology: A.H.; software: A.H. and L.P.; validation: A.H. and L.P.; formal analysis: A.H., L.P. and M.G. (Marco Götze); investigation: A.H. and M.G. (Maher Ghandour), L.P. and M.G (Marco Götze); resources: M.G. (Marco Götze) and A.H.; data curation: L.P. and A.H.; writing—original draft preparation: A.H., L.P. and M.G. (Maher Ghandour); writing—review and editing: A.H., C.P., M.G. (Marco Götze) and T.R.; visualization: L.P.; supervision: A.H.; project administration: A.H. All authors have read and agreed to the published version of the manuscript.

Funding: The authors have not declared a specific grant for this research from any funding agency in the public, commercial or not-for-profit sectors. For the publication fee we acknowledge financial support by Deutsche Forschungsgemeinschaft within the funding programme "Open Access Publikationskosten" as well as by Heidelberg University.

Institutional Review Board Statement: The study was conducted in accordance with the Declaration of Helsinki, and approved on 25 September 2018 by the Ethics Committee of Heidelberg University (protocol registration number: S-576/2018) for studies involving humans.

Informed Consent Statement: Patient consent was waived due to minimal risk.

Data Availability Statement: All the Data analyzed in this manuscript can be provided upon request by contacting the corresponding author.

Conflicts of Interest: None declared. There was no external funding for the study. Regardless, Tobias Renkawitz has received research support and personal fees from Arbeitsgemeinschaft Endoprothetik (AE), DGOU, DGOOC; BVOU, DePuy International, Otto Bock Foundation, Deutsche Arthrose Hilfe, Aesculap, Zimmer, Stiftung Oskar Helene Heim Berlin, Vielberth Foundation Regensburg, the German Ministry of Education and Research as well as the German Federal Ministry of Economic Cooperation and Development. Axel Horsch received research support from Arthrose Hilfe and Ipsen.

References

1. DeHeer, P.A. Equinus and Lengthening Techniques. *Clin. Podiatr. Med. Surg.* **2017**, *34*, 207–227. [CrossRef] [PubMed]
2. Chen, W.; Liu, X.; Pu, F.; Yang, Y.; Wang, L.; Liu, H.; Fan, Y. Conservative treatment for equinus deformity in children with cerebral palsy using an adjustable splint-assisted ankle-foot orthosis. *Medicine* **2017**, *96*, e8186. [CrossRef] [PubMed]
3. Goldstein, M.; Harper, D.C. Management of cerebral palsy: Equinus gait. *Dev. Med. Child Neurol.* **2001**, *43*, 563–569. [CrossRef] [PubMed]
4. Rutz, E.; McCarthy, J.; Shore, B.J.; Shrader, M.W.; Veerkamp, M.; Chambers, H.; Davids, J.R.; Kay, R.M.; Narayanan, U.; Novacheck, T.F.; et al. Indications for gastrocsoleus lengthening in ambulatory children with cerebral palsy: A Delphi consensus study. *J. Child. Orthop.* **2020**, *14*, 405–414. [CrossRef] [PubMed]
5. Shore, B.J.; White, N.; Kerr Graham, H. Surgical correction of equinus deformity in children with cerebral palsy: A systematic review. *J. Child. Orthop.* **2010**, *4*, 277–290. [CrossRef] [PubMed]
6. Gendy, S.; ElGebeily, M.; El-Sobky, T.A.; Khoshhal, K.I.; Jawadi, A.H. Current practice and preferences to management of equinus in children with ambulatory cerebral palsy: A survey of orthopedic surgeons. *Sicot-J.* **2019**, *5*, 3. [CrossRef]
7. Lovell, W.W.; Winter, R.B. *Lovell and Winter's Pediatric Orthopaedics*; Lippincott Williams & Wilkins: Philadelphia, PA, USA, 1990; Volume 1.
8. Horsch, A.; Götze, M.; Geisbüsch, A.; Beckmann, N.; Tsitlakidis, S.; Berrsche, G.; Klotz, M. Prevalence and classification of equinus foot in bilateral spastic cerebral palsy. *World J. Pediatrics* **2019**, *15*, 276–280. [CrossRef]
9. Dietz, F.R.; Albright, J.C.; Dolan, L. Medium-term follow-up of Achilles tendon lengthening in the treatment of ankle equinus in cerebral palsy. *Iowa Orthop. J.* **2006**, *26*, 27–32. [PubMed]
10. Ferreira, L.A.; Cimolin, V.; Costici, P.F.; Albertini, G.; Oliveira, C.S.; Galli, M. Effects of gastrocnemius fascia lengthening on gait pattern in children with cerebral palsy using the gait profile score. *Res. Dev. Disabil.* **2014**, *35*, 1137–1143. [CrossRef]
11. Firth, G.B.; Passmore, E.; Sangeux, M.; Thomason, P.; Rodda, J.; Donath, S.; Selber, P.; Graham, H.K. Multilevel surgery for equinus gait in children with spastic diplegic cerebral palsy: Medium-term follow-up with gait analysis. *J. Bone Jt. Surg. Am. Vol.* **2013**, *95*, 931–938. [CrossRef] [PubMed]
12. Franki, I.; De Cat, J.; Deschepper, E.; Molenaers, G.; Desloovere, K.; Himpens, E.; Vanderstraeten, G.; Van den Broeck, C. A clinical decision framework for the identification of main problems and treatment goals for ambulant children with bilateral spastic cerebral palsy. *Res. Dev. Disabil.* **2014**, *35*, 1160–1176. [CrossRef] [PubMed]
13. Steinwender, G.; Saraph, V.; Zwick, E.B.; Uitz, C.; Linhart, W. Fixed and dynamic equinus in cerebral palsy: Evaluation of ankle function after multilevel surgery. *J. Pediatric Orthop.* **2001**, *21*, 102–107. [CrossRef]
14. Horsch, A.; Klotz, M.C.M.; Platzer, H.; Seide, S.; Zeaiter, N.; Ghandour, M. Is the Prevalence of Equinus Foot in Cerebral Palsy Overestimated? Results from a Meta-Analysis of 4814 Feet. *J. Clin. Med.* **2021**, *10*, 4128. [CrossRef] [PubMed]
15. Galen, S.; Wiggins, L.; McWilliam, R.; Granat, M. A combination of Botulinum Toxin A therapy and Functional Electrical Stimulation in children with cerebral palsy–a pilot study. *Technol. Health Care Off. J. Eur. Soc. Eng. Med.* **2012**, *20*, 1–9. [CrossRef] [PubMed]
16. Hastings-Ison, T.; Sangeux, M.; Thomason, P.; Rawicki, B.; Fahey, M.; Graham, H.K. Onabotulinum toxin-A (Botox) for spastic equinus in cerebral palsy: A prospective kinematic study. *J. Child. Orthop.* **2018**, *12*, 390–397. [CrossRef] [PubMed]
17. Maas, J.; Dallmeijer, A.; Huijing, P.; Brunstrom-Hernandez, J.; van Kampen, P.; Bolster, E.; Dunn, C.; Herndon, K.; Jaspers, R.; Becher, J. A randomized controlled trial studying efficacy and tolerance of a knee-ankle-foot orthosis used to prevent equinus in children with spastic cerebral palsy. *Clin. Rehabil.* **2014**, *28*, 1025–1038. [CrossRef]
18. Nakagawa, S.; Mutsuzaki, H.; Mataki, Y.; Endo, Y.; Matsuda, M.; Yoshikawa, K.; Kamada, H.; Iwasaki, N.; Yamazaki, M. Safety and immediate effects of Hybrid Assistive Limb in children with cerebral palsy: A pilot study. *Brain Dev.* **2020**, *42*, 140–147. [CrossRef] [PubMed]
19. Putz, C.; Mertens, E.M.; Wolf, S.I.; Geisbüsch, A.; Niklasch, M.; Gantz, S.; Döderlein, L.; Dreher, T.; Klotz, M.C. Equinus Correction During Multilevel Surgery in Adults With Cerebral Palsy. *Foot Ankle Int.* **2018**, *39*, 812–820. [CrossRef]
20. Palisano, R.; Rosenbaum, P.; Walter, S.; Russell, D.; Wood, E.; Galuppi, B. Development and reliability of a system to classify gross motor function in children with cerebral palsy. *Dev. Med. Child Neurol.* **1997**, *39*, 214–223. [CrossRef] [PubMed]
21. Ramakrishnan, H.K.; Kadaba, M.P. On the estimation of joint kinematics during gait. *J. Biomech.* **1991**, *24*, 969–977. [CrossRef]
22. Perry, J.; Burnfield, J.M. *Gait Analysis Normal and Pathological Function*; Slack Incorporated: Thorofare, NJ, USA, 2010; Volume 2.
23. Lamm, B.M.; Paley, D.; Herzenberg, J.E. Gastrocnemius soleus recession: A simpler, more limited approach. *J. Am. Podiatr. Med. Assoc.* **2005**, *95*, 18–25. [CrossRef]
24. Southerland, J.T.; Boberg, J.S.; Downey, M.S.; Nakra, A.; Rabjohn, L.V. *McGlamry's Comprehensive Textbook of Foot and Ankle Surgery*; Lippincott Williams & Wilkins: Philadelphia, PA, USA, 2012.

25. Herzenberg, J.E.; Lamm, B.M.; Corwin, C.; Sekel, J. Isolated recession of the gastrocnemius muscle: The Baumann procedure. *Foot Ankle Int.* **2007**, *28*, 1154–1159. [CrossRef] [PubMed]
26. Digiovanni, C.W.; Holt, S.; Czerniecki, J.M.; Ledoux, W.R.; Sangeorzan, B.J. Can the presence of equinus contracture be established by physical exam alone? *J. Rehabil. Res. Dev.* **2001**, *38*, 335–340. [PubMed]
27. Sobel, E.; Caselli, M.A.; Velez, Z. Effect of persistent toe walking on ankle equinus. Analysis of 60 idiopathic toe walkers. *J. Am. Podiatr. Med. Assoc.* **1997**, *87*, 17–22. [CrossRef]
28. Orendurff, M.S.; Rohr, E.S.; Sangeorzan, B.J.; Weaver, K.; Czerniecki, J.M. An equinus deformity of the ankle accounts for only a small amount of the increased forefoot plantar pressure in patients with diabetes. *J. Bone Jt. Surg. Br. Vol.* **2006**, *88*, 65–68. [CrossRef]
29. DiGiovanni, C.W.; Kuo, R.; Tejwani, N.; Price, R.; Hansen, S.T., Jr.; Cziernecki, J.; Sangeorzan, B.J. Isolated gastrocnemius tightness. *J. Bone Jt. Surg. Am. Vol.* **2002**, *84*, 962–970. [CrossRef]
30. Perry, J.; Burnfield, J.M.; Gronley, J.K.; Mulroy, S.J. Toe walking: Muscular demands at the ankle and knee. *Arch. Phys. Med. Rehabil.* **2003**, *84*, 7–16. [CrossRef]
31. Meyer, D.C.; Werner, C.M.; Wyss, T.; Vienne, P. A mechanical equinometer to measure the range of motion of the ankle joint: Interobserver and intraobserver reliability. *Foot Ankle Int.* **2006**, *27*, 202–205. [CrossRef]
32. Ma, N.; Sclavos, N.; Passmore, E.; Thomason, P.; Graham, K.; Rutz, E. Three-Dimensional Gait Analysis in Children Undergoing Gastrocsoleus Lengthening for Equinus Secondary to Cerebral Palsy. *Medicina* **2021**, *57*, 98. [CrossRef] [PubMed]

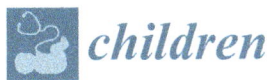

Systematic Review

Recurrence of Equinus Foot in Cerebral Palsy following Its Correction—A Meta-Analysis

Axel Horsch [1,*], Matthias Claus Michael Klotz [2], Hadrian Platzer [1], Svenja Elisabeth Seide [3] and Maher Ghandour [1]

1. Department of Orthopedics and Trauma Surgery, Heidelberg University Hospital, 69120 Heidelberg, Germany; hadrian.platzer@med.uni-heidelberg.de (H.P.); mghandourmd@gmail.com (M.G.)
2. Marienkrankenhaus Soest, Orthopedics and Trauma Surgery, 59494 Soest, Germany; mcmklotz@gmx.net
3. Institute of Medical Biometry, University of Heidelberg, 69117 Heidelberg, Germany; seide@imbi.uni-heidelberg.de
* Correspondence: axel.horsch@med.uni-heidelberg.de

Abstract: Background: Recurrence in cerebral palsy (CP) patients who have undergone operative or non-operative correction varies greatly from one study to another. Therefore, we conducted this meta-analysis to determine the pooled rate of equinus recurrence following its correction either surgically or non-surgically. Methods: Nine electronic databases were searched from inception to 6 May 2021, and the search was updated on 13 August 2021. We included all studies that reported the recurrence rate of equinus following its correction among CP patients. The primary outcome was recurrence, where data were reported as a pooled event (PE) rate and its corresponding 95% confidence interval (CI). We used the Cochrane's risk of bias (RoB-II) tool and ROBINS-I tool to assess the quality of included randomized and non-randomized trials, respectively. We conducted subgroup analyses to identify the sources of heterogeneity. Results: The overall rate of recurrence was 0.15 (95% CI: 0.05–0.18; $I^2 = 88\%$; $p < 0.01$). Subgroup analyses indicated that the laterality of CP, study design, and intervention type were significant contributors to heterogeneity. The recurrence rate of equinus differed among interventions; it was highest in the multilevel surgery group (PE = 0.27; 95% CI: 0.19–0.38) and lowest in the Ilizarov procedure group (PE = 0.10; 95% CI: 0.04–0.24). Twelve studies had a low risk of bias, eight had a moderate risk, and nine had a serious risk of bias. Conclusion: The recurrence of equinus following its correction, either surgically or non-surgically, in CP patients is notably high. However, due to the poor quality of available evidence, our findings should be interpreted with caution. Future studies are still warranted to determine the actual risk of equinus recurrence in CP.

Keywords: recurrence; equinus; surgery; meta-analysis

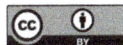

1. Introduction

Cerebral palsy (CP) is the result of a non-progressive brain injury which occurs during the early stages of development [1]. Equinus deformity is one of the most frequent gait abnormalities that is seen in patients with CP. It is characterized by excessive ankle plantarflexion, especially during the stance phase [2]. Equinus deformity occurs mainly due to the contracture of the gastrocsoleus muscle; however, it can occur due to abnormalities in other muscles of the ankle joint, including the tibialis anterior and peroneus longus muscles [3–5]. There are two major types of equinus: dynamic and fixed equinus. Although dynamic equinus is mainly treated through nonoperative options, such as physiotherapy, Botulinum toxin A injection, serial casting, or ankle foot orthoses, fixed equinus is treated surgically by the lengthening of the gastrocsoleus muscle-tendon unit through a wide variety of approaches [6]. These approaches include single-event multilevel surgery (SEMLS), Tendo-Achilles Lengthening (TAL), and the Ilizarov procedure.

Recurrence following equinus correction is reported in numerous studies with rates differing widely from one study to another (ranging from 4.7 to 28.2%). There is a wide discrepancy in the reported rates of recurrence, with no consistency in the rates reported in individual studies. In the same context, according to a recent systematic review, the recurrence rate of equinus deformity following TAL surgery was reported to range from 0 to 43% [7], with similar rates among unilateral and bilateral spastic CP patients who had undergone gastrocsoleus lengthening (0–38% and 0–35%, respectively) [8]. It is noteworthy that the rate of recurrence differs substantially among studies, and this warrants further investigation to determine the actual rate of recurrence of equinus following its correction. We hypothesize that the recurrence rate of equinus following its correction will be notably high, both in surgically and non-surgically treated CP patients.

Thus, we carried out this research to estimate the rate of equinus recurrence following its correction, either surgically or non-surgically, among CP patients. We also aimed to identify the current gaps in the literature regarding equinus recurrence following its correction.

2. Materials and Methods

2.1. Search Strategy and Study Selection

This study was carried out in accordance with the PRISMA guidelines for systematic reviews and meta-analyses, where registering a protocol is not considered mandatory [9]. We performed a database search through several databases: PubMed, Scopus, ScienceDirect, Clinicaltrials.gov (20 January 2022), CENTRAL, Virtual Health Library (VHL), Global Health Library (GHL), NYAM, and SIGLE. The search was originally carried out on 6 May 2021, and it was later updated on 13 August 2021, yielding no more relevant papers.

The following keywords were used when performing the search: (recurrence) AND (equinus) AND ("cerebral palsy"). Medical subject headings (MeSH) were also used to include a wider pool of studies. In an attempt to ensure that all relevant studies were included, we carried out a manual search of references through several approaches: searching for similar articles on PubMed, going through the reference list of included studies, and searching Google manually [10,11] (Supplementary File). The search process was conducted in accordance with the PICO framework: participants were patients with equinus who underwent operative or non-operative correction, the intervention was any type of management approach used for the correction of equinus, the comparison was any type of surgery or other treatment approaches (i.e., casting, injection), and recurrence was the outcome of interest.

We included all original studies that reported the recurrence of equinus following its correction (surgically or non-surgically), whether there was a comparison group or not. We excluded papers if they had one of the following criteria: (1) non-original research, (2) in vitro and animal research, (3) duplicates, (4) studies with overlapping datasets, (5) unextractable data due to selective reporting or unclear data, (6) studies with unavailable full texts, and (7) secondary research (i.e., reviews, editorials, commentaries, correspondence, etc.). Four authors carried out the title/abstract screening phase. Then, the full text of relevant articles was retrieved, and three authors screened the retrieved manuscripts. Any disagreements between authors were solved through thorough discussion, and if a solution was not reached a senior author was consulted. The PRISMA flow diagram of the study process is illustrated in Figure 1.

2.2. Data Extraction

A data extraction sheet was made using the Excel software. First, a pilot extraction was conducted to include all of the necessary components in the extraction sheet. In summary, the sheet included three parts, where each part was focused on a certain aspect of the included studies. The first part contained the baseline characteristics of included studies, such as the title of the study, authors' names, year of publication, journal, etc. The second part contained the demographic characteristics of patients included in the individual studies, such as sample size, age and gender, study design, type of equinus or

CP, type of intervention performed, etc. The third part focused on the outcome (i.e., rates of recurrence following correction). Two authors conducted the data extraction process, while a third author checked all of the extracted data to ensure their accuracy. Any disagreements between authors were solved by discussions and consensus.

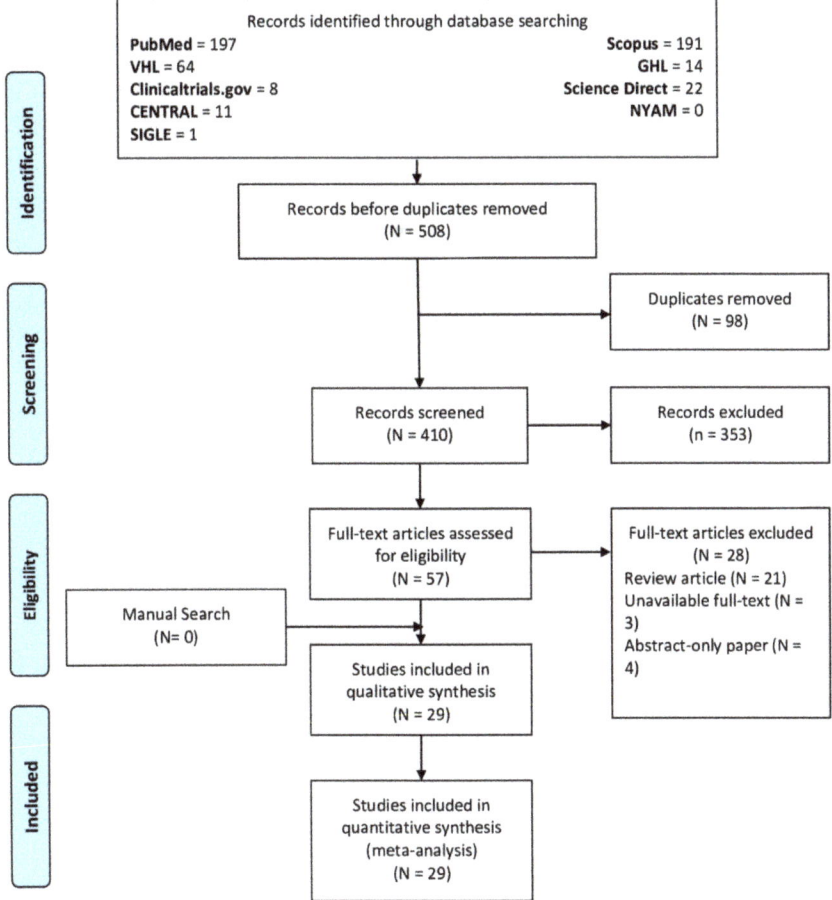

Figure 1. PRISMA flow diagram of the review process.

2.3. Risk of Bias

We checked the methodological quality of the included studies through the use of Cochrane's revised risk of bias tool [12] and the risk of bias in non-randomized studies of intervention (ROB 2) tool [13] for randomized and non-randomized trials, respectively. This process was carried out by three authors, and any discrepancy was solved by discussion amongst them.

2.4. Statistical Analysis

Overall pooled proportions were estimated using a generalized linear mixed model and a logit transformation to pool the recurrence rate [14]. The overall recurrence of equinus was reported in the form of the pooled estimate (PE) and its corresponding 95% confidence interval (CI). Meta-analyses were conducted using the random-effects model, where the DerSimonian–Laird estimator was used to report the between-trial heterogeneity [15]. In this study, between-trial heterogeneity is reported by using the estimated variance τ^2 and the I^2, and the meta-analysis results are visualized through forest plots. We further conducted several subgroup analyses based on a set of variables: laterality of CP, study design, definition of equinus, and type of intervention to correct equinus. Analyses were performed using R [16] version 4.0.3 and its extension, meta [17].

3. Results

3.1. Search Results

The initial database search yielded 508 articles, of which 410 were included in the title/abstract screening phase following the exclusion of duplicated articles through the EndNote software. Fifty-seven articles were eligible for full-text screening, of which twenty-eight articles were excluded for the following reasons: reviews (N = 21), unavailable full texts (N = 3), and abstract-only papers (N = 4). Ultimately, a total of 29 articles were included in our review and analysis.

3.2. Study Characteristics

The baseline characteristics of included studies are presented in Table 1.

Table 1. Baseline characteristics of studies included in the systematic review (N = 29).

Author/YOP	Design	Size	Laterality	CP Type	Equinus Type	Intervention	Control	Age: Mean (SD)	Male/Female	Follow up (Months)
Biedermann/2007 [18]	Case series	10	Both	Spastic	Fixed	Ilizarov external fixation	None	12.3	8/2	50
Boireau/2002 [19]	Case series	25	Both	NR	NR	Percutaneous lengthening of the Achilles tendon	None	NR	NR	NR
Sala/1997 [20]	Case series	27	Both	NR	NR	TAL	None	NR	15/12	66
El-Sobky/2011 [21]	Case series	21	Both	Spastic	Static	Open distal gastrocnemius recession	None	5–14 *	13/8	26
Throop/1975 [22]	Case series	48	NR	NR	NR	Murphy procedure	None	NR	NR	36
Uyttendaele/1989 [23]	Case series	9	NR	NR	NR	Combined Achilles and tibialis posterior lengthening	None	NR	NR	NR
Dreher/2012 [24]	Cohort	44	Bilateral	Spastic	NR	Multi-level surgery	None	9.8 (3.4)	NR	108
Matsuo/1994 [25]	Cohort study	92	Both	spastic/athetoid	Surgery	None	3–19 *	NR	50	18
Ahmad/2018 [26]	Prospective cohort	30	Both	NR	Fixed	Ilizarov external fixation	None	3–18 *	21/9	18
Al-Azzawi/2016 [27]	Prospective cohort	22	Both	NR	NR	Percutaneous TAL	Open TAL	4–10 *	14/8	12
Kay/2004 [28]	RCT	23	NR	Spastic	NR	Botox plus casting	serial casting alone	4.3–13.8 *	12/11	6
Gabor/2020 [29]	Retrospective Cohort	347	Both	NR	NR	Percutaneous (261 cases) and open TAL (86 cases)	None	2.8–15.1 *	NR	NR
Lee/1980 [30]	Retrospective Cohort	116	Both	Spastic	NR	Baker's method (tongue-in-groove incision in the gastrocnemius aponeurosis)	Hoke's method (tendo-calcaneus lengthening)	NR	NR	168
Firth/2013 [31]	Retrospective cohort	40	Bilateral	spastic	Fixed	Gastrocnemius lengthening	None	10	25/15	90
Kläusler/2017 [32]	Retrospective cohort	23	Both	spastic	Fixed	Tibialis Anterior Tendon Shortening plus TAL	None	14.9	13/8	70
Joo/2011 [33]	Retrospective Cohort	186	Both	NR	Fixed	Surgery	None	6.8	118/68	135.5
Rattey/1993 [34]	Retrospective Cohort	57	Both	NR	NR	TAL by open Z-plasty	None	NR	NR	120
Strecker/1990 [35]	Retrospective Cohort	100	NR	Spastic	NR	Anterior transposition of the Achilles tendon	None	NR	NR	30

Table 1. Cont.

Author/YOP	Design	Size	Laterality	CP Type	Equinus Type	Intervention	Control	Age: Mean (SD)	Male/Female	Follow up (Months)
Poul/2003 [36]	Retrospective Cohort	61	Both	NR	NR	Percutaneous aponeurectomy of the gastrocnemius	None	NR	NR	36
Chung/2015 [37]	Retrospective Cohort	243	Both	NR	NR	TAL	None	7.8 (2.7)	159/84	97
Vipulakom/2012 [38]	Retrospective Cohort	95	NR	NR	NR	TAL	Vulpius procedure	2–19.9 *	NR	NR
Borton/2000 [39]	Retrospective cohort	195	Both	NR	NR	Percutaneous TAL	Open TAL and Baker's method	2–18 *	113/82	NR
Grant/2015 [40]	Retrospective Cohort	27	Both	NR	NR	TAL	None	2–9 *	NR	120
Gaytan-Fernandez/2020 [41]	Retrospective Cohort	55	Both	Mixed	NR	Percutaneous TAL	Open TAL	1–16 *	45/19	72
Javors/1987 [42]	Retrospective Cohort	47	Both	NR	NR	Vulpius procedure	None	2–14 *	NR	68.4
Hiroshima/1988 [43]	Retrospective Cohort	21	Both	Spastic	NR	Surgery (Anterior transfer of long toe flexors)	None	NR	NR	NR
Katz/2000 [44]	Retrospective Cohort	36	Both	Spastic	NR	Below-knee cast plus early weight bearing without splint or orthosis	None	4–6 *	NR	75
Krupinski et al./2015 [45]	Retrospective Cohort	53	Both	Spastic	NR	Subcutaneous TAL	None	7	NR	121
Svehlik/2012 [46]	Retrospective Cohort	18	Both	NR	NR	Baumann's method (fractional lengthening of the gastrocnemii and soleus muscles)	None	NR	NR	120

* data provided in these studies refer to the range of age of participants included; TAL: Tendo-Achilles Lengthening; NR: Not Reported; SD: Standard Deviation; CP: Cerebral Palsy; YOP: Year of Publication.

In terms of study design, 18 articles were retrospective cohort studies [6,8,12,13,16–20,22,23,25,26,32,33,40,41,46], 6 were case series [18–23], 2 were cohort studies (unidentifiable as prospective or retrospective) [24,25], 2 were prospective cohort studies [26,27], and 1 was a randomized controlled trial [28]. The overall sample size was 2071 patients, ranging from 9 cases [23] to 347 cases [29]. Gender was reported in 12 studies, and males were predominant in all studies. The follow-up of patients varied among included studies, ranging from 6 months [28] to 168 months [30].

Individual studies reported different interventional approaches for the correction of equinus deformity, including Tendo-Achilles lengthening (TAL, both percutaneous and open), multilevel surgery, tibialis anterior tendon shortening, the Vulpius procedure, the aponeurectomy of gastrocnemius muscle, gastrocnemius recession, Ilizarov external fixation, Botox injections, casting, Baumann's method, and Baker's method. However, only six studies had a control or a comparison group [27,28,30,38,39,41].

The laterality of cerebral palsy was reported in 24 studies: bilateral in two studies [24,31] and both unilateral and bilateral in twenty-two studies [1,2,4–6,8,13,16–20,22,23,25,26,30,32,33,35,41,42]. The type of cerebral palsy was reported in thirteen studies, where one study reported a mixed CP type [41]. Twelve studies reported spastic CP [18,21,24,25,28,30–32,35,43–45], and one study reported athetoid CP [25]. The type of equinus was reported six studies, where one study reported static equinus [21] and five studies reported fixed equinus [18,26,31–33].

3.3. Risk of Bias

Based on the quality assessment of the single included RCT (based on five domains), the study was deemed to have a low risk of bias [28]. Based on the assessment of non-randomized studies of intervention (based on seven domains), eleven studies had a low risk of bias [18,21–23,25–27,35,36,38,42], eight studies had a moderate risk of bias [19,29,30,33,34,39,43,46], and nine studies had serious risk of bias [8,11–13,16,20,23,25,35]. The most common domain that had a serious risk of bias was confounding.

3.4. Overall Recurrence of Equinus

A total of 29 studies were included in the meta-analysis, and the overall rate of the recurrence of equinus following interventional correction of any type was 0.15 (95% CI: 0.10–0.20) (Figure 2). However, there was significant heterogeneity ($I^2 = 88\%$; $p < 0.01$). Six studies included a comparator group (Vulpius procedure, open TAL, serial casting, and Hoke's method), and, upon comparison of the intervention and comparator groups no significant difference in the rate of recurrence was noted (OR = 0.85; 95% CI: 0.36–2.06). Additionally, significant heterogeneity was encountered ($I^2 = 73\%$; $p < 0.01$) (Supplementary Figure S1). Due to the absence of a standard control group, no further discussion about the comparative risk/odds of equinus recurrence will be attempted.

3.5. Subgroup Analysis

In an attempt to determine the causes of heterogeneity in our analysis, various subgroup analyses were conducted based on laterality, study design, equinus definition, and intervention type.

3.6. Recurrence and Laterality

Laterality was a significant contributor to heterogeneity, where studies that reported both unilateral and bilateral disease were significantly heterogenous ($I^2 = 85\%$; $p < 0.01$), while studies reporting bilateral disease resulted in no heterogeneity ($I^2 = 0\%$; $p = 0.22$). That being said, the recurrence rate was different in studies reporting both laterality and bilaterality (pooled estimated (PE) = 0.16; 95% CI: 0.12–0.22) to those reporting bilateral disease alone (PE = 0.28; 95% CI: 0.21–0.36) (Figure 3).

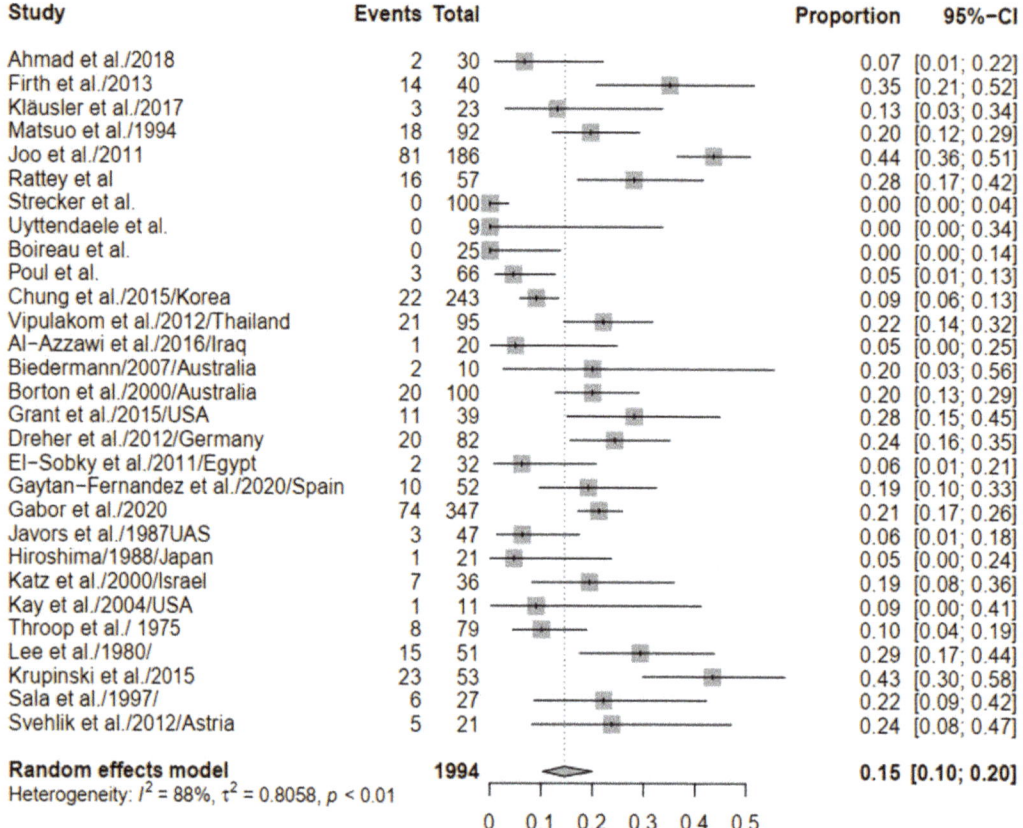

Figure 2. Forest plot of the overall recurrence of equinus.

3.7. Recurrence and Study Design

Study design was also a contributor to heterogeneity where case series did not result in significant heterogeneity ($I^2 = 38\%$; $p = 0.38$). In addition, the recurrence rate of equinus did not differ much between the different groups, where case series and retrospective cohort studies had an overall rate of 0.10 (95% CI: 0.05–0.18) and 0.17 (95% CI: 0.11–0.26) (Figure 4).

3.8. Recurrence and Equinus Definition

Equinus was defined in six studies [18,21,26,31–33], and even though the rate of recurrence was not different among studies that reported a definition of equinus (PE = 0.18; 95% CI: 0.09–0.34) and those that did not (PE = 0.14; 95% CI: 0.09–0.20), the heterogeneity remained significant ($I^2 = 82\%$; $p < 0.01$, $I^2 = 87\%$; $p < 0.01$, respectively) (Figure 5).

3.9. Recurrence and Intervention Type

Different interventions were reported in included studies, such as the Ilizarov procedure (N = 2 studies) [18,26], Tendo-Achilles Lengthening (N = 12 studies) [19,20,23,27,29,32,34,37,39–41,45], multilevel surgery (N = 4 studies) [24,25,33,38], and casting (N = 2 studies) [28,44].

The subgroup analysis based on the type of intervention (surgery) yielded no resultant heterogeneity in the Ilizarov method and casting subgroups ($I^2 = 0\%$; $p = 0.24$ and $I^2 = 0\%$; $p = 0.44$, respectively). That being said, the rate of the recurrence of equinus differed in different subgroups, where it was 0.10 (95% CI: 0.04–0.24), 0.17 (95% CI: 0.11–0.25), 0.27 (95% CI: 0.19–0.38), and 0.17 (95% CI: 0.09–0.31) in the Ilizarov, TAL, multilevel surgery, and casting subgroups, respectively (Figure 6).

Study	Events	Total		Proportion	95%–CI
Laterality = Both					
Ahmad et al./2018	2	30		0.07	[0.01; 0.22]
Kläusler et al./2017	3	23		0.13	[0.03; 0.34]
Matsuo et al./1994	18	92		0.20	[0.12; 0.29]
Joo et al./2011	81	186		0.44	[0.36; 0.51]
Rattey et al	16	57		0.28	[0.17; 0.42]
Boireau et al.	0	25		0.00	[0.00; 0.14]
Poul et al.	3	66		0.05	[0.01; 0.13]
Chung et al./2015/Korea	22	243		0.09	[0.06; 0.13]
Al-Azzawi et al./2016/Iraq	1	20		0.05	[0.00; 0.25]
Biedermann/2007/Australia	2	10		0.20	[0.03; 0.56]
Borton et al./2000/Australia	20	100		0.20	[0.13; 0.29]
Grant et al./2015/USA	11	39		0.28	[0.15; 0.45]
El-Sobky et al./2011/Egypt	2	32		0.06	[0.01; 0.21]
Gaytan-Fernandez et al./2020/Spain	10	52		0.19	[0.10; 0.33]
Gabor et al./2020	74	347		0.21	[0.17; 0.26]
Javors et al./1987UAS	3	47		0.06	[0.01; 0.18]
Hiroshima/1988/Japan	1	21		0.05	[0.00; 0.24]
Katz et al./2000/Israel	7	36		0.19	[0.08; 0.36]
Lee et al./1980/	15	51		0.29	[0.17; 0.44]
Krupinski et al./2015	23	53		0.43	[0.30; 0.58]
Sala et al./1997/	6	27		0.22	[0.09; 0.42]
Svehlik et al./2012/Astria	5	21		0.24	[0.08; 0.47]
Random effects model		1578		0.16	[0.12; 0.22]
Heterogeneity: I^2 = 85%, τ^2 = 0.5846, p < 0.01					
Laterality = Bilateral					
Firth et al./2013	14	40		0.35	[0.21; 0.52]
Dreher et al./2012/Germany	20	82		0.24	[0.16; 0.35]
Random effects model		122		0.28	[0.21; 0.36]
Heterogeneity: I^2 = 0%, τ^2 = 0, p = 0.22					
Random effects model		1700		**0.17**	**[0.13; 0.23]**
Heterogeneity: I^2 = 85%, τ^2 = 0.5490, p < 0.01					
Residual heterogeneity: I^2 = 81%, p < 0.01			0 0.1 0.2 0.3 0.4 0.5		

Figure 3. Forest plot of subgroup analysis of equinus recurrence based on the laterality of CP.

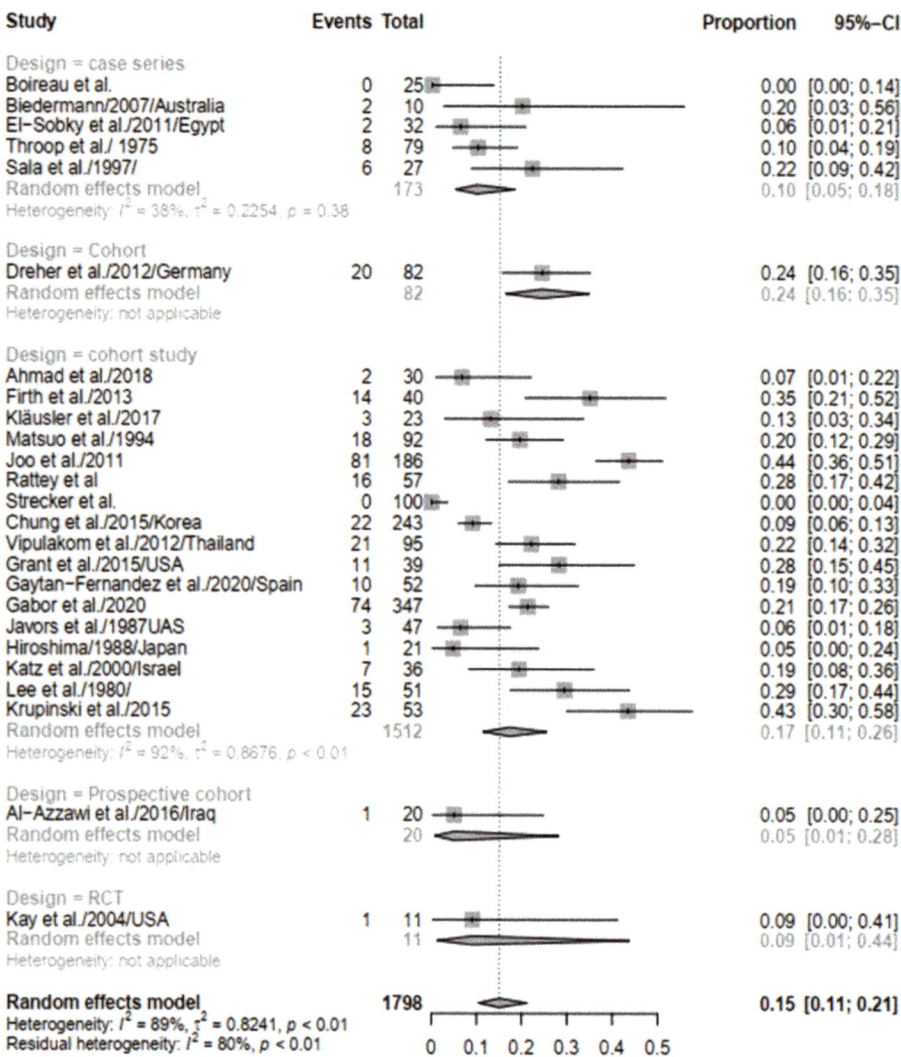

Figure 4. Forest plot of subgroup analysis of equinus recurrence based on study design.

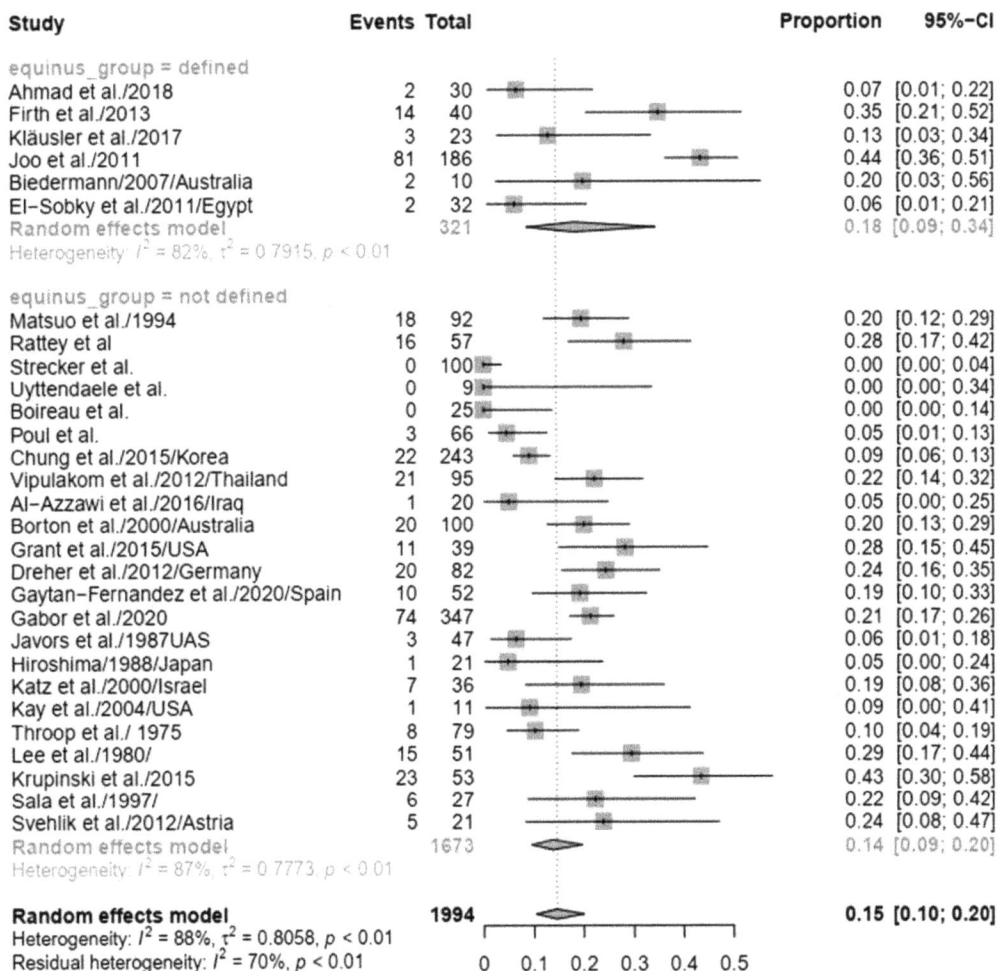

Figure 5. Forest plot of the subgroup analysis of equinus recurrence based on equinus definition.

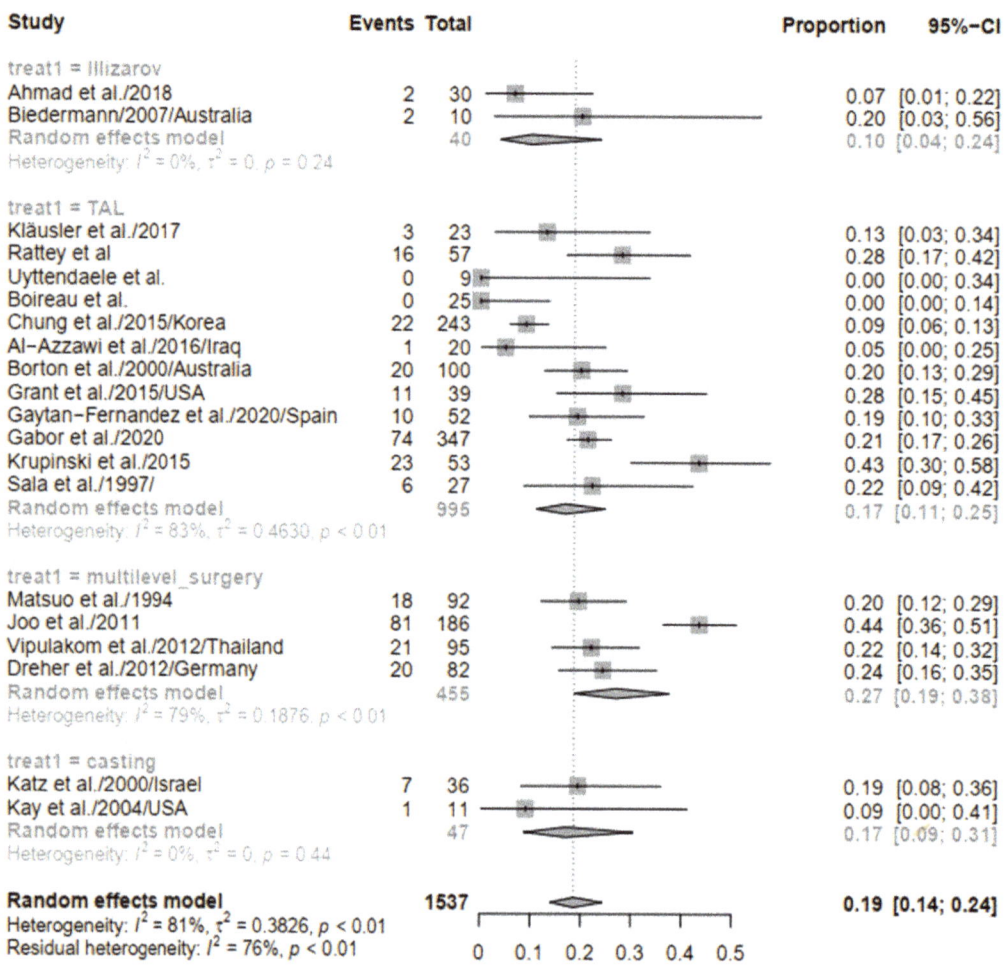

Figure 6. Forest plot of the subgroup analysis of equinus recurrence based on intervention type.

4. Discussion

This is the first systematic review and meta-analysis to examine the rate of equinus recurrence following its correction by different types of surgeries. This study is considered a hypothesis-generating review aimed at identifying the gaps in the current evidence in order to better determine the actual risk of the recurrence of equinus following its management. Four different interventional approaches are reported in this review: the Ilizarov procedure, Tendo-Achilles Lengthening (TAL), multilevel surgery, and casting. Multilevel surgery was defined as undergoing more than one procedure at the same time. For example, in the study of Matsuo et al. [25] patients underwent the following procedures: gastrocnemius aponeurotic lengthening, intramuscular lengthening of the peroneus longus and tabialis posterior, and sliding lengthening of the flexor hallucis longus and flexor digitorum longus.

Overall, the pooled recurrence rate in our meta-analysis was 15%, which differed substantially based on laterality, study design, equinus definition (yes/no), and the type of intervention. For instance, the pooled rate of recurrence of equinus was higher in bilateral disease (28%) compared to both unilateral and bilateral disease (16%). Case series had lower rates of recurrence compared to retrospective cohort design (10% vs. 17%). The difference between studies that reported a clear definition of equinus and those that did not, in terms of recurrence rates, was minimal (18% vs. 14%, respectively). It is of note that casting and TAL had the same recurrence rate of 17%, while the Ilizarov procedure resulted in a lower rate (10%) and multilevel surgery was associated with the highest rate of recurrence (27%).

That being said, we encountered significant substantial heterogeneity in our analyses. Therefore, we conducted several subgroup analyses to determine the causes of the resultant heterogeneity. We carried out a subgroup analysis based on laterality, study design, equinus definition (defined/not), and intervention type. It is worth noting that laterality, study design, and intervention types were significant contributors to heterogeneity where bilateral disease, case series, the Ilizarov method, and casting procedures had no significant heterogeneity ($I^2 < 40\%$).

It is noteworthy that the follow-up duration of equinus patients varied remarkably between individual studies, ranging from 6 months to as long as 168 months after the interventional correction of equinus. Moreover, based on the qualitative assessment of retrieved data from individual studies, we noted a tendency towards higher recurrence rates in studies with longer follow-up durations. This further complicates the issue of the actual recurrence rate after equinus correction in CP patients. Therefore, we recommend future studies report the recurrence rate in both the short and long term.

Our findings are quite different from what has been reported in the literature. In 2011, Shore et al. [7] conducted a systematic review aimed at determining the different operative options for the correction of equinus in patients with cerebral palsy. A total of 23 studies reported the use of TAL for the correction of equinus deformity, of which 14 studies reported the recurrence rate of equinus after surgery, which ranged from 0% to 43%. Similarly, in the recently published systematic review of Ma et al. [8], the authors investigated the recurrence rates of equinus in patients with cerebral palsy who underwent gastrocsoleus lengthening. The authors reported recurrence rates of 0–38% and 0–35% among patients with unilateral spastic and bilateral spastic cerebral palsy, respectively. In our study, the recurrence rate of TAL was 17%. This difference could be related to numerous factors. For instance, studies that had longer follow-up times reported much higher recurrence rates [33,45]. Other factors include age at the index date (time of undergoing surgery), the typographical distribution of CP, and the use of postoperative casting [47].

5. Limitations

Our study is the first to examine the rate of equinus recurrence in different interventions for the correction of equinus in patients with cerebral palsy. We highlight that many factors could play a role in the rate/risk of equinus recurrence following its correction, including clinicodemographic characteristics, such as laterality and the type of intervention used. However, our review encountered several limitations. First, there is a clear lack of randomized controlled trials that investigate the recurrence rate of equinus following either intervention (surgical or non-surgical), and this may be, in part, due to the long follow up period that is required to diagnose recurrence. That being said, available cohort studies are of poor quality, with 17 studies having a moderate to serious risk of bias. Notably, the investigation of potential confounders is lacking in most studies. Therefore, future work should take into consideration the potential confounding variables that might affect the recurrence rate. Second, there is no standardized definition or diagnostic criteria for equinus recurrence, which could potentially contribute to the wide variability in recurrence rates among studies. Therefore, scholars are advised to clearly state the criteria they used for defining recurrence. Third, due to the absence of a standardized control group, we could not analyze the comparative risk of developing recurrence among different treatment groups. This needs to be addressed in future randomized controlled trials. Fourth, the resultant heterogeneity in our analysis limits the validity and generalizability of our findings; therefore, more work is needed to investigate the potential patient- or intervention-related sources of heterogeneity. Finally, due to the lack of relevant data, we could not analyze the predictors of the recurrence of equinus. Notably, only four studies in our review classified patients with CP according to their GMFCS levels [21,24,29,45], despite the value of GMFCS being the best approach in deciding for the correction of equinus in CP patients. We hypothesize that outcomes, particularly recurrence, could vary considerably across different GMFCS levels; therefore, future studies are warranted to investigate this matter.

6. Conclusions

The rate of recurrence of equinus following surgery in CP patients is notably high. However, due to the poor quality of available evidence and the presence of multiple limitations, our findings should be interpreted with caution. Our review can be used for hypothesis generation, and more studies are still needed to determine the actual rate of equinus recurrence in CP.

Supplementary Materials: The following supporting information can be downloaded at: https://www.mdpi.com/article/10.3390/children9030339/s1. Figure S1. Forest plot of the risk of equinus recurrence among studies with two comparison groups.

Author Contributions: Conceptualization, A.H. and M.G.; methodology, A.H. and M.G.; software, M.G.; validation, A.H., M.C.M.K., H.P., S.E.S. and M.G.; formal analysis, A.H., M.C.M.K., H.P. and M.G.; investigation, A.H., M.C.M.K., H.P., S.E.S. and M.G.; resources, M.G., A.H.; data curation, M.G., A.H.; writing—original draft preparation A.H. and M.G.; writing—review and editing, A.H. and M.G.; visualization, M.G.; supervision, A.H.; project administration, A.H. All authors have read and agreed to the published version of the manuscript.

Funding: This research received no external funding.

Institutional Review Board Statement: Ethical approval will not be required because this study will retrieve and synthesise data from already published studies.

Informed Consent Statement: Not required.

Conflicts of Interest: The authors declare no conflict of interest.

References

1. Lovell, W.W.; Winter, R.B.; Morrissy, R.T.; Weinstein, S.L. *Lovell and Winter's Pediatric Orthopaedics*; Lippincott Williams & Wilkins: Philadelphia, PA, USA, 2006.
2. Rethlefsen, S.A.; Blumstein, G.; Kay, R.M.; Dorey, F.; Wren, T.A. Prevalence of specific gait abnormalities in children with cerebral palsy revisited: Influence of age, prior surgery, and Gross Motor Function Classification System level. *Dev. Med. Child Neurol.* **2017**, *59*, 79–88. [CrossRef] [PubMed]
3. Boulay, C.; Pomero, V.; Viehweger, E.; Glard, Y.; Castanier, E.; Authier, G.; Halbert, C.; Jouve, J.L.; Chabrol, B.; Bollini, G.; et al. Dynamic equinus with hindfoot valgus in children with hemiplegia. *Gait Posture* **2012**, *36*, 108–112. [CrossRef] [PubMed]
4. Davids, J.R.; Rogozinski, B.M.; Hardin, J.W.; Davis, R.B. Ankle dorsiflexor function after plantar flexor surgery in children with cerebral palsy. *J. Bone Jt. Surg. Am. Vol.* **2011**, *93*, e138. [CrossRef]
5. Gracies, J.M. Pathophysiology of spastic paresis. II: Emergence of muscle overactivity. *Muscle Nerve* **2005**, *31*, 552–571. [CrossRef]
6. Panteliadis, C.P. *Cerebral Palsy: A Multidisciplinary Approach*; Springer: Berlin/Heidelberg, Germany, 2018.
7. Shore, B.J.; White, N.; Kerr Graham, H. Surgical correction of equinus deformity in children with cerebral palsy: A systematic review. *J. Child. Orthop.* **2010**, *4*, 277–290. [CrossRef]
8. Ma, N.; Sclavos, N.; Passmore, E.; Thomason, P.; Graham, K.; Rutz, E. Three-Dimensional Gait Analysis in Children Undergoing Gastrocsoleus Lengthening for Equinus Secondary to Cerebral Palsy. *Medicina* **2021**, *57*, 98. [CrossRef] [PubMed]
9. Liberati, A.; Altman, D.G.; Tetzlaff, J.; Mulrow, C.; Gøtzsche, P.C.; Ioannidis, J.P.; Clarke, M.; Devereaux, P.J.; Kleijnen, J.; Moher, D.; et al. The PRISMA statement for reporting systematic reviews and meta-analyses of studies that evaluate health care interventions: Explanation and elaboration. *PLoS Med.* **2009**, *6*, e1000100. [CrossRef]
10. Ghozy, S.; Nam, N.H.; Radwan, I.; Karimzadeh, S.; Tieu, T.M.; Hashan, M.R.; Abbas, A.S.; Eid, P.S.; Vuong, N.L.; Khang, N.V.; et al. Therapeutic efficacy of hepatitis B virus vaccine in treatment of chronic HBV infections: A systematic review and meta-analysis. *Rev. Med. Virol.* **2020**, *30*, e2089. [CrossRef]
11. Vassar, M.; Atakpo, P.; Kash, M.J. Manual search approaches used by systematic reviewers in dermatology. *J. Med. Libr. Assoc. JMLA* **2016**, *104*, 302. [CrossRef]
12. Sterne, J.A.; Savović, J.; Page, M.J.; Elbers, R.G.; Blencowe, N.S.; Boutron, I.; Cates, C.J.; Cheng, H.Y.; Corbett, M.S.; Eldridge, S.M.; et al. RoB 2: A revised tool for assessing risk of bias in randomised trials. *BMJ* **2019**, *366*, l4898. [CrossRef]

13. Sterne, J.A.; Hernán, M.A.; Reeves, B.C.; Savović, J.; Berkman, N.D.; Viswanathan, M.; Henry, D.; Altman, D.G.; Ansari, M.T.; Boutron, I.; et al. ROBINS-I: A tool for assessing risk of bias in non-randomised studies of interventions. *BMJ* **2016**, *355*, i4919. [CrossRef] [PubMed]
14. Stijnen, T.; Hamza, T.H.; Ozdemir, P. Random effects meta-analysis of event outcome in the framework of the generalized linear mixed model with applications in sparse data. *Stat. Med.* **2010**, *29*, 3046–3067. [CrossRef] [PubMed]
15. DerSimonian, R.; Laird, N. Meta-analysis in clinical trials. *Control. Clin. Trials* **1986**, *7*, 177–188. [CrossRef]
16. R Core Team. *R: A Language and Environment for Statistical Computing*; R Foundation for Statistical Computing: Vienna, Austria, 2013.
17. Balduzzi, S.; Rücker, G.; Schwarzer, G. How to perform a meta-analysis with R: A practical tutorial. *Evid.-Based Ment. Health* **2019**, *22*, 153–160. [CrossRef]
18. Biedermann, R.; Kaufmann, G.; Lair, J.; Bach, C.; Wachter, R.; Donnan, L. High recurrence after calf lengthening with the Ilizarov apparatus for treatment of spastic equinus foot deformity. *J. Pediatric Orthop. Part B* **2007**, *16*, 125–128. [CrossRef]
19. Boireau, P.; Laville, J.M. Percutaneous lengthening of the Achilles tendon in children with cerebral palsy. Technique and results. *Rev. Chir. Orthop. Reparatrice L'appareil Mot.* **2002**, *88*, 705–709.
20. Sala, D.A.; Grant, A.D.; Kummer, F.J. Equinus deformity in cerebral palsy: Recurrence after tendo Achillis lengthening. *Dev. Med. Child Neurol.* **1997**, *39*, 45–48. [CrossRef]
21. Tamer, E.-S. Gastrocnemius recession in children with cerebral palsy. *Egypt. Orthop. J.* **2012**, *47*, 399–402.
22. Throop, F.B.; DeRosa, G.P.; Reeck, C.; Waterman, S. Correction of equinus in cerebral palsy by the Murphy procedure of tendo calcaneus advancement: A preliminary communication. *Dev. Med. Child Neurol.* **1975**, *17*, 182–185. [CrossRef]
23. Uyttendaele, D.; Burssens, P.; Pollefliet, A.; Claessens, H. Simultaneous Achilles and tibialis posterior tendon lengthening in cerebral palsy. *Acta Orthop. Belg.* **1989**, *55*, 62–66.
24. Dreher, T.; Buccoliero, T.; Wolf, S.I.; Heitzmann, D.; Gantz, S.; Braatz, F.; Wenz, W. Long-term results after gastrocnemius-soleus intramuscular aponeurotic recession as a part of multilevel surgery in spastic diplegic cerebral palsy. *J. Bone Jt. Surg. Am.* **2012**, *94*, 627–637. [CrossRef] [PubMed]
25. Matsuo, T.; Kawada, N.; Tomishige, O. Combined lengthening of the plantar flexors of the ankle and foot for equinus gait in cerebral palsy. *Foot* **1994**, *4*, 136–144. [CrossRef]
26. Ahmad, K.; Ahmad Bhat, S.; Avtar Agrawal, R.; Agrawal, R. Results of Ilizarov External Fixation in Rigid Equinus Deformity: An Experience of 30 Patients. *Ortop. Traumatol. Rehabil.* **2018**, *20*, 25–30. [CrossRef]
27. Al-Azzawi, I.; Mohammed, A.A. Open Versus Percutaneous Lengthening Of Tendo Achilles In Spastic Cerebral Palsy: A Prospective Study Of Tendo Achilles Lengthening Trauma In Spastic Cerebral Palsy In Al-Yarmouk Teaching Hospital In Iraq. *IRAQI J. Community Med.* **2016**, *29*, 53–59.
28. Kay, R.M.; Rethlefsen, S.A.; Fern-Buneo, A.; Wren, T.A.; Skaggs, D.L. Botulinum toxin as an adjunct to serial casting treatment in children with cerebral palsy. *J. Bone Jt. Surg. Am. Vol.* **2004**, *86*, 2377–2384. [CrossRef]
29. Kérő, G.; Frigyesi, L.; Szabó, T.; Than, P.; Vermes, C. Long-term follow-up of achillotenotomy in patients with cerebral palsy. *Orv. Hetil.* **2020**, *161*, 306–312. [CrossRef]
30. Lee, C.L.; Bleck, E.E. Surgical correction of equinus deformity in cerebral palsy. *Dev. Med. Child Neurol.* **1980**, *22*, 287–292. [CrossRef]
31. Firth, G.B.; Passmore, E.; Sangeux, M.; Thomason, P.; Rodda, J.; Donath, S.; Selber, P.; Graham, H.K. Multilevel surgery for equinus gait in children with spastic diplegic cerebral palsy: Medium-term follow-up with gait analysis. *J. Bone Jt. Surg. Am. Vol.* **2013**, *95*, 931–938. [CrossRef]
32. Kläusler, M.; Speth, B.M.; Brunner, R.; Tirosh, O.; Camathias, C.; Rutz, E. Long-term follow-up after tibialis anterior tendon shortening in combination with Achilles tendon lengthening in spastic equinus in cerebral palsy. *Gait Posture* **2017**, *58*, 457–462. [CrossRef]
33. Joo, S.Y.; Knowtharapu, D.N.; Rogers, K.J.; Holmes, L., Jr.; Miller, F. Recurrence after surgery for equinus foot deformity in children with cerebral palsy: Assessment of predisposing factors for recurrence in a long-term follow-up study. *J. Child. Orthop.* **2011**, *5*, 289–296. [CrossRef]
34. Rattey, T.E.; Leahey, L.; Hyndman, J.; Brown, D.C.; Gross, M. Recurrence after Achilles tendon lengthening in cerebral palsy. *J. Pediatric Orthop.* **1993**, *13*, 184–187.
35. Strecker, W.B.; Via, M.W.; Oliver, S.K.; Schoenecker, P.L. Heel cord advancement for treatment of equinus deformity in cerebral palsy. *J. Pediatric Orthop.* **1990**, *10*, 105–108. [CrossRef]
36. Poul, J.; Pesl, M.; Pokorná, M. Percutaneous aponeurotomy of the triceps surae muscle in cerebral palsy in children. *Acta Chir. Orthop. Traumatol. Cechoslov.* **2003**, *70*, 292–295.
37. Chung, C.Y.; Sung, K.H.; Lee, K.M.; Lee, S.Y.; Choi, I.H.; Cho, T.J.; Yoo, W.J.; Park, M.S. Recurrence of equinus foot deformity after tendo-achilles lengthening in patients with cerebral palsy. *J. Pediatric Orthop.* **2015**, *35*, 419–425. [CrossRef] [PubMed]
38. Vipulakorn, K.; Prichanond, S.; Kharnwan, S. Recurrence of Equinus Deformity in Cerebral Palsy Children after Orthopaedics Surgery, Long Term Follow-up Study. *Srinagarind Med. J.* **2012**, *27*, 272–278.
39. Borton, D.C.; Walker, K.; Pirpiris, M.; Nattrass, G.R.; Graham, H.K. Isolated calf lengthening in cerebral palsy. Outcome analysis of risk factors. *J. Bone Jt. Surg. Br. Vol.* **2001**, *83*, 364–370. [CrossRef]

40. Grant, A.D.; Feldman, R.; Lehman, W.B. Equinus deformity in cerebral palsy: A retrospective analysis of treatment and function in 39 cases. *J. Pediatric Orthop.* **1985**, *5*, 678–681. [CrossRef]
41. Gaytán-Fernández, S.; Chaidez, P.; García-Galicia, A.; Martínez-Asención, P.; Barragán-Hervella, R.G.; Corpus-Mariscal, E.; Jiménez-Reyes, M.; Montiel-Jarquín, A.J. Analysis to determine optimal age for surgical management of equinus foot in patients with childhood cerebral palsy. *Acta Ortop. Mex.* **2020**, *34*, 2–5.
42. Javors, J.R.; Klaaren, H.E. The Vulpius procedure for correction of equinus deformity in cerebral palsy. *J. Pediatric Orthop.* **1987**, *7*, 191–193. [CrossRef]
43. Hiroshima, K.; Hamada, S.; Shimizu, N.; Ohshita, S.; Ono, K. Anterior transfer of the long toe flexors for the treatment of spastic equinovarus and equinus foot in cerebral palsy. *J. Pediatric Orthop.* **1988**, *8*, 164–168. [CrossRef]
44. Katz, K.; Arbel, N.; Apter, N.; Soudry, M. Early mobilization after sliding achilles tendon lengthening in children with spastic cerebral palsy. *Foot Ankle Int.* **2000**, *21*, 1011–1014. [CrossRef] [PubMed]
45. Krupiński, M.; Borowski, A.; Synder, M. Long Term Follow-up of Subcutaneous Achilles Tendon Lengthening in the Treatment of Spastic Equinus Foot in Patients with Cerebral Palsy. *Ortop. Traumatol. Rehabil.* **2015**, *17*, 155–161. [CrossRef] [PubMed]
46. Svehlík, M.; Kraus, T.; Steinwender, G.; Zwick, E.B.; Saraph, V.; Linhart, W.E. The Baumann procedure to correct equinus gait in children with diplegic cerebral palsy: Long-term results. *J. Bone Jt. Surg. Br. Vol.* **2012**, *94*, 1143–1147. [CrossRef]
47. Koman, L.A.; Smith, B.P.; Barron, R. Recurrence of equinus foot deformity in cerebral palsy patients following surgery: A review. *J. South. Orthop. Assoc.* **2003**, *12*, 125–133, quiz 134. [PubMed]

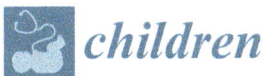

Article

Clinical Follow-Up without Radiographs Is Sufficient after Most Nonoperatively Treated Distal Radius Fractures in Children

Marja Perhomaa [1,2,*], Markus Stöckell [1], Tytti Pokka [3], Justus Lieber [4], Jaakko Niinimäki [2] and Juha-Jaakko Sinikumpu [1]

[1] Research Unit of Clinical Medicine, Medical Research Center, Oulu Childhood Fracture and Sports Injury Study, Division of Pediatric Surgery and Orthopedics, Department of Children and Adolescents, (MRC) Oulu, Oulu University Hospital, Oulu University, 90220 Oulu, Finland
[2] Research Unit of Health Sciences and Technology, Department of Radiology, Oulu University Hospital, Oulu University, 90220 Oulu, Finland
[3] Research Service Unit, Research Unit of Clinical Medicine, Oulu University Hospital, 90220 Oulu, Finland
[4] Department of Pediatric Surgery and Pediatric Urology, University Children's Hospital of Tübingen, 72076 Tübingen, Germany
* Correspondence: marja.perhomaa@pohde.fi

Abstract: Distal forearm fractures are common in children and are usually treated nonoperatively. No consensus has been reached on how to perform clinical and radiographic follow-up of these fractures. Our aim was to study whether radiographic and clinical follow-up is justified. We included 100 consecutive patients with non-operatively treated distal forearm fractures who were treated at Oulu University Hospital in 2010–2011. The natural history of the fractures during the nonoperative treatment was analyzed by measuring the potential worsening of the alignment during the follow-up period. The limits of acceptable fracture position were set according to the current literature using "strict" or "wide" criteria for alignment. We determined the rate of worsening fracture position (i.e., patients who reached the threshold of unacceptable alignment). In relation to splinting, we evaluated how many patients benefited from clinical follow-up. Most of the fractures (98%) preserved acceptable alignment during the entire follow-up period when wide criteria were used. The application of stricter criteria for alignment in radiographs showed loss of reduction in 19% of the fractures. Worsening of the alignment was recognized at a mean of 13 days (range 5–29) after the injury. One in three (32%) patients needed some intervention due to splint loosening or failure. Radiographic follow-up of nonoperatively treated distal forearm fractures remains questionable. Instead, clinical follow-up is important, as 32% of patients needed their splints fixed.

Keywords: distal forearm fractures; pediatric; non-operative treatment; radiographic follow-up

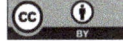

1. Introduction

Distal radius fractures are the most common fractures in children, accounting for 20–30% of all pediatric fractures [1–6]. The highest incidence rates are observed in older school-age boys (10–16 years) [3,4,7,8] due to a pubertal growth spurt, when the skeleton is weaker, and increased physical activity [7]. Fractures of the distal radial physis and metaphysis show a great capacity for spontaneous correction of injury-related deformity [9–12]; however, the remodeling capacity depends on the location of the fracture and the child's age. Fractures near the physis in young children have the greatest potential to remodel. Most pediatric distal forearm fractures can be treated nonoperatively [13] by casting or splinting [14] with or without a closed reduction. Loss of alignment of distal radius fractures after nonoperative treatment is common, with a rate reported between 7% and 91% [13,15–18]. Fracture-related and treatment-related risk factors for secondary displacement are presented in Table 1.

Table 1. Risk factors for secondary displacement of nonoperatively treated distal forearm fractures in children.

Fracture-related	Complete/high-grade initial displacement [1]
	Both-bone fracture [2]
	Obliquity of the fracture line [3]
	Initial angulation and shortening [4]
Treatment-related	Quality of reduction [5]
	Three-Point Index [6]
	Cast Index [7]
	Padding Index [7]
	Canterbury Index [7]
Patient-related	Age ≥ 11 years [8]
	Obesity [9]

References: [1] [13,18–21]; [2] [19]; [3] [20]; [4] [21]; [5] [18,21–25]; [6] [20]; [7] [26]; [8] [27]; [9] [28].

Much controversy exists regarding the acceptable degree of angular deformity [29,30]. Up to 30–35° of angular deformity in the sagittal plane and 10° in the coronal plane are suggested for adequate remodeling if the patient has at least 5 years of growth left [11,31].

Conventional radiographs of children's nonoperatively treated forearm fractures are usually taken 1 and 2 weeks after the injury and again at the time of completion of immobilization (4–5 weeks) [17,32] to evaluate the alignment. During this follow-up, the clinician also assesses the condition of the splint.

The aim of the present study was to determine the clinical importance of radiographic follow-up of pediatric distal forearm fractures after splinting. We hypothesized that less than 20% of children with a distal forearm fracture treated with non-operative means would show worsening of the alignment or increasing displacement that would meet the wide reduction criteria. Another aim was to determine the importance of clinical follow-up in detecting the need for splint repairing. We hypothesized that more than 50% of the patients would require splint correction or renewal.

2. Materials and Methods

This study included 100 children less than 16 years old who were consecutively treated for distal forearm fracture in the pediatric orthopedic outpatient clinic of Oulu University Hospital, Finland from January 2010 to December 2011. Acute distal radius fractures, with or without distal ulna fractures, were included if they were considered suitable for nonoperative treatment. Only fractures with the potential for displacement were accepted. For the coherence of the study patients, we excluded a few patients who had circumferential casts and included only patients treated with a splint. Stable buckle fractures and patients who were referred for operative treatment were excluded. The fracture types were classified according to the AO pediatric comprehensive classification of long bone fractures [33]. All clinical and radiological data concerning the injuries in question were retrieved from hospital medical records.

Most children with acute fractures, including forearm fractures, receive primary treatment in the emergency room at Oulu University Hospital. The treating physician can be a family doctor or a surgeon. The conservative treatment protocol includes the application of a splint with or without manipulation. The reduction, if needed, is performed under local or general anesthesia. We mainly use a custom-made below-elbow padded dorsal or volar splint of plaster of Paris, which is curved to the other side of the forearm to give three-point support. The splint reaches distally to the metacarpophalangeal joint. Post-reduction radiographs are taken before discharge. The first follow-up visit is scheduled 7–10 days later and includes a radiograph and evaluation by a pediatric orthopedic surgeon, a pediatric surgeon familiarized with childhood trauma or a resident in these specialties. Subsequent visits with radiographs usually occur at 2 weeks and 4 weeks following the injury. Undisplaced or minimally displaced fractures may have only one follow-up visit with radiographs at 1–2 weeks after the injury without further actions. Follow-up is decided on an individual basis for every patient, and no obligatory follow-up schema is applied for these patients.

In accordance with the study protocol, the patients' radiographic and clinical follow-up findings were studied at every follow-up visit. The radiographs included anteroposterior and lateral projections taken via a digital radiograph system. The angulation degree was defined as the angle between the central longitudinal axis of the proximal and distal fragments of the distal radius. The anterior–posterior and lateral displacement was expressed in millimeters. One researcher (MP), with 20 years of experience in pediatric radiology and childhood trauma imaging, performed all radiographic analyses.

Two criteria, "strict" and "wide" (Table 2), were defined according to the current literature [11–13,19,29,34,35] prior to the study to evaluate the course of the nonoperatively treated distal forearm fractures and their alignment. The 2 criteria included the upper limits for the angulation in the anterior–posterior and coronal directions and for translational displacement in any direction, expressed in millimeters. We adjusted for the age and gender of the patients regarding these criteria (Table 2). Institutional approval for the study was obtained prior to its initiation (21 October 2019, 146/2009).

Table 2. Limits of acceptable alignment according to the "strict" and "wide" criteria.

Treatment Protocol	Age	Sagittal Plane		Coronal Plane	Displacement
		Boys	Girls		
"Strict"					
	0–5	>25°	>25°	>10°	>10 mm
	6–10	>20°	>20°	>10°	>10 mm
	≥11	>15°	>10°	>5°	>5 mm
"Wide"					
	0–5	>35°	>35°	>20°	>10 mm
	6–10	>30°	>30°	>15°	>10 mm
	≥11	>25°	>20°	>15°	>10 mm

The main outcome of the study was a worsening fracture alignment beyond the accepted limits (Table 2) during the follow-up period. In total, 2 separate analyses were performed to analyze the worsening alignment in relation to the 2 limits of acceptance (wide and strict). As a secondary outcome, the importance of clinical follow-up was determined based on the frequency of splint repair or new casting at every follow-up visit.

Statistical Analysis

Based on prior prospective studies of Asadollahi et al. and Alemdaroğlu et al. [18,36], we hypothesized that 20% of the fractures would lose their alignment during follow-up. An odds ratio of 10 for the loss of alignment of children's distal radial fractures was considered clinically significant when using strict criteria. This was reasonable given that the occurrence of re-displacement in this self-controlled case study was 2% among non-operative children. With a statistical power of 80% and a two-sided α error of 0.05, we calculated that the required sample size was 87 children. To overcome the potential missing data of the individual consecutive cases in this research, we conducted a sample size analysis prior to the study initiation, and we opted for the study population size of 100 to exceed the minimum sample size. The quantitative data are described as the mean and range for categorical variables and as frequencies and proportions with 95% confidence intervals constructed using the exact Clopper–Pearson method. Basic statistics were calculated using IBM SPSS Statistics for Windows, Version 27 (Armonk, NY, USA, IBM Corp.) statistical software. Confidence intervals of the proportions were calculated using StatsDirect Statistical Software, version 3.3.5 (Wirral, England, StatsDirect Ltd. 2008).

3. Results

3.1. Study Sample and Patients' Characteristics

Altogether, 100 patients were included in the study. Of these, one patient received their primary treatment at another hospital, but their follow-up visits were carried out at the study institution. Of the original one hundred thirteen patients, thirteen patients were excluded from the analysis. Overall, five of these thirteen patients did not have post-reduction radiographs for follow-up, one patient had a primary fracture that was missed, and one patient with a Salter–Harris type 1 fracture was excluded because the fracture was one of a kind. The other six patients were excluded because they were treated with a circumferential cast.

The mean age of the patients was 11.7 years (range 4–16 years). Overall, 70% of the patients were aged 11–16 years, and 60% of the patients were male. The most common injury cause (73%) was a fall from a standing height. Snowboarding, downhill skiing, scootering, and skateboarding were the most common recreational activities related to distal forearm fractures in this population. The radius fractures comprised 18% complete metaphyseal fractures, 32% incomplete metaphyseal fractures, and 50% physeal Salter–Harris type 2 fractures. The fracture types, according to the AO pediatric comprehensive classification of long bone fractures, were 23r-E/2, 23r-M/2, and 23r-M/3. The baseline characteristics of the patients, their injury types, and their treatments are presented in Table 3.

Table 3. Baseline characteristics of the patients, their injury types, and treatments.

		n = 100
Age, years		11.7 ± 2.8
Age distribution		
	0–5 years	3
	6–10 years	27
	11–16 years	70
Gender		
	males	60
	females	40
Fracture side		
	left	70
	right	30
Type of injury		
	Fall	73
	Fall > 1 m	12
	Traffic incident	3
	other	12
Fracture type		
	Salter–Harris II	50
	Incomplete metaphyseal	32
	Complete metaphyseal	18
Treatment *		
	Immobilization in situ	44
	Reduction with LA **	43
	Reduction with GA ***	12
Treating physician on admission *		
	Family doctor	57
	Junior Surgeon	39
	Senior Surgeon	3
Time of treatment		
	Day, 6 a.m.–9 p.m.	72
	Night 9 p.m.–6 a.m.	28

* n = 99, ** Local anesthesia (LA), *** General anesthesia (GA).

Altogether, 226 follow-up visits with radiographs took place. Follow-up visit one occurred 2–10 days after the injury in 95 patients. The second follow-up visits took place between 11 and 20 days (41 patients) and the third between 21 and 41 days (83 patients) after injury. Only seven patients had a later follow-up visit, occurring between 42 and 212 days after the injury.

In terms of reduction, 55% of the fractures were reduced on admission and 44% were immobilized without reduction. The fracture alignment after the primary treatment is presented in Table 4.

Table 4. Fracture position during primary care.

Treatment on Admission	Immobilization In Situ ($n = 44$)	Reduction ($n = 55$)	Post Reduction ($n = 55$)
Angulation on sagittal plane *	8.6	22.9	5.4
range	0–17	5–57	0–18
Angulation on coronal plane *	0.5	5.2	0.7
range	0–10	0–26	0–16
Displacement **	0.5	5.1	1.4
range	0–5	0–24	0–7

* Mean, degrees; ** mean, millimeters.

3.2. Occurrence of Loss of Alignment

A total of 84 (84%) of the fractures showed acceptable alignment after primary treatment according to the strict criteria, and 99 (99%) fractures were acceptably aligned according to the wide criteria. The only case exceeding the wide criterion of coronal angulation after primary treatment was an 11-year-old girl, who had a complete metaphyseal fracture. Most (97/99) of the fractures (98%, 95% confidence interval [CI] 93–100%) showed acceptable alignment during the entire follow-up period according to the wide criteria (Table 5).

Table 5. Fracture alignment after primary care and during follow-up visits No 1–4.

Protocol	Alignment	Primary Care	Visit 1	Visit 2	Visit 3	Visit 4
Strict	Accepted	84	88	36	79	7
	Not accepted	16	7	5	4	0
Wide	Accepted	99	95	41	81	7
	Not accepted	1	0	0	2	0
	Current practice *	100	95	41	83	7

* True number of patients at every visit.

In total, two patients dropped out during the follow-up period; these were two girls aged 12 and 14 years with complete metaphyseal fractures. Deterioration of the sagittal alignment in the radial fractures was detected 4 weeks after the injury (Figure 1).

Altogether 16/84 (19%, 95% CI 11–29%) of the patients lost acceptable alignment during the follow-up when the strict criteria were used. According to the different fracture types, loss of alignment occurred in 18% (9/50) of the SH 2 fractures, 13% (4/32) of the incomplete metaphyseal fractures, and 17% (3/18) of the complete metaphyseal fractures. Worsening of the alignment was recognized at a mean of 13 days (range 5–29).

3.3. Rate of Reduction during Follow-Up

In total, one patient of the 100 (1%, 95% CI 0.03–5%) was re-treated during the follow-up period. She was a 12-year-old girl who had a complete metaphyseal fracture with dorsal angulation (17°), and she was primarily treated with immobilization without manipulation. At 12 days after the injury, the angulation was similar, but the first reduction was determined. However, the fracture malalignment of 17° was within the limit of acceptable alignment, and no intervention was needed according to the wide criteria.

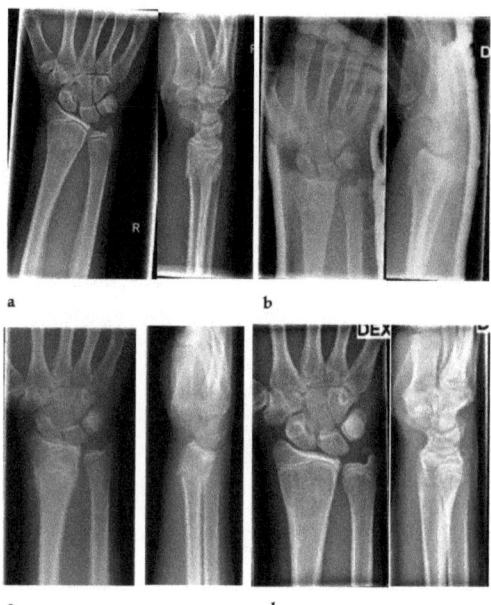

Figure 1. A 14-year-old girl injured her right wrist in downhill skiing. A complete metaphyseal fracture was detected and treated by immobilization without manipulation (**a**). In a follow-up visit at one-week mark, the alignment was good (**b**), but four weeks later a worsening alignment in radius was revealed with 24° dorsal angulation (**c**). A six-month follow-up visit was arranged showing good fracture position (**d**).

3.4. Need for Splint Repair

The clinical evaluation of the patients resulted in repairs of splints in 32 (32%, 95% CI 23–42%) of the cases. Most of the cases (24, 24%) required repairs within 10 days after injury, whereas seven casts were fixed at the second follow-up visit. One patient received a removable splint 3 weeks after the trauma. The intervention with the splint was a consequence of loosening or failure of the splint, irritative reactions, or other inconvenience caused by the splint.

4. Discussion

Distal radius fractures are the most common pediatric fractures, but due to their good remodeling capacity, they can mostly be treated nonoperatively [13]. No consensus has yet been reached regarding the limits of acceptable angular and translational displacement for decisions on whether to reduce the fracture or to leave correction of the position to remodeling during growth. Therefore, in this study, we retrospectively used two different criteria, "strict" and "wide", to evaluate the course of 100 consecutive pediatric nonoperatively treated distal forearm fractures and their alignments. Instead, we decided not to use the (re-)reduction as the primary variable of treatment failure because it depends on the particular decision of each particular treating physician rather than on the evidence-based guidelines for this injury. We found that 16/84 (19%) of the fractures showed secondary displacement beyond the acceptable alignment when the strict criteria were used. When the wide criteria were applied, only two (2%) of ninety-nine fractures benefited from radiographic follow-up. Maccagnano et al. have evaluated accordingly predetermined radiographic parameters for failure predictors of conservative treatment in pediatric forearm shaft fractures in their study [37].

Consideration of the benefit of radiographic follow-up in accordance with the patient's age depends on how much remodeling potential is available should a displacement occur [29,38]. Van der Sluijs found that a malunion of 15° had a mean remodeling time of 12 months, and this increased to 36 months for a malunion of 30° [39]. In metaphyseal fractures, a mean remodeling rate of 2.5° per month and up to 7.6° of correction per month has been reported in children [40]. A positive correlation between the remodeling speed and malunion angulation and a negative correlation between remodeling speed and remodeling time have been found [40,41]. The coronal remodeling potential in distal radius fractures of skeletally immature patients is remarkable. A mean coronal angulation remodeling rate of 2.3° per month was detected by Lynch et al. in 2020 among 36 pediatric patients aged from 4 to 12 years [35]. In Australia, Roth et al. studied 66 children suffering from nonoperatively treated distal forearm fractures that had failed and undergone re-displacement: 24 were re-manipulated, and 42 were left to heal in the position of the angular deformity. Re-manipulation of the distal forearm fractures in the children < 12 years did not improve their outcomes [34]. Therefore, Roth et al. suggest the following acceptance criteria when re-angulation occurs: up to 30° of angulation in children < 9 years, 25° of angulation in children aged 9–12 years, and 20° of angulation in children ≥ 12 years. They also encourage clinicians to be more reluctant to perform re-reductions. A Norwegian prospective study reported that 12 patients out of 88 showed more than 15 degrees of malangulation after nonoperative treatment. Of these twelve, seven participated for 7 years of follow-up visits and demonstrated complete remodeling [42]. Similar long-term outcomes have been found among children under 10 years of age independent of residual fracture deformity during fracture healing [12,20,23,35].

In addition to the displacement criteria and the patient's maturity, the age and location of the fracture, any clinical deformity, and the clinicians' judgement can influence the treatment options [18]. Complete fracture displacement [13,18], translation of more than half the bone diameter, volar angulation, and a simultaneous ulnar fracture at the same level as the radius fracture have been identified as predictors of instability [36]. In their study, Asadollahi et al. reported a secondary displacement rate of 28.8%, but only 7.4% of the patients needed a second procedure [18]. Their criteria for displacement were even tighter than the strict criteria used in the present study. Notably, the use of strict radiographic displacement criteria alone may increase the number of unnecessary interventions and follow-up visits for fractures with a high potential to remodel. An internet-based survey conducted by Bernthal et al., (2015) on the management of pediatric distal radius fractures revealed that, in addition to the fracture displacement and the patient's age, the surgeon's subspecialty and the practice environment affected the treatment recommendations. Pediatric orthopedic surgeons favored the most conservative management [30].

In the present study, 32 (32%) of the patients needed clinical interventions during follow-up, namely fixing or renewing the splint. In most of these cases (24/32; 75%) the need arose in the first 10 days after the injury. The need to fix a splint can be the result of the splint loosening when post-traumatic edema in soft tissues decreases. Some of the required clinical interventions may have been due to the quality of the splint and the experience of the personnel in the emergency department, which is not dedicated to treating children's fractures. This finding supports the idea of routine clinical follow-up of distal forearm fracture patients during the early follow-up period. An option for later clinical assessment could be to interview the patient and the parent(s) by phone and, if necessary, to the arrange an outpatient clinic visit. Routine clinical follow-up could be performed by trained orthopedic nurses without intervention by a surgeon.

Because of the high frequency of pediatric distal radius fractures, the expenses related to the treatment of these fractures are not trivial. Godfrey et al. [43] retrospectively investigated the treatment-related costs of closed distal radius fractures in 5640 children treated at a large academic children's hospital in the USA. The median costs of closed reductions without manipulation, closed reductions in the emergency department or radiology procedure suite, and percutaneous pinning in the operating room were USD 1390, USD 4263, and USD 9389, respectively. This included only medical services. The fracture management approach and use of the operating room had the greatest influence on the treatment costs. They concluded that choosing not to perform a closed reduction in patients whose fractures will adequately remodel during their growth could reduce treatment costs. Considering the primary treatment of distal radial metaphyseal fractures, Orland et al. [44] estimated that in children younger than 10 years of age 27% of closed reduction procedures were unnecessary. The costs of closed reduction and manipulation using procedural sedation in the emergency department were estimated to be eight times higher than the costs of cast immobilization in an outpatient clinic. Cost saving of up to 12% of the total cost of nonoperatively treated pediatric forearm fractures can be achieved by eliminating the radiographic follow-up visit at 4 weeks after the injury, according to Luther et al. [32].

Health care resources could be optimized by employing wide criteria for acceptable alignment in the primary treatment of children's distal forearm fractures, favoring splinting/casting in an outpatient clinic without manipulation, and conducting rigorous casting. As most activity concerning loose, unfit, or broken splints appeared in the one follow-up visit at 1 week after the injury, clinical inspection at the one-week mark seems justifiable. Informing the patient and the parents about the good natural course of fracture healing, even with moderate displacement, and encouraging them to contact the treating unit with any concerns about splint impairment will increase compliance.

Strengths and Limitations

The retrospective nature of this study did not produce systematic long-term outcomes. The number and timing of follow-up visits were also inconsistent in the study population. We do not have available information for all risk factors for the displacement of distal forearm fractures. Because no widely accepted guidelines are available concerning acceptable alignment of children's distal forearm fractures, the effect of the treating physician's preferences may have influenced the treatment choices. Although we included 100 fractures, 70% of the patients were aged 11–16 years and the number of patients in the younger age groups was quite small. However, the risk for loss of reduction is higher in children ≥ 11 years old. Accordingly, when the fractures were classified by fracture type, only 18 patients had fractures with the greatest potential for dislocation (i.e., complete metaphyseal fractures). A strength of this study is its design with an objective measurable outcome, namely the malalignment beyond a predetermined threshold, despite the dependence of the rate of (re-)reduction on the decision by the treating surgeon for every single patient.

5. Conclusions

We evaluated 100 consecutive nonoperatively treated distal forearm fractures with the potential to displace. One in five of the fractures (16/84, 19%) that were acceptable after primary treatment were found to lose reduction when strict criteria for reduction were applied. Worsening alignment was found in two patients (2%) with complete metaphyseal fractures when the wide criteria were applied. However, only one of the one hundred fractures underwent a reduction during follow-up in real life. The use of strict criteria for acceptable alignment would have increased the number of fracture reductions and follow-up visits with radiographs. Nevertheless, this study does not resolve whether these potential (re-)reductions would have been important in achieving any long-term benefits regarding the clinical outcomes of the patients. Another important finding was that one in three of the patients needed their splint repaired, and this mostly occurred 1 week after the injury.

Author Contributions: Conceptualization, J.-J.S.; methodology J.-J.S.; software, T.P.; validation, T.P., M.P. and J.-J.S.; formal analysis, T.P., M.P. and J.-J.S.; investigation, M.P. and M.S.; resources, J.N. and J.-J.S.; data curation, M.S. and M.P.; writing—original draft preparation, M.P.; writing—review and editing, all authors; visualization, M.P. and T.P.; supervision, J.-J.S. and J.N.; project administration, J.-J.S. All authors have read and agreed to the published version of the manuscript.

Funding: This research received no external funding.

Institutional Review Board Statement: The study was conducted in accordance with the Declaration of Helsinki and approved by the Institutional Review Board of Oulu University Hospital prior to its initiation (21 October 2019, 146/2009).

Informed Consent Statement: Patient consent was waived due to retrospective study design.

Data Availability Statement: Research data available on request from the authors.

Acknowledgments: Licensed material: Abstract. 40. Jahrestagung der Sektion Kindertraumatologie der Deutschen Gesellschaft für Unfallchirurgie e. V. Varia A-37 Clinical follow-up without radiographs is sufficient after most non-operatively treated distal radius fractures in children. *Eur J Trauma Emerg Surg* 48, 3387 (2022). Springer Nature. https://doi.org/10.1007/s00068-022-01977-0. License Number 5480360989201, Copyright Clearance Center.

Conflicts of Interest: Juha-Jaakko Sinikumpu: Research grants from Alma and KA Snellman Foundation, Emil Aaltonen Foundation, Foundation of Pediatric Research, and national VTR-funding. The funders had no role in the design of the study; in the collection, analyses, or interpretation of data; in the writing of the manuscript; in the decision to publish the results. All other authors declare no conflict of interest.

References

1. Rennie, L.; Court-Brown, C.M.; Mok, J.Y.Q.; Beattie, T.F. The epidemiology of fractures in children. *Injury* **2007**, *38*, 913–922. [CrossRef] [PubMed]
2. Jones, I.E.; Cannan, R.; Goulding, A. Distal forearm fractures in New Zealand children: Annual rates in a geographically defined area. *N. Z. Med. J.* **2000**, *113*, 443–445. [PubMed]
3. Brudvik, C.; Hove, L.M. Childhood fractures in Bergen, Norway: Identifying high-risk groups and activities. *J. Pediatr. Orthop.* **2003**, *23*, 629–634. [CrossRef] [PubMed]
4. Hedström, E.M.; Svensson, O.; Bergström, U.; Michno, P. Epidemiology of fractures in children and adolescents. *Acta Orthop.* **2010**, *81*, 148–153. [CrossRef] [PubMed]
5. Lempesis, V.; Jerrhag, D.; Rosengren, B.E.; Landin, L.; Tiderius, C.J.; Karlsson, M.K. Pediatric Distal Forearm Fracture Epidemiology in Malmö, Sweden—Time Trends During Six Decades. *J. Wrist Surg.* **2019**, *8*, 463–469. [CrossRef]
6. Monget, F.; Sapienza, M.; McCracken, K.L.; Nectoux, E.; Fron, D.; Andreacchio, A.; Pavone, V.; Canavese, F. Clinical Characteristics and Distribution of Pediatric Fractures at a Tertiary Hospital in Northern France: A 20-Year-Distance Comparative Analysis (1999–2019). *Medicina* **2022**, *58*, 610. [CrossRef]
7. Khosla, S.; Melton, L.J., 3rd; Dekutoski, M.B.; Achenbach, S.J.; Oberg, A.L.; Riggs, B.L. Incidence of childhood distal forearm fractures over 30 years: A population-based study. *JAMA* **2003**, *290*, 1479–1485. [CrossRef]
8. Mamoowala, N.; Johnson, N.A.; Dias, J.J. Trends in paediatric distal radius fractures: An eight-year review from a large UK trauma unit. *Ann. R. Coll. Surg. Engl.* **2019**, *101*, 297–303. [CrossRef]
9. Noonan, K.J.; Price, C.T. Forearm and distal radius fractures in children. *J. Am. Acad. Orthop. Surg.* **1998**, *6*, 146–156. [CrossRef]
10. Johari, A.N.; Sinha, M. Remodeling of forearm fractures in children. *J. Pediatr. Orthop. B.* **1999**, *8*, 84–87.
11. Wilkins, K.E. Principles of fracture remodeling in children. *Injury* **2005**, *36* (Suppl. 1), A3–A11. [CrossRef] [PubMed]
12. Zimmermann, R.; Gschwentner, M.; Kralinger, F.; Arora, R.; Gabl, M.; Pechlaner, S. Long-term results following pediatric distal forearm fractures. *Arch Orthop. Trauma Surg.* **2004**, *124*, 179–186. [CrossRef] [PubMed]
13. van Delft, E.A.K.; Vermeulen, J.; Schep, N.W.L.; van Stralen, K.J.; van der Bij, G.J. Prevention of secondary displacement and reoperation of distal metaphyseal forearm fractures in children. *J. Clin. Orthop. Trauma.* **2020**, *11* (Suppl. 5), S817–S822. [CrossRef]
14. Murphy, R.F.; Sleasman, B.; Osborn, D.; Barfield, W.R.; Dow, M.A.; Mooney, J.F., III. A Single Sugar-Tong Splint Can Maintain Pediatric Forearm Fractures. *Orthopedics (Thorofare N.J.)* **2021**, *44*, e178–e182. [CrossRef]
15. Voto, S.J.; Weiner, D.S.; Leighley, B. Redisplacement after closed reduction of forearm fractures in children. *J. Pediatr. Orthop.* **1990**, *10*, 79–84. [CrossRef] [PubMed]
16. van Egmond, P.W.; Schipper, I.B.; van Luijt, P.A. Displaced distal forearm fractures in children with an indication for reduction under general anesthesia should be percutaneously fixated. *Eur. J. Orthop. Surg. Traumatol.* **2012**, *22*, 201–207. [CrossRef]
17. Colaris, J.W.; Allema, J.H.; Biter, L.U.; de Vries, M.R.; van de Ven, C.P.; Bloem, R.M.; Kerver, A.J.; Reijman, M.; Verhaar, J.A. Re-displacement of stable distal both-bone forearm fractures in children: A randomised controlled multicentre trial. *Injury* **2013**, *44*, 498–503. [CrossRef]
18. Asadollahi, S.; Ooi, K.S.; Hau, R.C. Distal radial fractures in children: Risk factors for redisplacement following closed reduction. *J. Pediatr. Orthop.* **2015**, *35*, 224–228. [CrossRef]
19. Sengab, A.; Krijnen, P.; Schipper, I.B. Risk factors for fracture redisplacement after reduction and cast immobilization of displaced distal radius fractures in children: A meta-analysis. *Eur. J. Trauma Emerg. Surg.* **2020**, *46*, 789–800. [CrossRef]

20. Crawford, S.N.; Lee, L.S.; Izuka, B.H. Closed treatment of overriding distal radial fractures without reduction in children. *J. Bone Jt. Surg. Am.* **2012**, *94*, 246–252. [CrossRef]
21. Proctor, M.T.; Moore, D.J.; Paterson, J.M. Redisplacement after manipulation of distal radial fractures in children. *J. Bone Jt. Surg. Br.* **1993**, *75*, 453–454. [CrossRef]
22. McQuinn, A.G.; Jaarsma, R.L. Risk factors for redisplacement of pediatric distal forearm and distal radius fractures. *J. Pediatr. Orthop.* **2012**, *32*, 687–692. [CrossRef] [PubMed]
23. Houshian, S.; Holst, A.K.; Larsen, M.S.; Torfing, T. Remodeling of Salter-Harris type II epiphyseal plate injury of the distal radius. *J. Pediatr. Orthop.* **2004**, *24*, 472–476. [CrossRef]
24. Sankar, W.N.; Beck, N.A.; Brewer, J.M.; Baldwin, K.D.; Pretell, J.A. Isolated distal radial metaphyseal fractures with an intact ulna: Risk factors for loss of reduction. *J. Child Orthop.* **2011**, *5*, 459–464. [CrossRef] [PubMed]
25. Constantino, D.M.C.; Machado, L.; Carvalho, M.; Cabral, J.; Sá Cardoso, P.; Balacó, I.; Ling, T.P.; Alves, C. Redisplacement of paediatric distal radius fractures: What is the problem? *J. Child Orthop.* **2021**, *15*, 532–539. [CrossRef] [PubMed]
26. Ravier, D.; Morelli, I.; Buscarino, V.; Mattiuz, C.; Sconfienza, L.M.; Spreafico, A.A.; Peretti, G.M.; Curci, D. Plaster cast treatment for distal forearm fractures in children: Which index best predicts the loss of reduction? *J. Pediatr. Orthop. B.* **2020**, *29*, 179–186. [CrossRef]
27. Dittmer, A.J.; Molina, D., 4th; Jacobs, C.A.; Walker, J.; Muchow, R.D. Pediatric Forearm Fractures Are Effectively Immobilized with a Sugar-Tong Splint Following Closed Reduction. *J. Pediatr. Orthop.* **2019**, *39*, e245–e247. [CrossRef]
28. Auer, R.T.; Mazzone, P.; Robinson, L.; Nyland, J.; Chan, G. Childhood Obesity Increases the Risk of Failure in the Treatment of Distal Forearm Fractures. *J. Pediatr. Orthop.* **2016**, *36*, e86–e88. [CrossRef]
29. Ploegmakers, J.J.; Verheyen, C.C. Acceptance of angulation in the non-operative treatment of paediatric forearm fractures. *J Pediatr. Orthop. B.* **2006**, *15*, 428–432. [CrossRef]
30. Bernthal, N.M.; Mitchell, S.; Bales, J.G.; Benhaim, P.; Silva, M. Variation in practice habits in the treatment of pediatric distal radius fractures. *J. Pediatr. Orthop. B.* **2015**, *24*, 400–407. [CrossRef]
31. Wilkins, K.E.; O'Brien, E. Fractures of the distal radius and ulna. In *Fractures in Children*, 4th ed.; Rockwood, C.A., Jr., Wilkins, K.E., Beaty, J.H., Eds.; Lippincott-Raven: Philadelphia, PA, USA, 1996; Volume 3, pp. 451–515.
32. Luther, G.; Miller, P.; Waters, P.M.; Bae, D.S. Radiographic Evaluation during Treatment of Pediatric Forearm Fractures: Implications on Clinical Care and Cost. *J. Pediatr. Orthop.* **2016**, *36*, 465–471. [CrossRef]
33. Slongo, T.; Audigé, L.; Schlickewei, W.; Clavert, J.M.; Hunter, J. International Association for Pediatric Traumatology. Development and validation of the AO pediatric comprehensive classification of long bone fractures by the Pediatric Expert Group of the AO Foundation in collaboration with AO Clinical Investigation and Documentation and the International Association for Pediatric Traumatology. *J. Pediatr. Orthop.* **2006**, *26*, 43–49. [CrossRef]
34. Roth, K.C.; Denk, K.; Colaris, J.W.; Jaarsma, R.L. Think twice before re-manipulating distal metaphyseal forearm fractures in children. *Arch Orthop. Trauma Surg.* **2014**, *134*, 1699–1707. [CrossRef] [PubMed]
35. Lynch, K.A.; Wesolowski, M.; Cappello, T. Coronal Remodeling Potential of Pediatric Distal Radius Fractures. *J. Pediatr. Orthop.* **2020**, *40*, 556–561. [CrossRef] [PubMed]
36. Alemdaroğlu, K.B.; Iltar, S.; Cimen, O.; Uysal, M.; Alagöz, E.; Atlihan, D. Risk factors in redisplacement of distal radial fractures in children. *J. Bone Jt. Surg. Am.* **2008**, *90*, 1224–1230. [CrossRef]
37. Maccagnano, G.; Notarnicola, A.; Pesce, V.; Tafuri, S.; Mudoni, S.; Nappi, V.; Moretti, B. Failure Predictor Factors of Conservative Treatment in Pediatric Forearm Fractures. *BioMed Res. Int.* **2018**, *2018*, 5930106. [CrossRef] [PubMed]
38. Laaksonen, T.; Puhakka, J.; Stenroos, A.; Kosola, J.; Ahonen, M.; Nietosvaara, Y. Cast immobilization in bayonet position versus reduction and pin fixation of overriding distal metaphyseal radius fractures in children under ten years of age: A case control study. *J. Child Orthop.* **2021**, *15*, 63–69. [CrossRef]
39. van der Sluijs, J.A.; Bron, J.L. Malunion of the distal radius in children: Accurate prediction of the expected remodeling. *J. Child Orthop.* **2016**, *10*, 235–240. [CrossRef]
40. Jeroense, K.T.; America, T.; Witbreuk, M.M.; van der Sluijs, J.A. Malunion of distal radius fractures in children. *Acta Orthop.* **2015**, *86*, 233–237. [CrossRef]
41. Friberg, K.S. Remodelling after distal forearm fractures in children. I. The effect of residual angulation on the spatial orientation of the epiphyseal plates. *Acta Orthop. Scand.* **1979**, *50*, 537–546. [CrossRef]
42. Hove, L.M.; Brudvik, C. Displaced paediatric fractures of the distal radius. *Arch Orthop. Trauma Surg.* **2008**, *128*, 55–60. [CrossRef] [PubMed]
43. Godfrey, J.M.; Little, K.J.; Cornwall, R.; Sitzman, T.J. A Bundled Payment Model for Pediatric Distal Radius Fractures: Defining an Episode of Care. *J. Pediatr. Orthop.* **2019**, *39*, e216–e221. [CrossRef] [PubMed]
44. Orland, K.J.; Boissonneault, A.; Schwartz, A.M.; Goel, R.; Bruce, R.W., Jr.; Fletcher, N.D. Resource Utilization for Patients With Distal Radius Fractures in a Pediatric Emergency Department. *JAMA Netw. Open.* **2020**, *3*, e1921202. [CrossRef] [PubMed]

Disclaimer/Publisher's Note: The statements, opinions and data contained in all publications are solely those of the individual author(s) and contributor(s) and not of MDPI and/or the editor(s). MDPI and/or the editor(s) disclaim responsibility for any injury to people or property resulting from any ideas, methods, instructions or products referred to in the content.

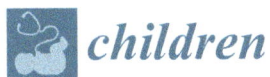

Article

The Variable Influence of Orthotic Management on Hip and Pelvic Rotation in Children with Unilateral Neurogenic Equinus Deformity

Domenic Grisch [1], Manuela Stäuble [1], Sandra Baumgartner [2], Hubertus J. A. van Hedel [2], Andreas Meyer-Heim [2], Thomas Dreher [1,3,*] and Britta Krautwurst [1,3]

[1] Department of Pediatric Orthopedics, Neuroorthopedics and Traumatology, University Children's Hospital Zurich, 8032 Zurich, Switzerland
[2] Swiss Children's Rehab, University Children's Hospital Zurich, 8910 Affoltern am Albis, Switzerland
[3] Pediatric Orthopedics, Balgrist University Hospital, University of Zurich, 8008 Zürich, Switzerland
* Correspondence: thomas.dreher@kispi.uzh.ch; Tel.: +41-44-266-75-35

Abstract: Background: Equinus deformity with or without concomitant drop foot is a common finding in children with unilateral spastic cerebral palsy and spastic hemiplegia of other causes. Hypothetically, these deformities may lead to pelvic retraction and hip internal rotation during gait. Orthoses are used to reduce pes equinus during gait and to restore hindfoot first contact. Objective: We aimed to investigate whether the use of orthotic equinus correction reduces rotational hip and pelvic asymmetries. Methods: In a retrospective study, 34 children with unilateral spastic cerebral palsy or spastic hemiplegia of other causes underwent standardized instrumented 3D gait analysis with and without orthotic equinus management. We analyzed the differences in the torsional profile during barefoot walking and while wearing orthoses, as well as investigated the influence of ankle dorsiflexion and femoral anteversion on pelvic and hip kinematics and hip kinetics. Results: Wearing orthoses corrected pes equinus and pelvic internal rotation at the end of the stance phase and in the swing phase compared to barefoot walking. Hip rotation and the rotational moment did not significantly change with orthoses. Orthotic management or femoral anteversion did not correlate to pelvic and hip asymmetry. Conclusion: The findings indicate that the correction of the equinus by using orthoses had a variable effect on the asymmetry of the hip and pelvis and internal rotation; both appear to have a multifactorial cause that is not primarily driven by the equinus component.

Keywords: hemiplegia; cerebral palsy; pelvic asymmetry; hip asymmetry; pes equinus; orthotic management

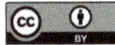

1. Introduction

The most common gait abnormalities in children with unilateral spastic cerebral palsy and spastic hemiplegia of other causes are pes equinus with or without drop foot, in-toeing, and stiff knee in the swing phase. Other manifestations are hip flexion, hip internal rotation, and pelvic retraction [1–3]. As a consequence of these abnormalities, children are prone to developing lever arm dysfunction and clearance problems, such as dripping and falling [1]. The standard treatment for in-toeing gait is femoral derotation osteotomy (FDO). The surgically improved hip centration results in reduced internal rotation of the hip and pelvic retraction [4,5]. Nevertheless, FDO carries the risk of over- or under-correction of rotational abnormalities [6]. To date, the pathogenetic mechanisms of internal rotation gait are not fully understood, and dynamic factors need to be discussed. Dynamic components can include muscular imbalance, increased muscle tone, spasticity, and altered moment arms [7]. It was hypothesized that hip internal rotation might be a result of high femoral anteversion or increased hip flexion present in children with unilateral spastic cerebral palsy [8,9]. However, it is still unclear whether this is a cause or a consequence of other factors. This might explain the variability of results after femoral derotation osteotomies. Based on computerized modeling, Brunner et al. showed a significant correlation between ankle plantar flexion and hip internal rotation in children with unilateral spastic cerebral palsy as a direct functional effect. Hence, an equinus position changes the torsional forces in the hip joint and, thus, increases hip internal rotation and pelvic retraction. This mechanism may represent a driving factor for the persistence of increased femoral anteversion during growth. Furthermore, it was suggested that the effects at the hip and knee are related to the function of the triceps surae and are not directly dependent on neuromuscular control [10]. In addition, Pasin Neto et al. found a combined improvement of ankle dorsiflexion and internal rotation of the hip through postural insoles in children with bilateral spastic cerebral palsy [11]. However, the body of literature lacks studies that underline the hypothesis that increased plantar flexion is a relevant factor leading to internal rotation gait.

Orthotic management is typically applied to correct pes equinus during walking and restore heel contact at initial contact (IC) in children with unilateral spastic cerebral palsy or spastic hemiplegia of other causes [12–14]. This results in an improvement of the first and second ankle rocker, increased dorsiflexion, and reduced drop foot [12,13,15–17]. Furthermore, orthotic management to correct pes equinus decreases energy cost, increases speed and stride length, enlarges hip and ankle range of motion, and improves the kinematics and kinetics of the knee [12,15–19].

In addition to conservative treatment with orthotics or the surgical rotation correction of the femur described above, various other treatment approaches are used for spasticity management, the improvement of foot elevation, or the correction of contractures. These include oral spasmolytics, selective dorsal rhizotomy, oral or intrathecal baclofen [20], botulinum toxin injections [21], muscular strengthening and stretching through physiotherapy, neuromuscular electrical stimulation [22], lengthening of the calf muscles, and shortening of the anterior tibialis tendon with or without split transfer to peroneus brevis [23]. The latter contributes to the balanced, active foot elevation or at least leads to a supporting tenodesis.

If pes equinus plays a central role as a driving factor for internal rotation gait, torsional moments of the hip, hip internal rotation, and pelvic asymmetry [1–3,10,24], these patterns should vanish or at least be significantly reduced by the orthotic management of equinus foot deformity. However, to the best knowledge of the authors, this was not previously investigated.

We hypothesized that the rotational effects and asymmetry of the hip and pelvis are significantly reduced by using orthoses to correct pes equinus in children with unilateral spastic cerebral palsy and spastic hemiplegia of other causes. As a secondary research question, this study aimed to investigate whether a high femoral anteversion reduces the corrective effect of the orthoses on hip and pelvic asymmetry.

2. Materials and Methods

2.1. Participants

Gait analysis data from children with unilateral spastic cerebral palsy and spastic hemiplegia of other causes and equinus foot deformity were investigated in this study. Furthermore, these patients needed to have orthotics for the management of equinus deformity. The exclusion criteria were the absence of dynamic pelvic or hip asymmetry, botulinum toxin therapy of the leg conducted within three months prior to gait analysis, or a history of selective dorsal rhizotomy (See Figure 1). None of the children had a previous derotating femoral osteotomy. The inclusion criteria were the neurological disorder due to cerebral palsy, post-stroke, post-trauma, neoplasia, syndrome or post-infection, between 4 and 18 years old, and Gross Motor Function Classification System (GMFCS) I or II. Further inclusion criteria based on the gait analysis parameters were pes equinus of the affected side (ankle plantar flexion at IC and/or < 5° ankle dorsiflexion in the single support phase); $\geq 4°$ transversal hip internal rotation (>1 standard deviation (SD) of typically developing reference group); and $\geq 5°$ asymmetry of the hip or pelvis (>1 SD of typically developing reference group). Only one gait analysis per patient was included. The examination was carried out barefoot and with orthotic support of the equinus foot. The type of orthosis was based on the individual need of the patient and varied from heel wedges, insoles, and foot drop bandages to ankle–foot orthosis and supramalleolar orthosis, according to Nancy Hilton. All orthotics shared the goal of correcting the equinus position during walking to reduce the effects of increased plantar flexion on proximal segments and planes.

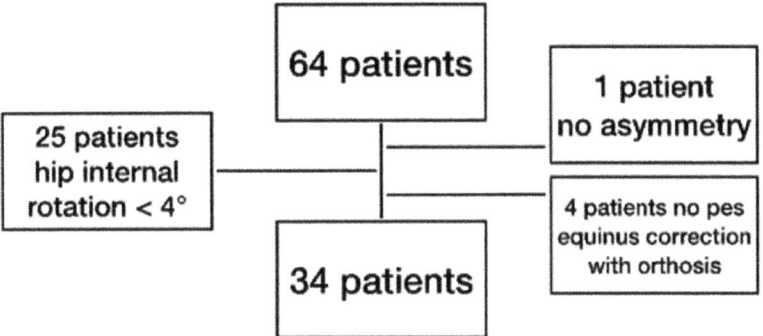

Figure 1. Schematic illustration of the inclusion of the patients. Middle row: number of patients; right and left row: number of and reason for excluded patients.

2.2. Measurements

All 3D gait analyses were carried out by the same experienced physiotherapists and pursuant to standardized procedures [25]. The participants were asked to walk along a 10-m walkway at a self-selected speed. Two gait analyses were performed in succession: the first barefoot and the second wearing their individual orthosis. Reflective markers were transferred from the foot to the orthosis according to a standardized protocol. At least three valid strides per patient and per condition were analyzed. A clinical examination was carried out as a standard part of each gait analysis. As a part of the clinical examination, femoral anteversion was measured using the TPAT (trochanteric prominence angle test).

2.3. Data Analysis

Several parameters for pelvic, hip, and ankle motion were derived from the gait analysis data. The pelvic motion in the transverse plane was calculated over the entire gait cycle (GC) due to the interdependent motion of the left and right pelvic hemispheres. Hip rotation was calculated as a mean during the stance phase (ST) and specifically at initial contact (IC). Furthermore, the internal hip rotational moments were calculated and used for further analysis. The ankle joint position was calculated at IC and as a mean during the stance phase. Furthermore, manually measured femoral torsion was used to determine a possible influence on pelvic and hip asymmetry. To determine any possible influences of the pes equinus and the femoral torsion on the pelvic and hip movements, differences in the joint angles between barefoot and orthotic management were calculated (See Table 1). They represent the change in joint angles while wearing the orthoses.

To study the dynamic effect of equinus position over the first half of the stance phase (30%) on the hip rotation angle (See Figure 2), the Δ hip rotation was calculated with and without orthotics (See Figure 3). This difference was then correlated with the femoral anteversion angle to evaluate whether patients with a high anteversion angle showed significantly less Δ hip rotation during this phase.

Table 1. Description of the calculation of the used variables.

Variable	Calculation
Pelvic asymmetry barefoot [°]	| mean pelvic rotation GC affected/unaffected side |
Pelvic asymmetry with orthosis [°]	| mean pelvic rotation GC affected/unaffected side |
Δ pelvic asymmetry [°]	barefoot affected side/orthotic affected side
Hip asymmetry barefoot [°]	| mean hip rotation ST affected/unaffected side |
Hip asymmetry with orthosis [°]	| mean hip rotation ST affected/unaffected side |
Δ hip asymmetry [°]	barefoot affected side/orthotic affected side
Δ mean hip rotation ST [°]	orthotic affected side/barefoot affected side
Δ hip rotation IC [°]	orthotic affected side/barefoot affected side
Δ hip rotational moments ST [°]	orthotic affected side/barefoot affected side
Barefoot Δ hip rotation [°]	hip rotation midstance/hip rotation initial contact
Orthotic Δ hip rotation [°]	hip rotation midstance/hip rotation initial contact
Δ ankle dorsi/plantar flexion IC [°]	orthotic affected side/barefoot affected side

Δ = delta; \| \| = absolute value; GC = gait cycle; ST = stance phase; IC = initial contact.

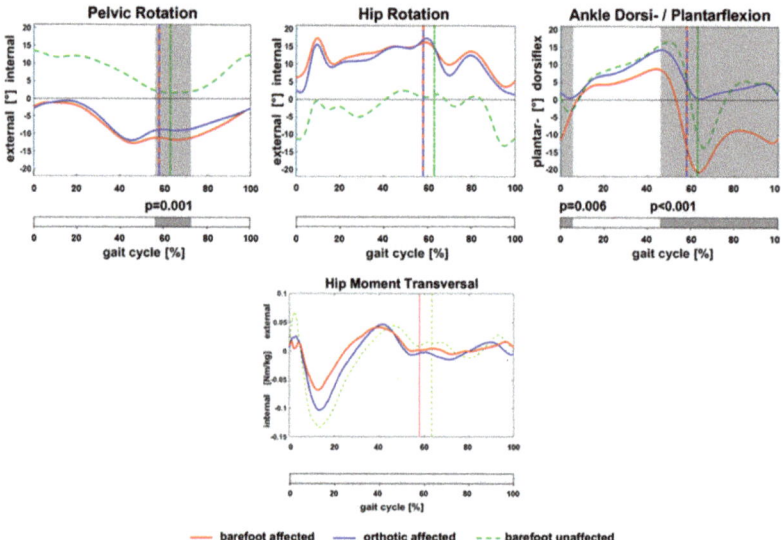

Figure 2. Statistic parametric mapping of kinematics of pelvic rotation, hip rotation, ankle flexion, and hip movement during gait. Grey area: significant changes on affected side between barefoot (red curve) and walking wearing orthoses (blue curve). The kinematics of the unaffected side (green curve) are shown as a reference.

2.4. Statistical Analysis

The data were tested for normal distribution using the Shapiro–Wilk test. Based on normally distributed data, for each parameter, descriptive statistics were calculated with means and SD. Paired sample t-tests and statistical parametric mapping (SPM), including the Bonferroni method, were used to investigate differences between barefoot and orthotic management. The influence of Δ ankle dorsi/plantar flexion IC and femoral anteversion on Δ pelvic and hip asymmetries and Δ hip rotation ST were analyzed by linear regression analyses. The significance level was set at $\alpha \leq 0.05$.

2.5. Sample Size

Due to a retrospective study design, out of 64 patients with unilateral spastic cerebral palsy and spastic hemiplegia of other causes who underwent a gait analysis, 34 were included in this study, according to the inclusion and exclusion criteria (See Figure 1).

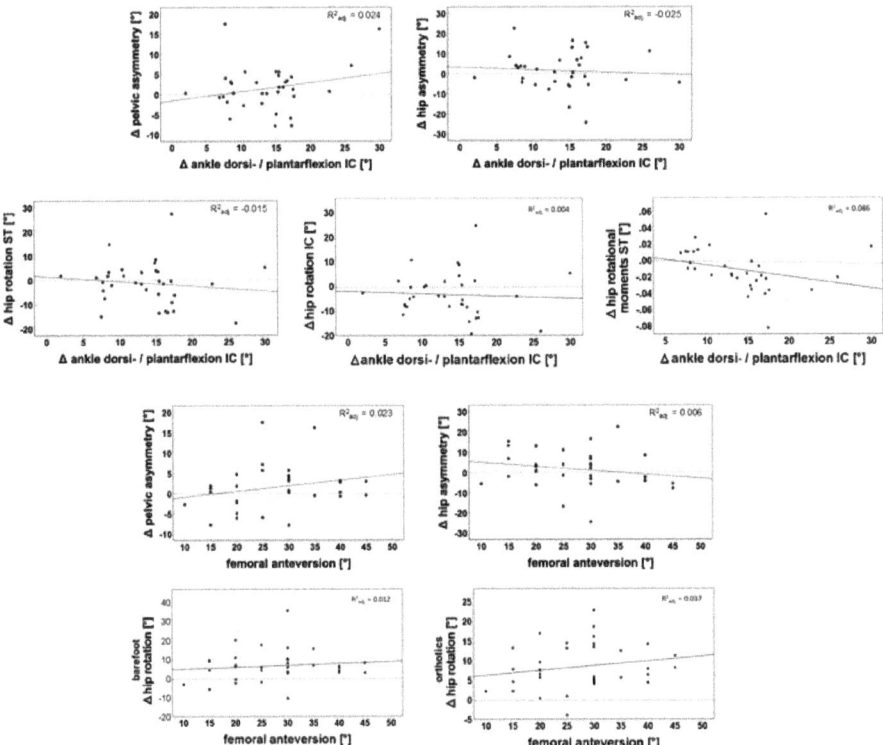

Figure 3. Linear regression of femoral anteversion or changes in pes equinus on changes in pelvic and hip asymmetry, hip rotation, and hip rotational moments. Δ pelvic asymmetry = barefoot affected side/orthotic affected side; Δ hip asymmetry = barefoot affected side/orthotic affected side; Δ hip rotation ST = orthotic affected side/barefoot affected side; Δ hip rotation IC = orthotic affected side/barefoot affected side; Δ hip rotational moments ST = orthotic affected side/barefoot affected side; Δ ankle dorsi/plantar flexion IC = orthotic affected side/barefoot affected side; barefoot Δ hip rotation = hip rotation 30%/hip rotation IC; orthotics Δ hip rotation = hip rotation 30%/hip rotation IC; R^2_{adj} = R^2 adjusted. Dotted line: zero line; continuous line: regression line.

3. Results

Sixty-four children with unilateral spastic cerebral palsy and spastic hemiplegia of other causes were found in our database. A total of thirty patients were excluded due to the inclusion and exclusion criteria from the gait analysis data.

The selection process resulted in 34 children (17 females, 17 males) with unilateral spastic (n = 24) or spastic-dystonic (n = 10) hemiplegia of different causes. Reasons for the movement disorder were cerebral palsy (n = 24), post-stroke (n = 6), post-traumatic (n = 1), neoplastic (n = 1), syndromal (n = 1), and post-infectious (n = 1) disease. Twenty-seven patients had GMFCS-level I and 7 GMFCS-level II. The patients' mean age at examination was 10 ± 4 years (4 to 17 years old). Individual orthotic management was used for pes equinus correction and compensation for leg length discrepancy. In the clinical examination, the participants showed a femoral anteversion from 10° to 45° (mean = 27.65° ± 9.07°).

Pelvic and hip asymmetry did not significantly change with orthoses (each by approx. 2°) (See Table 2). There was a significant difference in mean pelvic rotation during GC. With orthotic management, the pelvis rotated approx. 1° more inwards. When walking barefoot, the group showed an ankle plantar flexion at IC of around 12°, which was significantly reduced with orthoses (by approx. 14°) and resulted in a mean dorsiflexion at IC around 2°.

Table 2. Comparison of kinematic gait data barefoot and with orthoses.

Parameter	Barefoot (Mean ± SD) [°]	Orthoses (Mean ± SD) [°]	p-Value
Pelvic rotation GC (mean)	−7.4 ± 5.5	−6.1 ± 4.7	0.018
Pelvic rotation GC (ROM)	16.6 ± 4.3	16.3 ± 4.9	0.657
Pelvic asymmetry	15.5 ± 9.8	13.9 ± 7.2	0.106
Hip rotation ST (mean)	12.9 ± 6.3	11.6 ± 8.4	0.398
Hip rotation ST (ROM)	21.1 ± 8.2	25.1 ± 9.4	<0.001
Hip asymmetry	16.2 ± 10.2	14.6 ± 9.3	0.326
Ankle dorsi/plantar flexion IC	−11.5 ± 6.0	2.2 ± 4.1	<0.001
Ankle dorsi/plantar flexion ST (mean)	3.2 ± 8.8	8.0 ± 4.6	<0.001

GC: gait cycle, ROM: range of motion, ST: stance phase, IC: initial contact. Pelvic rotation: protraction = +/retraction = −; hip rotation: internal = +/external = −; pelvic asymmetry = |affected/unaffected pelvic rotation GC (mean)|; hip asymmetry = |affected/unaffected hip rotation ST (mean)|; ankle: dorsiflexion = +/plantar flexion = −.

With orthotic equinus management, there was a significant pelvic internal rotation at the end of ST and the beginning of the swing phase compared to barefoot (See Figure 2). There was a visible but not significant deviation of hip rotation with orthoses compared to barefoot at IC but no longer in midstance (MST). Hip moments during ST showed no significant changes. Pes equinus was corrected at IC, the end of ST, and during the swing phase using orthoses.

The changes in the ankle position at IC did not relate to the changes in pelvic asymmetry ($\beta = 0.222$, $p = 0.189$), hip asymmetry ($\beta = -0.128$, $p = 0.662$), Δ hip rotation at ST ($\beta = -0.195$, $p = 0.486$) and at IC ($\beta = -0.096$, $p = 0.731$), or Δ hip rotational moments at ST ($\beta = -0.001$, $p = 0.109$) (See Figure 3). Femoral anteversion did not show a relationship with rotational asymmetries (pelvis: $\beta = 0.139$, $p = 0.190$) (hip: $\beta = -0.196$, $p = 0.280$). The changes in the hip rotation at IC to MST did not relate to the femoral anteversion. This could be shown with orthoses ($\beta = 0.124$, $p = 0.278$) and barefoot ($\beta = 0.98$, $p = 0.542$).

The hip asymmetry increased in 15 participants and decreased in 19 participants while wearing their orthosis (See Figure 4). Twenty-three children showed a reduced pelvic asymmetry when wearing the orthosis, while 11 children had an increased pelvic asymmetry with the orthosis.

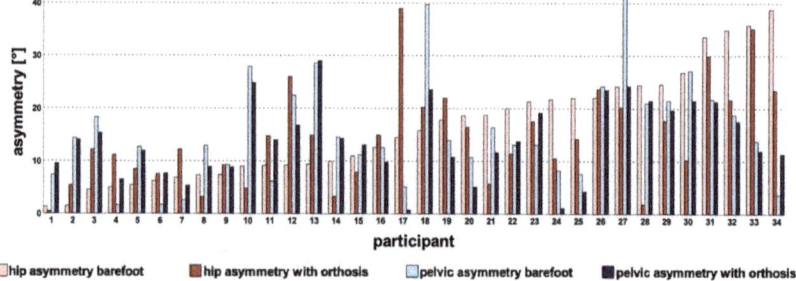

Figure 4. Illustration of hip (red) and pelvic (blue) asymmetry barefoot (light colored) and with orthosis (dark colored). X-axis: 34 patients (4 bars per participant), in order of ascending hip asymmetry barefoot. Y-axis: absolute value of difference in affected and unaffected sides.

4. Discussion

The current study investigated the influence of orthotic equinus correction in children with unilateral spastic cerebral palsy and spastic hemiplegia of other causes on hip and pelvic rotation and associated asymmetries. All the participants showed a significant reduction in plantar flexion when wearing orthotics, underlining that there was a functional correction of pes equinus during gait and corroborating the findings of previous investigations [14,16,17,26].

However, this correction of pes equinus showed variable effects on hip and pelvic rotation, even though pes equinus has been associated with pelvic retraction and internal hip rotation in the previous literature [10,27]. From this global evaluation, the clinical relevance of these effects seems only to be relevant for some children, or other factors mask this association.

On average, only a significant difference in mean pelvic rotation at the end of the stance phase and the beginning of the swing phase of 1° toward the internal rotation could be found, which we consider not to be clinically relevant. This reduction could be explained by the reduction in leg extension due to the orthosis and, therefore, the reduction in pelvic retraction movement and the lifting of the foot is no longer delayed. According to Aminian et al., the retraction on the affected side was also seen as compensation for the stride length of the opposite side, which is impaired by the weakness of the hip extensors on the affected side [28].

There was a trend in the linear regression analysis that when the pes equinus was corrected while wearing orthoses, there was a marginal decrease in the hip asymmetry, and the asymmetry of the pelvis slightly increased. The hip rotation at initial contact and hip rotational moments during the stance phase showed no significant relationship with the ankle position. Furthermore, the amount of femoral anteversion did not significantly affect rotational asymmetries when wearing an orthosis. However, there was also a slight opposite trend as the femoral anteversion increased, the pelvic asymmetry also increased, and the hip asymmetry decreased (See Figure 3).

In line with the results of Brunner et al. [5], Figure 2 shows a visible but not significant deviation of hip rotation with orthoses compared to barefoot at initial contact, but no longer during midstance. This may explain why the dynamic effect is most relevant during the early stance phase or why static torsional or lever arm preconditions are the more relevant factors for torsional positioning after the loading response.

For a better understanding, we additionally correlated the dynamic change in hip rotation during the first 30% of the gait cycle with the clinically measured femoral anteversion angle (See Figure 3). There, we could not find a significant relationship either with orthoses or barefoot. This may have several explanations. First, if there is remaining passive internal rotation in the hip despite an increased femoral anteversion, the dynamic effects of equinus foot position on hip rotation may still work. Another explanation may be that other dynamic effects could be relevant and mask the dependence between this suggested effect. Furthermore, clinical evaluation of the femoral anteversion angle shows only a weak correlation with the anatomical anteversion, which may also mask this effect. This will be further addressed in the limitations section.

Figure 4 further illustrates that there was a very variable effect of the orthoses on the rotational asymmetries. About half of the patients saw improved hip asymmetry, and about two-thirds saw improved pelvic asymmetry (See Figure 4). However, the effects on asymmetries were highly inconsistent, and possible reasons need to be further discussed.

Weak hip abductors [29] or increased hip flexion, which contribute to an increase in the internal rotating movement of the hips, may also play a role [9]. There is some limited evidence that soft tissue surgery of the hip flexors and adductors, in addition to femoral derotational osteotomy, improves pelvic retraction, as well as internal hip rotation [30].

A potential leg length difference was compensated with orthotic management. The influence of leg length differences on rotational asymmetries is possible; however, to conclude this, the exact calculation would be beneficial. Furthermore, malalignment, altered tibial torsion, and a structural or functional pointed foot may influence a possible correction of the asymmetries.

In summary, we recommend a correction of the pes equinus through orthoptic management for a proven significant reduction in ankle plantar flexion and, thus, functional correction. Multiple factors seem to influence rotational asymmetry. Our results underline that other factors need to be considered to understand internal rotation hip and pelvic retraction patterns in children with unilateral spastic cerebral palsy and spastic hemiplegia of other causes. We suggest that a more comprehensive dynamic and static investigation is needed, taking into account various additional confounding factors, such as tibia torsion, muscular weaknesses, and joint contractures, in order to improve our understanding of the mechanisms underlying rotational asymmetries. Since internal rotation is one of the most disturbing aspects of gait impairment in these children, it is crucial to inform the children and their parents that the internal rotation of the hip and pelvic asymmetry may persist despite orthotic management of the equinus foot position and potentially needs to be addressed by other means, such as rotational orthotics or surgical correction through rotational osteotomy.

There are several limitations to mention. One reason for a pronounced internal rotation gait is increased femoral anteversion. This was manually measured in the current study with the commonly used Craig's test. Measured in the prone position, the hip is rotated until the greater trochanter can be palpated most prominently. The amount of torsion corresponds to the angle of the flexed lower leg to the vertical. Several studies have compared the widely used Craig's test and computed tomography to measure femoral anteversion without significant correlation [31,32]. Therefore, the analysis of whether a higher femoral anteversion produces a smaller effect on correcting asymmetry in walking is limited. However, in our study, the differences in gait parameters between barefoot and wearing orthoses were the main parameters not affected by femoral anteversion measurement.

The type of orthosis was based on the individual need of the patient. Due to the individual orthotic management, it was not possible to create subgroups of orthotic type. However, to answer the main question, it was only relevant that the orthosis corrected the equinus foot functionally, which was the case in all participants.

Our retrospective study population included children with spastic and spastic–dystonic hemiplegia with variable causes, which resulted in a rather inhomogeneous population. For a more detailed analysis investigating further possible influencing factors, such as further stratification, e.g., on the influence of spastic or dyskinesia (dystonia) or on the influence of structural or functional pes equinus—a larger number of patients should be included.

All participants walked first barefoot and then with orthoses. The changes in gait pattern between the two examinations could have occurred due to muscular and/or mental fatigue. No studies have investigated the effect of fatigue on physical function. A prospective study randomizing the order of walking with a larger sample size could outweigh some of the limitations of the current study.

The variability of dynamic effects of orthotic management on the hip and pelvic rotation, which was found in our study, clearly shows that there is a need to further investigate these mechanisms. A major limitation of this retrospective approach is the limited number of patients, which did not allow for further subgroup analysis.

5. Conclusions

Orthotic management of pes equinus significantly reduced ankle plantar in children with unilateral spastic cerebral palsy or spastic hemiplegia of other causes and is, therefore, recommended for functional correction. However, there was a variable effect on the hip and pelvic asymmetry. The increased hip internal rotation problem appears to be multifactorial. Children and their parents need to be informed that rotational asymmetries may persist when using orthoses.

Author Contributions: Conceptualization and methodology, all authors; ethical approval, M.S., H.J.A.v.H. and A.M.-H.; data curation, M.S., S.B. and B.K.; analysis, M.S., B.K. and H.J.A.v.H.; project administration, D.G., B.K. and T.D.; writing—original draft, D.G., M.S. and B.K.; writing—review and editing, T.D., S.B., H.J.A.v.H. and A.M.-H. All authors have read and agreed to the published version of the manuscript.

Funding: This research received no external funding.

Institutional Review Board Statement: This study was conducted according to the guidelines of the Declaration of Helsinki and approved by the Ethics Committee Zurich, Switzerland (2011-0404, PB_2016-01843), date of approval 21 June 2018.

Informed Consent Statement: Informed consent was signed by each patient involved in this study or by their statutory representative.

Data Availability Statement: All data are stored at the University Children's Hospital Zurich.

Conflicts of Interest: The authors declare no conflict of interest.

References

1. Aiona, M.D.; Sussman, M.D. Treatment of spastic diplegia in patients with cerebral palsy: Part II. *J. Pediatr. Orthop. B* **2004**, *13*, S13–S38.
2. Wren, T.A.; Rethlefsen, S.; Kay, R.M. Prevalence of specific gait abnormalities in children with cerebral palsy: Influence of cerebral palsy subtype, age, and previous surgery. *J. Pediatr. Orthop.* **2005**, *25*, 79–83.
3. Gage, J. *The Treatment of Gait Problems in Cerebral Palsy. Section 3: Gait Pathology in Cerebral Palsy*; Mac Keith: London, UK, 2004; ISBN 1898683379.
4. Carty, C.P.; Walsh, H.P.; Gillett, J.G.; Phillips, T.; Edwards, J.M.; Delacy, M.; Boyd, R.N. The effect of femoral derotation osteotomy on transverse plane hip and pelvic kinematics in children with cerebral palsy: A systematic review and meta-analysis. *Gait Posture* **2014**, *40*, 333–340. [CrossRef]
5. Brunner, R.; Baumann, J.U. Long-term effects of intertrochanteric varus-derotation osteotomy on femur and acetabulum in spastic cerebral palsy: An 11- to 18-year follow-up study. *J. Pediatr. Orthop.* **1997**, *17*, 585–591. [CrossRef]
6. Kim, H.; Aiona, M.; Sussman, M. Recurrence After Femoral Derotational Osteotomy in Cerebral Palsy. *J. Pediatr. Orthop.* **2005**, *25*, 739–743. [CrossRef]
7. Arnold, A.S.; Delp, S.L. Rotational moment arms of the medial hamstrings and adductors vary with femoral geometry and limb position: Implications for the treatment of internally rotated gait. *J. Biomech.* **2001**, *34*, 437–447. [CrossRef]
8. Arnold, A.S.; Komallu, A.V.; Delp, S.L. Internal rotation gait: A compensatory mechanism to restore abduction capacity decreased by bone deformity? *Dev. Med. Child Neurol.* **1997**, *39*, 40–44. [CrossRef]
9. Delp, S.L.; Hess, W.E.; Hungerford, D.S.; Jones, L.C. Variation of rotation moment arms with hip flexion. *J. Biomech.* **1999**, *32*, 493–501. [CrossRef] [PubMed]
10. Brunner, R.; Dreher, T.; Romkes, J.; Frigo, C. Effects of plantarflexion on pelvis and lower limb kinematics. *Gait Posture* **2008**, *28*, 150–156. [CrossRef]
11. Pasin Neto, H.; Grecco, L.A.C.; Ferreira, L.A.B.; Duarte, N.A.C.; Galli, M.; Oliveira, C.S. Postural insoles on gait in children with cerebral palsy: Randomized controlled double-blind clinical trial. *J. Bodyw. Mov. Ther.* **2017**, *21*, 890–895. [CrossRef]
12. Romkes, J.; Brunner, R. Comparison of a dynamic and a hinged ankle–foot orthosis by gait analysis in patients with hemiplegic cerebral palsy. *Gait Posture* **2002**, *15*, 18–24. [CrossRef] [PubMed]
13. Altschuck, N.; Bauer, C.; Nehring, I.; Böhm, H.; Jakobeit, M.; Schröder, A.S.; Mall, V.; Jung, N.H. Efficacy of prefabricated carbon-composite ankle foot orthoses for children with unilateral spastic cerebral palsy exhibiting a drop foot pattern. *J. Pediatr. Rehabil. Med.* **2019**, *12*, 171–180. [CrossRef] [PubMed]
14. Boudarham, J.; Pradon, D.; Roche, N.; Bensmail, D.; Zory, R. Effects of a dynamic-ankle-foot orthosis (Liberté®) on kinematics and electromyographic activity during gait in hemiplegic patients with spastic foot equinus. *Neurorehabilitation* **2014**, *35*, 369–379. [CrossRef] [PubMed]
15. Desloovere, K.; Molenaers, G.; Van Gestel, L.; Huenaerts, C.; Van Campenhout, A.; Callewaert, B.; Van de Walle, P.; Seyler, J. How can push-off be preserved during use of an ankle foot orthosis in children with hemiplegia? A prospective controlled study. *Gait Posture* **2006**, *24*, 142–151. [CrossRef]
16. Balaban, B.; Yasar, E.; Dal, U.; Yazicioglu, K.; Mohur, H.; Kalyon, T.A. The effect of hinged ankle-foot orthosis on gait and energy expenditure in spastic hemiplegic cerebral palsy. *Disabil. Rehabil.* **2007**, *29*, 139–144. [CrossRef]
17. Lintanf, M.; Bourseul, J.-S.; Houx, L.; Lempereur, M.; Brochard, S.; Pons, C. Effect of ankle-foot orthoses on gait, balance and gross motor function in children with cerebral palsy: A systematic review and meta-analysis. *Clin. Rehabil.* **2018**, *32*, 1175–1188. [CrossRef]
18. Butler, P.B.; Farmer, S.E.; Stewart, C.; Jones, P.W.; Forward, M. The effect of fixed ankle foot orthoses in children with cerebral palsy. *Disabil. Rehabil. Assist. Technol.* **2007**, *2*, 51–58. [CrossRef]
19. Aboutorabi, A.; Arazpour, M.; Bani, M.A.; Saeedi, H.; Head, J.S. Efficacy of ankle foot orthoses types on walking in children with cerebral palsy: A systematic review. *Ann. Phys. Rehabil. Med.* **2017**, *60*, 393–402. [CrossRef]
20. Novacheck, T.F.; Gage, J.R. Orthopedic management of spasticity in cerebral palsy. *Child's Nerv. Syst.* **2007**, *23*, 1015–1031. [CrossRef]

21. Sapienza, M.; Kapoor, R.; Alberghina, F.; Maheshwari, R.; McCracken, K.L.; Canavese, F.; Johari, A.N. Adverse Effects Following Botulinum Toxin A Injections in Children with Cerebral Palsy. Journal of Pediatric Orthopaedics B. 2023. Available online: https://journals.lww.com/jpo-b/Abstract/9900/Adverse_effects_following_botulinum_toxin_A.85.aspx (accessed on 1 February 2023).
22. Hong, Z.; Sui, M.; Zhuang, Z.; Liu, H.; Zheng, X.; Cai, C.; Jin, D. Effectiveness of Neuromuscular Electrical Stimulation on Lower Limbs of Patients with Hemiplegia After Chronic Stroke: A Systematic Review. *Arch. Phys. Med. Rehabil.* **2018**, *99*, 1011–1022.e1. [CrossRef]
23. Wong, P.; Fransch, S.; Gallagher, C.; Francis, K.L.; Khot, A.; Rutz, E.; Graham, H.K. Split anterior tibialis tendon transfer to peroneus brevis for spastic equinovarus in children with hemiplegia. *J. Child. Orthop.* **2021**, *15*, 279–290. [CrossRef] [PubMed]
24. Rodda, J.; Graham, H.K. Classification of gait patterns in spastic hemiplegia and spastic diplegia: A basis for a management algorithm. *Eur. J. Neurol.* **2001**, *8* (Suppl. S5), 98–108. [CrossRef] [PubMed]
25. Kadaba, M.P.; Ramakrishnan, H.K.; Wootten, M.E. Measurement of lower extremity kinematics during level walking. *J. Orthop. Res.* **1990**, *8*, 383–392. [CrossRef] [PubMed]
26. Martins, E.; Cordovil, R.; Oliveira, R.; Pinho, J.; Diniz, A.; Vaz, J.R. The Immediate Effects of a Dynamic Orthosis on Gait Patterns in Children with Unilateral Spastic Cerebral Palsy: A Kinematic Analysis. *Front. Pediatr.* **2019**, *7*, 42. [CrossRef]
27. Park, K.-B.; Park, H.; Park, B.K.; Abdel-Baki, S.W.; Kim, H.W. Clinical and Gait Parameters Related to Pelvic Retraction in Patients with Spastic Hemiplegia. *J. Clin. Med.* **2019**, *8*, 679. [CrossRef]
28. Aminian, A.; Vankoski, S.J.; Dias, L.; Novak, R.A. Spastic Hemiplegic Cerebral Palsy and the Femoral Derotation Osteotomy: Effect at the Pelvis and Hip in the Transverse Plane During Gait. *J. Pediatr. Orthop.* **2003**, *23*, 314–320. [CrossRef]
29. Arnold, A.S.; Asakawa, D.J.; Delp, S.L. Do the hamstrings and adductors contribute to excessive internal rotation of the hip in persons with cerebral palsy? *Gait Posture* **2000**, *11*, 181–190. [CrossRef]
30. Rutz, E.; Passmore, E.; Baker, R.; Graham, K.H. Multilevel Surgery Improves Gait in Spastic Hemiplegia but Does Not Resolve Hip Dysplasia. *Clin. Orthop. Relat. Res.* **2012**, *470*, 1294–1302. [CrossRef]
31. Ito, I.; Miura, K.; Kimura, Y.; Sasaki, E.; Tsuda, E.; Ishibashi, Y. Retraction: Differences between the Craig's test and computed tomography in measuring femoral anteversion in patients with anterior cruciate ligament injuries. *J. Phys. Ther. Sci.* **2020**, *32*, 365–369. [CrossRef]
32. Uota, S.; Morikita, I.; Shimokochi, Y. Validity and clinical significance of a clinical method to measure femoral anteversion. *J. Sports Med. Phys. Fit.* **2019**, *59*, 1908–1914. [CrossRef]

Disclaimer/Publisher's Note: The statements, opinions and data contained in all publications are solely those of the individual author(s) and contributor(s) and not of MDPI and/or the editor(s). MDPI and/or the editor(s) disclaim responsibility for any injury to people or property resulting from any ideas, methods, instructions or products referred to in the content.

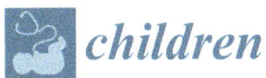

Article

Partial Remodeling after Conservative Treatment of Trampoline Fractures in Children

Laura Zaccaria [1,*], Enno Stranzinger [2], Theodoros Xydias [3], Sabine Schaedelin [4], Kai Ziebarth [5], Mike Trück [6], Vivienne Sommer-Joergensen [7], Christoph Aufdenblatten [8] and Peter Michael Klimek [9]

1. Department of Pediatric Surgery, Hospital Center Biel, 2501 Biel, Switzerland
2. Department of Diagnostic, Interventional and Pediatric Radiology, Inselspital, Bern University Hospital, University of Bern, 3010 Bern, Switzerland
3. Pediatric Radiology, Cantonal Hospital Aarau, 5001 Aarau, Switzerland
4. Department of Clinical Research and Data Analysis, University Hospital Basel, 4031 Basel, Switzerland
5. Department of Pediatric Orthopaedics and Traumatology, University Children's Hospital Bern, Inselspital Bern, 3010 Bern, Switzerland
6. Department of Pediatric Surgery, Cantonal Hospital Lucerne, 6002 Lucerne, Switzerland
7. Department of Pediatric Surgery, University Children's Hospital Basel, 4056 Basel, Switzerland
8. Department of Pediatric Orthopaedics and Traumatology, University Children's Hospital Zurich, 8032 Zurich, Switzerland
9. Department of Pediatric Surgery, Kantonsspital Aarau, 5001 Aarau, Switzerland
* Correspondence: laura.zaccaria@szb-chb.ch; Tel.: +41-323241383

Abstract: (1) Background: Trampoline fractures (proximal tibia fracture with positive anterior tilt) are increasing. This study represents the first attempt to determine the extent of remodeling in these fractures after conservative treatment (2) Methods: This Swiss prospective multicenter study included children aged 2 to 5 years with a trampoline fracture who were radiologically examined on the day of the accident and after one year. In addition, the anterior tilt angle was compared between the injured and unaffected tibia. Remodeling was defined as complete (final anterior tilt angle $\leq 0°$), incomplete (smaller but still >0°), or no remodeling. (3) Results: The mean extent of remodeling was $-3.5°$ (95% CI: $-4.29°$, $-2.66°$, $p < 0.001$). Among the 89 children included in the study, 26 (29.2%) showed complete, 63 (70.8%) incomplete, and 17 patients (19.1%) no remodeling. Comparison of the anterior tilt angles between the fractured and healthy tibia showed that the anterior tilt angle on the fractured leg was, on average larger by $2.82°$ (95% CI: $2.01°$, $3.63°$; $p < 0.001$). (4) Conclusions: Although the anterior tilt angle decreased during the study period, the majority of patients showed incomplete remodeling. In contrast, children with radiological examinations >1 year after the trauma showed advanced remodeling, suggesting that one year is too short to observe complete remodeling.

Keywords: trampoline; trampoline fracture; proximal tibia; positive anterior tilt angle; remodeling

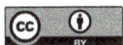

1. Introduction

The popularity of backyard trampolines in Switzerland has been increasing over the past two decades. Jumping on the trampoline has positive effects on the development of physical strength, coordination, and psychological well-being and is an excellent opportunity to improve the perception of body and space. Unfortunately, we noticed a remarkable increase in trampoline fractures [1–7]. Among these injuries, fractures of the proximal tibia are particularly common in children under 5 years of age [1,8–10]. A recent retrospective study [2] at our institution showed increased anterior tilt angles of the proximal tibia in children who had sustained a trampoline injury compared with tilt angles in an age-matched cohort of healthy children.

Trampoline fractures are typically caused by bouncing on the trampoline, especially when the child jumps with an older or heavier child without parental supervision [1–3,5,6]. When two children of unequal weight jump on the trampoline, the jump net follows the heavier child. When the lighter child is in the air, while the heavier one is jumping off, the net hits the leg of the lighter child with full force from below. The fracture pattern results from axial compression of the leg (especially the proximal tibia) and concomitant hyperextension of the knee joint in young children with open growth plates. Other forces, such as torsion, varus, or valgus, are usually not present. However, these fractures are not at risk of progressive valgus deformity after fracture healing, as described by the Cozen phenomenon [3,11–13]. Crucial to the diagnosis of a trampoline fracture is the combination of an appropriate medical history, typical symptoms (i.e., pain in the proximal tibia after jumping on a trampoline, refusal to walk), and radiologically, an increased anterior tilt angle at the proximal tibia. Measurement of the anterior tilting of the proximal tibia in the lateral plane is an important, valuable radiological tool for the diagnosis of suspected trampoline fractures, even when no fracture line is evident [2]. Other obvious radiological signs of a trampoline fracture include a buckle, torus, or transverse hairline fracture of the proximal tibial metaphysis or scooping of the tibial tubercle notch. Before radiographic measurement of the positive anterior tilt angle at the tibia, it was difficult to diagnose a trampoline fracture [2], and we must assume that these fractures may have been overlooked in the past. Trampoline fractures are typically treated conservatively [10] in a long leg cast for 3–4 weeks.

However, the long-term effects in terms of functionality and stability of the knee joint after a trampoline fracture remains unclear, and currently, there is nothing in the literature on bone remodeling after trampoline fractures in children.

The aim of this study was to investigate the extent of tibial remodeling after trampoline fracture over the course of at least one year. For this purpose, we documented the anterior tilt angle during follow-up, with a focus on checking for the uplift of the tibial plateau with correction of the anterior tilt angle to values $\leq 0°$ (range $-2°$ to $+2°$).

Based on our observations, we proposed two hypotheses:

Hypothesis I (main hypothesis). *In children with a trampoline fracture, the bone might remodel within one year, and the pathologically positive anterior tilt angle might become ≤ 0.*

Hypothesis II. *In children with a trampoline fracture, the anterior tilt angle may reach the same angle measured on the healthy leg after conservative therapy in a long leg cast.*

2. Materials and Methods

The hospital ethics committees of the five participating national children's hospitals (Aarau, Basel, Bern, Lucerne, and Zurich) approved this prospective observational multi-center study with a retrospective component. The study was sponsored by the Research Council of the Cantonal Hospital Aarau. One statistician from the clinical trial unit in Basel evaluated the blinded radiological measurements and assessed their statistical relevance. This study was registered at: ClinicalTrials.gov, identifier: NCT04028908.

Parents were informed about the study during normal follow-ups. Participation was voluntary and free of charge for the families. Before study initiation, a specific information pamphlet was created and approved by the ethics committees. The families were required to sign it before participating in the study.

The study included children aged 2 to 5 years who had sustained a fracture of the proximal tibia while jumping on a trampoline and who had radiographs of the injured leg taken on the day of the accident and at least one year after the trauma. Clinical examination included assessment of gait, leg length, and axes such as varus, valgus, and ante- or retro-curvature of the lower leg. For the present study, we prospectively enrolled patients that had sustained a new trampoline fracture in 2016. We also retrospectively enrolled some children (13 of 89 patients) of the same age who had sustained a trampoline fracture between 2011 and 2016 to analyze the remodeling of trampoline fractures even more than one year after trauma. In some cases (72 of 89 patients), we had obtained formal consent to x-ray the opposite healthy tibia (only lateral plane) at least one year after trauma. This was performed exclusively on a voluntary basis with the idea of documenting the uplift of the tibial plateau and comparing the anterior tilt angles between the own injured and healthy leg. All children were treated conservatively in a long leg cast with the knee in full extension or 15–20 degrees of flexion for 3–4 weeks.

The initial and follow-up radiographs were evaluated separately by two specialized pediatric radiologists. Fractures were classified as complete fractures or torus fractures. The anterior tilt angle of the tibia was measured according to our previous study [2] in a lateral radiograph of the lower leg. For this purpose, a tangent was drawn through the proximal and distal ends of the tibial epiphyseal plate. The proximal line of the angle was defined by drawing a tangent between the dorsal and middle points of the physis (the anterior point of the physis can be used if the line also intersects the middle point or two lines of the plate were visible, in which case the lower line was used for measurement). The distal part of the angle was determined by drawing a tangent between the dorsal and ventral epiphyseal plates of the distal physis (Figure 1). Strict or standardized lateral images are not necessary for the measurements of the anterior tilt angles. Measurements were performed with an angle measurement tool on a Sectra AB picture archiving and communication system (PACS IDS7TM, Version 19.3, Teknikringen 20, SE-58330 Linkoping, Sweden).

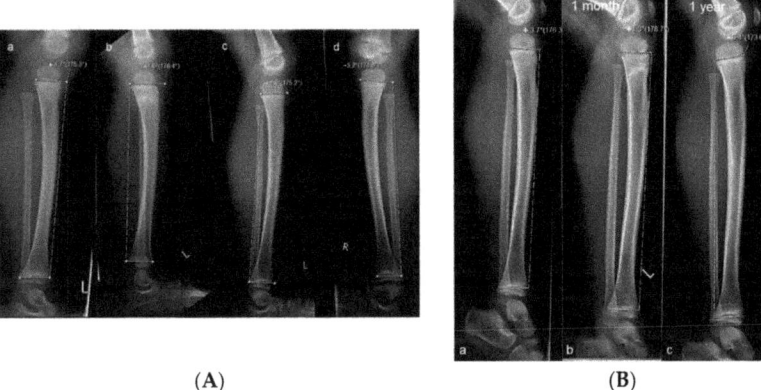

(A)   (B)

Figure 1. Measurements of the anterior tilt angle of the proximal tibia in children with trampoline fracture. (**A**) Radiographs of a child with a torus fracture. Measurements were taken (a) on the day of the accident; (b) after one month, and (c) after one year; (d) x-ray of the healthy opposite leg. The negative anterior tilt angle (−4.8°) at one year indicates complete remodeling. (**B**) Radiographs of a child with a complete fracture. Measurements were taken (a) on the day of the accident, (b) after one month, and (c) after one year. The negative anterior tilt angle at one year (−6.4°) shows complete remodeling.

Before and during the study, we searched the literature for anterior tilt angle values, but to date, no normative pediatric anterior tilt angle values have been defined; therefore, we based our evaluations on results from a previous study [2] and defined a physiological angle as ≤0° (range −2° to +2°). All analyses were performed with R Version 3.6.2 (Vienna, Austria).

Statistics

Continuous variables are expressed as the arithmetic mean, standard deviation (SD), and categorical variables are expressed as the absolute and relative frequencies. The measurements of the two radiologists were averaged prior to analysis, and their agreement was quantified with the intraclass correlation coefficient (ICC). The ICC is calculated based on an analysis of variance. The ICC is estimated by dividing the variation, which was due to the subject-to-subject difference, through the total variance seen in these data. An ICC of

1 indicates that all differences in the measurements are explainable by differences in the subjects and, therefore, that the method is completely reproducible. The Student's t-test was performed to estimate the extent of remodeling. We defined complete remodeling as an anterior tilt angle $\leq 0°$ at the end of the exam. We defined incomplete remodeling as any remodeling that resulted in an anterior tilt angle that was less positive than the initial angle measured after the fracture. Risk factors for incomplete remodeling were assessed with a logistic model.

To evaluate our second hypothesis, we assessed the difference between the healthy and broken legs based on a paired t-test. Results are expressed as the odds ratio (OR) and 95% confidence interval (95% CI).

3. Results

We identified 93 children, aged 2 to 5 years, that had sustained a trampoline fracture during the period of October 2011 to December 2019 (Figure 2). Four children had to be excluded from the study: two children because their parents refused to participate in the study and two other children because they could not provide a lateral radiograph of the lower leg at the final examination. Therefore, the study included 89 children with an evaluable radiograph of the tibia on the day of the injury and a final examination at least one year (range 11–16 months, median 12 months) after the trauma. In addition, 13/89 patients (14.6%) had a final x-ray taken between 2 and 5 years (range 20–64 months, median 36 months) after the injury. The cohort included 40 males (45%) and 49 (55%) females. The mean age was 3.3 years (SD 1.2). In 72/89 patients (80.9%), we could compare anterior tilt angles between the affected and healthy legs.

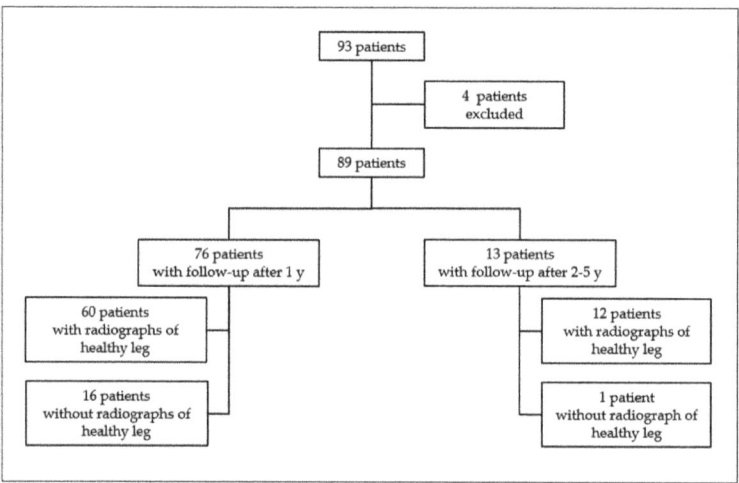

Figure 2. Distribution of our study population.

Hypothesis I. *Anterior tilt angle might show remodeling within one year.*

Among the 89 patients, the mean anterior tilt angle at the time of injury was 5.8° (SD 3.7°), and the average value at the final examination was 2.3° (95% CI: 1.41°, 3.26°, $p < 0.001$; Table 1). Thus, the mean extent of remodeling was −3.5° (95% CI: −4.29°, −2.66°, $p < 0.001$) during the observation period. Overall, 26/89 patients showed complete remodeling with a final anterior tilt angle $\leq 0°$. However, 17/89 patients showed no remodeling at all. In 63/89 children with remodeling, the anterior tilt angle remained positive at the final examination, which indicated incomplete remodeling after the trampoline fracture (Table 2 and Figure 3).

Table 1. Measurements of anterior tilt angles after trampoline fracture in our study population (N = 89) on the day of the injury and one year after trauma.

Time	Anterior Tilt Angle [a]			
	Min	Max	Mean	Sd
Day of injury	−4.45°	16.60°	5.751°	3.734°
Final exam (fractured leg)	−8.45°	11.85°	2.298°	4.394°

[a] Values are averages of measurements performed by two radiologists.

Table 2. Characteristics of children with trampoline fractures of the tibia, defined by remodeling (complete/incomplete/no remodeling) and the anterior tilt angle value at the final examination.

Characteristic	Any Remodeling?		Complete Remodeling? Final Anterior Tilt Angle ≤ 0°	
	yes	no	yes	no
n (%)	72 (80.9)	17 (19.1)	26 (29.2)	63 (70.8)
Mean age, y (SD)	3.2 (1.1)	3.5 (1.4)	2.8 (1.1)	3.5 (1.2)
male sex, n (%)	30 (41.7)	10 (58.8)	7 (26.9)	33 (52.4)
Mean initial tilt, degree (SD)	6.3 (3.6)	3.8 (3.7)	3.5 (3.6)	6.8 (3.4)
Type of fracture, n (%)				
- complete	18 (25.0)	4 (23.5)	2 (7.7)	20 (31.7)
- torus	54 (75.0)	13 (76.5)	24 (92.3)	43 (68.3)

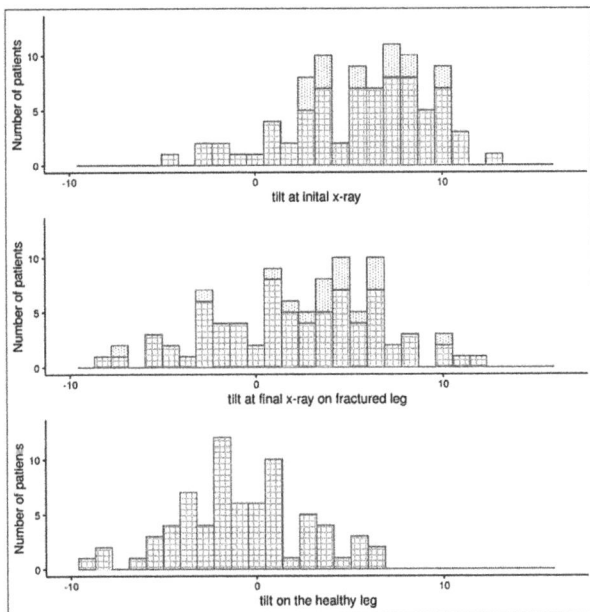

Figure 3. Anterior tilt angles of the proximal tibia in fractured and healthy legs of children with trampoline fractures. The fractured legs were measured in the initial x-ray, taken at the time of the injury, and final x-rays were taken at least one year later. The tilt scale ranges from rather normal (negative) to rather pathological (positive) values. *Dotted bars*: children without an x-ray of the healthy leg (17/89 patients); *checked bars*: children with an x-ray of the healthy leg at the final examination (72/89 patients).

Hypothesis II. *Anterior tilt angle might reach the same value as on the healthy leg.*

At least one year after the trauma, 72/89 patients received a radiograph of the healthy leg. The anterior tilt angles at the final examination between the fractured and healthy legs were comparable. However, after remodeling, the anterior tilt angle on the fractured leg remained 2.82° (95% CI: 2.01°, 3.63°, $p < 0.001$; Figure 3) larger than on the healthy leg. The anterior tilt angles measured on the healthy proximal tibia in our study population ranged from −9.4° to +6.2° (mean −0.7336°, Table 3).

Table 3. Summary statistics of anterior tilt angle measurements in children with trampoline fracture of the tibia who received radiographs of the healthy leg on the day of the injury and at least one year after trauma ($n = 72/89$).

Time	Anterior Tilt Angle [a]			
	Min	Max	Mean	Sd
Day of injury	−4.45°	16.60°	5.6926°	3.853°
Final exam (fractured leg)	−8.45°	11.85°	1.9554°	4.382°
Final exam (healthy leg)	−9.40°	6.20°	−0.7336°	3.453°

[a] Values are averages of measurements performed by two radiologists.

In 30/72 patients, the anterior tilt angle was ≥0° at the final examination. In these children, the initial anterior tilt angle was significantly larger than in children with an anterior tilt angle ≤0° at the final exam (7.2° vs. 4.8°, $p = 0.008$; Table 4), despite similar age and sex distributions between groups. Similarly, patients with a large tilt angle on the healthy leg also tended to have a large tilt angle on the fractured leg at the final examination, and thus, they were more often classified as incomplete remodeling (Figure 4).

Table 4. Characteristics of children with trampoline fractures of the tibia also had radiographs of the healthy leg ($n = 72/89$), categorized by the tilt angle measured at the final exam.

Characteristic	Final Tilt > 0°	Final Tilt ≤ 0°
n (%)	30 (41.7)	42 (58.3)
Mean age, y (SD)	3.2 (1.1)	3.1 (1.2)
Male sex, n (%)	14 (46.7)	18 (42.9)
Mean initial tilt on the fractured leg, degrees (SD)	7.2 (3.7)	4.8 (3.7)
Type of fracture, n (%)		
- complete	6 (20.0)	9 (21.4)
- torus	24 (80.0)	33 (78.6)

In our study population, torus fractures were clearly more frequent than complete fractures (Tables 2 and 4).

We found three significant risk factors associated with a lack of remodeling (final anterior tilt angle >0°, Table 5): male sex (OR: 0.82 compared to females, $p = 0.0252$); large anterior tilt angle on the initial x-ray ($p < 0.001$); and complete fracture (OR torus versus a complete fracture was 1.28, $p = 0.0193$).

None of our patients developed a valgus (Cozen phenomenon) or varus deformity. All patients retained a normal gait and an unaffected leg length.

The average ICC was between 0.68 and 0.82, indicating that the anterior tilt angle measurements were highly congruent between the two radiologists (Table 6).

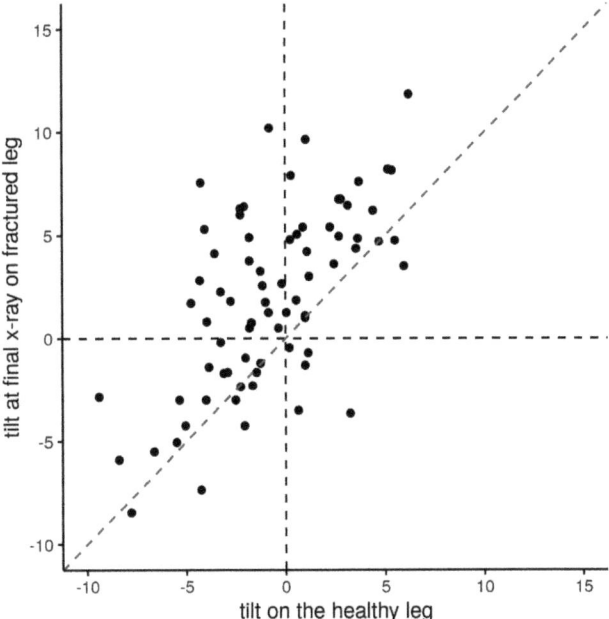

Figure 4. Comparison of the anterior tilt angles between the fractured and the healthy leg at the final x-ray among children with trampoline fractures of the tibia. After remodeling, the anterior tilt angle in the injured leg is still larger than on the opposite healthy leg, as shown here by the majority of anterior tilt angle values (*black dots*) above the bisecting blue line.

Table 5. Factors associated with lack of remodeling at one year (anterior tilt angle > 0° at the final exam) after a trampoline fracture of the tibia.

Variable	OR	CI	*p*-Value
Age at final x-ray	0.95	[0.88, 1.02]	0.1885
Male (vs. female)	0.82	[0.70, 0.97]	0.0252
Tilt at initial x-ray	0.96	[0.93, 0.98]	<0.001
Torus (vs. complete fracture)	1.28	[1.05, 1.57]	0.0193

Table 6. Inter-rater agreement between the two radiologists that evaluated radiographs of trampoline fractures of the tibia based on intraclass coefficient (ICC). Only the tilt angle values of patients measured independently by both radiologists were considered.

Time of Measurement	ICC	Patients, *n*	Measurements, *n*
Day of Injury	0.81	89	178
Final x-ray (fractured leg)	0.82	86	172
Final x-ray (healthy leg)	0.68	71	142

4. Discussion

This is the first study to determine the extent of remodeling in trampoline fractures in children. Our data demonstrated that most fractures showed signs of remodeling on radiographs taken at least one year after the injury. During the study period, we observed an average correction at the tibial plateau of −3.5°. Nevertheless, the anterior tilt angles remained larger (pathologic positive values) than the tilt angles in the healthy legs at the final examination. Due to the values of the anterior tilt angle not reaching negative physiological values or the values of the opposite healthy leg, we concluded that remodeling was largely incomplete (Figure 3 and Table 3).

Our observation time was too short to observe complete remodeling, which was confirmed by the fact that most children who had a final examination > 1 year after the trauma showed, on average, advanced remodeling (most anterior tilt angles < 0°) than children who had a final examination one-year post-trauma (Figure 5).

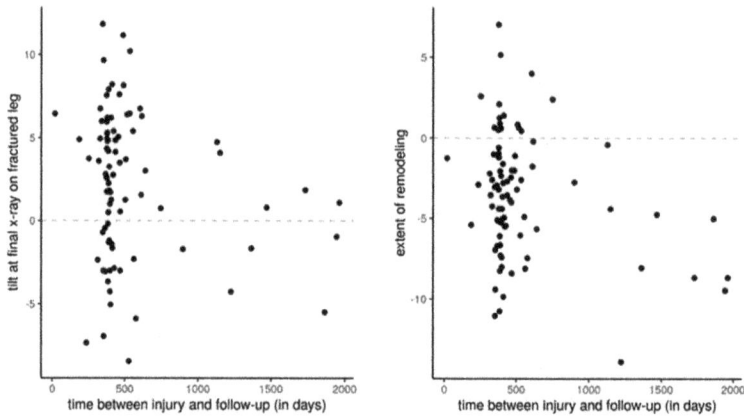

Figure 5. Extent of remodeling over time in children with trampoline fracture of the tibia. Based on the extent of remodeling and the anterior tilt angle at the final examination, we can conclude that patients in whom the final examination was performed >1 year after trauma had better remodeling.

Summarizing, we can say that remodeling occurs, and the conservative treatment is sufficient. However, we cannot predict how long complete remodeling will take. Therefore, we could not reject either of our two hypotheses.

Unfortunately, we were unable to demonstrate which values of anterior tilt angle predict complete, incomplete, or no remodeling and ultimately determine at which anterior tilt angle the fracture should be treated surgically. Our data suggested that a lack of remodeling was associated with the male sex, a large tilt angle at the initial radiological examination, and a complete fracture (Table 5). Moreover, torus fractures occurred more frequently in our cohort, indicating that fracture severity did not affect remodeling (Tables 2 and 4).

In our study population, the anterior tilt angles of the proximal tibia of the healthy legs ranged from −9.4° to +6.2° (mean −0.7336°, Table 3). This finding suggests that children of this age might have a physiologically positive anterior tilt angle in the absence of a fracture or have been exposed to repetitive trauma to the proximal tibia while jumping on the trampoline (Tables 3 and 4). In our previous study, we found chronic repetitive changes such as sclerosis of the metaphysis, growth arrest lines (Harris lines), and widening of the growth plates in children who regularly jump on the trampoline [1]. The latter would at least explain why in our previous work [2], the values of the anterior tilt angle in healthy children who had not suffered any trauma on the trampoline were smaller (3.2°, SD 2.8°). An alternative explanation for the positive anterior tilt angles could be that children with physiologically positive anterior tilt angles, a priori, are more vulnerable or predisposed to trampoline fractures than children with less positive or negative anterior tilt angles. In contrast, the large negative anterior tilt angles indicate that a large normal variation is possible at this young age. In turn, our values reflect the normal ranges of the anterior tilt angles in adults, where the tibial slope averages approximately 10° (SD 3°) [14,15]. Due to the current lack of normative data on proximal tibial tilt angles in children, all these possibilities are speculative. This once again underlines the need to collect more data on normal tilt angles for the child population.

As claimed in the previous study [2], our data indicates that an anterior tilt angle $\geq 0°$ does not necessarily indicate a fracture. To diagnose a trampoline fracture with certainty, the clinical presentation and the trauma mechanism must be considered.

All children received conservative treatment for the fractures, and the clinical courses were uneventful. We observed no disturbances in the gait and no angular deformities such as varus, valgus, ante- or retro-curvature of the lower leg during follow-up. In contrast to our work, some previous studies reported growth disturbances related to proximal tibial injuries in children [16–18] or angular deformities described by Tuten and Cozen [11,19,20]. These findings suggest that trampoline fracture may be a subtype of proximal tibia fracture that occurs in early childhood and does not affect the growth plate. However, it is still unclear whether persistent ventral tilt of the tibial plateau could lead to altered biomechanics in the knee joint in the future. As shown in previous publications [21], an increase in the tibial slope in teenagers might be a risk factor for ACL (anterior cruciate ligament) injuries, especially in adolescents participating in high-risk activities. This phenomenon is attributed to the fact that increased tibial slope affects the biomechanics of the knee in terms of the anterior translation of the tibia relative to the femur, increasing the load on the ACL and creating a tibial shear force that results in ACL injury [22]. Currently, the future effects of positive tilt angles after trampoline fractures on biomechanics in the knee joint are unknown. In general, we recommend a clinical examination 1–2 years after trauma to avoid overlooking patients who have angular deformities, ante- or retro-curvature, and possibly even no remodeling. Especially in children who do not show remodeling, we recommend clinical and radiological follow-up at the latest before the end of growth in order to intervene in time in case of increasing anterior tilt of the proximal tibia.

This study had some major limitations. First, the low number of patients. Despite our substantial number of cases ($n = 89$ patients), we achieved a power of 0.7, which was below the pre-calculated power of 0.8, for which we needed to include at least 125 patients in the study. Second, a major limitation is the time factor. After at least one year, our data showed mostly incomplete remodeling, suggesting that one year is too short for complete remodeling. Third, the anterior tilt angle was measured indirectly by the growth plate, which does not necessarily represent the tibial slope. The angle values were also not verified by MRI or CT scans. Another limitation was that we only compared injured legs with healthy legs within the same study population. Unfortunately, we did not have data for a large control group or normative data.

5. Conclusions

In summary, this study represented the first attempt to understand and show the remodeling of trampoline fractures in children. We could demonstrate that conservative treatment was sufficient and that the post-traumatic course was mainly uneventful. In most of our cases, we could show partial remodeling after one year. However, we cannot determine how long complete remodeling will take. In children who do not show remodeling, we recommend prolonged clinical and possibly radiologic follow-up because the consequences of incomplete remodeling and its effects on biomechanics in the knee joint remain unclear to date.

Our findings should encourage further studies to establish the normal range of anterior tilt angles in the proximal tibias of children to better understand this mechanism in the future.

Author Contributions: Conceptualization, L.Z., P.M.K. and S.S.; methodology, L.Z., P.M.K. and S.S.; software, S.S.; resources, L.Z., P.M.K., K.Z., M.T., V.S.-J. and C.A.; validation, E.S., T.X. and S.S.; formal analysis, L.Z., E.S., T.X., P.M.K. and S.S.; investigation, L.Z. and S.S.; resources, L.Z. and P.M.K.; data curation, L.Z. and S.S.; writing—original draft preparation, L.Z., P.M.K. and K.Z.; writing—review and editing, L.Z. and P.M.K.; visualization, L.Z. and P.M.K.; supervision, P.M.K. and K.Z.; project administration, L.Z.; funding acquisition, P.M.K. All authors have read and agreed to the published version of the manuscript.

Funding: This research was funded by Kantonsspital Aarau, Department for Pediatric Surgery, Funded by Research Council KSA. Project number 1410.000.075.

Institutional Review Board Statement: This study was registered at: ClinicalTrials.gov, identifier: NCT04028908, Approval Date: 10 August 2016.

Informed Consent Statement: Informed consent was obtained from all subjects involved in the study.

Acknowledgments: We would like to thank all participating Children's Hospitals, their study leaders, and the Directors of the Departments of Pediatric Surgery (Aarau: Valerié Oesch; Basel: Stefan Holland-Cunz; Bern: Steffen Berger; Lucerne: Philipp Szavay; Zurich: Martin Meuli), the radiologists: Enno Stranzinger, Theodoros Xydias, and Georg Eich (Pediatric Radiology Cantonal Hospital Aarau), the CTU statistician: Sabine Schaedelin, our Sponsor from the Research Council of the Cantonal Hospital Aarau, Henrik Köhler for supporting us in the submission of this paper, and especially the parents of the patients for their contribution to this prospective multicenter study. Finally, we would like to express our sincere gratitude to our family, who supported us throughout our study.

Conflicts of Interest: The authors declare no conflict of interest.

References

1. Klimek, P.M.; Juen, D.; Stranzinger, E.; Wolf, R.; Slongo, T. Trampoline related injuries in children: Risk factors and radiographics findings. *World J. Pediatr.* **2013**, *9*, 169–174. [CrossRef]
2. Stranzinger, E.; Leidolt, L.; Eich, G.; Klimek, P.M. The anterior tilt angle of the proximal tibia epiphyseal plate: A significant radiological finding in young children with trampoline fractures. *Eur. J. Radiol.* **2014**, *83*, 1433–1436. [CrossRef] [PubMed]
3. Boyer, R.S.; Jaffe, R.B.; Nixon, G.W.; Condon, V.R. Trampoline fracture of the proximal tibia in children. *Am. J. Roentgen.* **1986**, *146*, 83–85. [CrossRef] [PubMed]
4. Hurson, C.; Browne, K.; Callender, O.; O'donnell, T.; O'Neill, A.; Moore, D.P.; Fogarty, E.E.; Dowling, F.E. Pediatric trampoline injuries. *J. Pediatr. Orthop.* **2007**, *27*, 729–732. [CrossRef]
5. Menelaws, S.; Bogacz, A.R.; Drew, T.; Paterson, B.C. Trampoline-related injuries in children: A preliminary biomechanical model of multiple users. *Emerg. Med. J.* **2011**, *28*, 594–598. [CrossRef]
6. Bruyeer, E.; Geusens, E.; Catry, F.; Vanstraelen, L.; Vanhoenacker, F. Trampoline fracture of the proximal tibia in children: Report of 3 cases and review of literature. *JBR-BTR* **2012**, *95*, 10–12. [CrossRef] [PubMed]
7. Mubarak, S.J.; Kim, J.R.; Edmonds, E.W.; Pring, M.E.; Bastrom, T.P. Classification of proximal tibial fractures in children. *J. Child. Orthop.* **2009**, *3*, 191–197. [CrossRef]
8. Königshausen, M.; Gothner, M.; Kruppa, C.; Dudda, M.; Godry, H.; Schildhauer, T.A.; Seybold, D. Trampoline-related injuries in children, an increasing problem. *Sportverl. Sportschad.* **2014**, *28*, 69–74.
9. Huynh, A.N.; Andersen, M.M.; Petersen, P.; Hansen, T.B.; Kirkegaard, H.; Weile, J.B. Childhood trampoline injuries. *Dan. Med. J.* **2018**, *65*, A5512.
10. Choi, E.S.; Hong, J.H.; Sim, J.A. Distinct features of trampoline-related orthopedic injuries in children aged under 6 years. *Injury* **2018**, *49*, 443–446. [CrossRef]
11. Cozen, L. Fracture of the proximal portion of the tibia in children followed by valgus deformity. *Surg. Gynecol. Obst.* **1953**, *97*, 183–188.
12. Kakel, R. Trampoline fracture of the proximal tibial metaphysis in children may not progress into valgus: A report of seven and a brief review. *Orthop. Traumatol. Surg. Res.* **2012**, *98*, 446–449. [CrossRef]
13. Murray, D.W.; Wilson-MacDonald, J.; Morscher, E.; Rahn, B.A.; Käslin, M. Bone growth and remodeling after fracture. *J. Bone. Joint Surg. Br.* **1996**, *78*, 42–50. [CrossRef]
14. Genin, P.; Weill, G.; Julliard, R. The tibial slope. Proposal for a measurement method. *J. Radiol.* **1993**, *74*, 27–33.
15. Giffin, J.R.; Vogrin, T.M.; Zantop, T.; Woo, S.L.; Harner, C.D. Effects of increasing tibial slope on the biomechanics of the knee. *Am. J. Sports Med.* **2004**, *32*, 376–382. [CrossRef]
16. Vrettakos, A.N.; Evaggelidis, D.C.; Kyrkos, M.J.; Tsatsos, A.V.; Nenopoulos, A.; Beslikas, T. Lower limb deformity following proximal tibia physeal injury: Long-term follow-up. *J. Orthopaed. Traumatol.* **2012**, *13*, 7–11. [CrossRef]
17. Nenopoulos, S.; Vrettakos, A.; Chaftikis, N.; Beslikas, T.; Dadoukis, D. The effect of proximal tibial fractures on the limb axis in children. *Acta Orthop. Belg.* **2007**, *73*, 345–353.
18. Müller, I.; Muschol, M.; Mann, M.; Hassenpflug, J. Results of proximal metaphyseal fractures in children. *Arch. Orthop. Trauma. Surg.* **2002**, *122*, 331–333. [CrossRef]

19. Tuten, H.R.; Keeler, K.A.; Gabos, P.G.; Zionts, L.E.; MacKenzie, W.G. Posttraumatic tibia valga in children. A long-term follow-up note. *J. Bone Joint Surg. Am.* **1999**, *81*, 799–810. [CrossRef]
20. Jackson, D.W.; Cozen, L. Genu valgum as a complication of proximal tibial metaphyseal fractures in children. *J. Bone Joint Surg. Am.* **1971**, *53*, 1571–1578. [CrossRef]
21. Vyas, S.; Van Eck, C.F.; Vyas, N.; Fu, F.H.; Otsuka, N.Y. Increased medial tibial slope in teenage pediatric population with open physes and anterior cruciate ligament injuries. *Knee Surg. Sport. Traumatol. Arthrose.* **2011**, *19*, 372–377. [CrossRef] [PubMed]
22. Shelburne, K.B.; Kim, H.J.; Sterett, W.I.; Pandy, M.G. Effect of posterior tibial slope on knee biomechanics during functional activity. *J. Orthop. Res.* **2011**, *29*, 223–231. [CrossRef] [PubMed]

Disclaimer/Publisher's Note: The statements, opinions and data contained in all publications are solely those of the individual author(s) and contributor(s) and not of MDPI and/or the editor(s). MDPI and/or the editor(s) disclaim responsibility for any injury to people or property resulting from any ideas, methods, instructions or products referred to in the content.

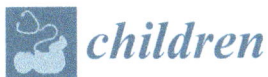

Article

Concentric Circles: A New Ultrasonographic Sign for the Diagnosis of Normal Infantile Hip Development

Nikolaos Laliotis *, Chrysanthos Chrysanthou and Panagiotis Konstandinidis

Orthopaedic Department, Inter Balkan Medical Center, Asklipiou 10 Pilea, 57001 Thessaloniki, Greece
* Correspondence: nicklaliotis@gmail.com

Abstract: Ultrasound (US) of the infant hip is used to diagnose developmental dysplasia of the hip (DDH). We present a new sonographic sign that describes the periphery of the femoral head and the acetabulum as two concentric circles. During 2008–2019, 3650 infants were referred for diagnosis of DDH. All underwent a clinical and US examination. We recorded the femoral head as the inner circle, within a fixed external circle, which was identified as the acetabulum. We analysed the clinical signs and risk factors. The US sign of two concentric circles was normal in 3522 infants and was classified as normal hip development. The alpha angle was >60° in 3449 (95%) infants. For the remaining 73 (5%) infants, the alpha angle was 50–60° and underwent further follow-up examination until the alpha angle was normalised. In 128 babies (3.5%), we detected the disruption of the concentric circle sign; the femoral head was found outside the acetabulum, which appeared with an upward sloping roof and the alpha angle was <50°. These infants had DDH and received appropriate treatment. Infants with a concentric circle sign and normal alpha angle are normal, whereas those with a disrupted sign are considered as having DDH.

Keywords: hip ultrasound; developmental dysplasia of the hip; concentric circle sign; hip dysplasia; diagnostic imaging

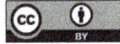

1. Introduction

Developmental dysplasia of the hip (DDH) is the most common disorder of the infant hip. A clinical examination is an essential part of diagnosis for infants with potential hip dysplasia. The main clinical features are a positive Ortolani sign, reduced hip abduction, and apparent leg length discrepancy. A variety of risk factors for hip dysplasia have been reported and the most common include breech presentation, positive family history, and multiple pregnancies. Congenital foot abnormalities, congenital muscular torticollis, prematurity, low birth weight, and oligohydramnios are among other risk factors [1–3]. A definite diagnosis for the normal or dysplastic hip is established with ultrasound examination (US) and, if required, is followed by an X-ray examination [4–6]. Hip joint sonography, as described by Graf, describes the hip anatomy with an area of immature hip development between that of the normal and dysplastic hip [7]. Rosendahl et al. described hip stability during the US examination using the term "concentric" with the dynamic Barlow manoeuvre and measured the gap between the femoral head and the acetabulum. She proposed the division of the infant hip into four types as stable, minor instability, major instability, and dislocated hips [8,9].

Our study presents a new sign during sonography of the infantile hip. We recorded in the standard coronal plane, the spherical periphery of the femoral head lying inside the concentric spherical acetabulum, which forms a double concentric circle figure. When hip development is abnormal, as in dysplasia or dislocation, this sign is not detected. The acetabulum appears as an elliptic surface, there is clear disruption of the concentric circle sign, and the head appears as a sphere in a sloping roof.

2. Patients and Methods

2.1. Study Group

A cohort of clinical and ultrasound (US) data were prospectively collected during the decade 2008–2019. In our paediatric orthopaedic department, 3650 neonates and infants were referred from their attending paediatricianfor a hip evaluation. The infants presented with suspicious clinical signs or risk factors for hip dysplasia. Their ages ranged from 10 days to 12 months. This selective cohort of patients was specifically referred from their community or hospital paediatricians and did not represent a screening cohort.

Initially, we formulated an evaluation data collection form to record the sex, name and date of birth, and aetiology of the referral. We recorded as risk factors the positive family history for hip dysplasia, breech presentation, twins, or multiple birth. We have not evaluated other risk factors such as prematurity or low birth weight.

Positive family history referred to babies with a first-degree relative that required an intervention, such as orthotic treatment or surgery, excluding a history of double nappies.

2.2. Clinical Examination

Clinical signs suspicious for DDH were reduced hip abduction (bilateral or unilateral), asymmetry of gluteal creases, leg length discrepancy, or pelvic tilt. The asymmetry of gluteal creases was also recorded in the prone position. Infants with foot disorders and torticollis were included in the group of children that were referred from the clinical examination.

Ortolani and Barlow tests were used to evaluate the stability of the infant's hip. We recorded the test as negative or positive, indicating the possible presence of dysplasia. We were careful with the strength used for performing the test, especially in neonates during the first month of age. Infants referred for clicky hips were evaluated in the clinical examination and scored only as showing positive or negative Ortolani test findings.

2.3. Ultrasound Examination

US examination was performed during the same referral examination. We performed the scans according to Graf's principles, trying to identify the lower limb, iliac bony rim, and prominent acetabular labrum. Examination was performed along the coronal plane. We measured the alpha angle. US was performed using a GE Logiq 100 system with a 7.5-MHz linear transducer (GE-Healthcare, Milwaukee, IL, USA).

We defined the periphery of the femoral head and the subchondral part of the acetabulum. The acetabulum was recorded from the labrum to the triradiate cartilage, at the boundary of the growth plate of the femoral head. Thesigns formed an image resembling double concentric circles, clearly incorporated one in the other. The observation was clear, and it was not necessary to draw lines. The presence of the ossification nucleus was recorded and compared to the size in each leg.

A dynamic US examination followed, which was performed by internal and external rotation of the limbto evaluate the movement of the inner circle, the femoral head, while the external circle, the acetabulum, remained rigid. The inner circle was rotated without losing contact with the acetabulum. In the presence of dysplasia or dislocation, the round femoral head was detected but the acetabulum appeared with an upward sloping roof and we could not define its spherical shape. The inner acetabulum presented an elliptic shape, and the round femoral head was at a distance from the triradiate cartilage. A spherical femoral head lying on an elliptically shaped acetabulum could be detected. For all unilateral cases, when the ossific nucleus appeared on the normal side, there was a distinct difference in the size of the affected nucleus in contrast to the normal nucleus. The average time required for the entire evaluationin calm babies was 10 min (Figures 1–5).

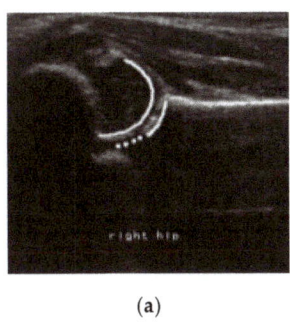 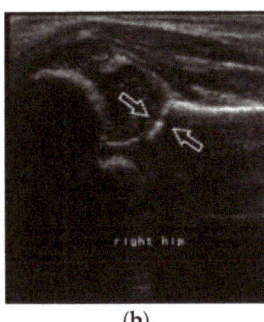

(a) (b)

Figure 1. Representative image of a concentric double circle. (**a**): The inner circle is the femoral head and the outer circle is the acetabulum. (**b**): The arrows point to the boundaries of the head and the acetabulum.

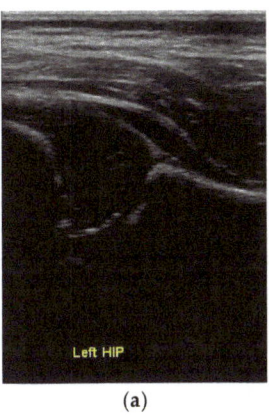 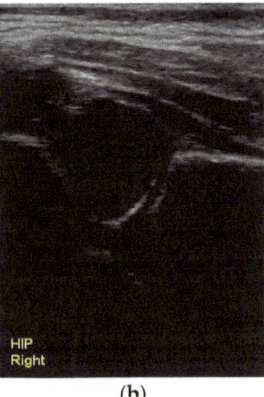

(a) (b)

Figure 2. Normal concentric circles with the spherical femoral head lying inside the spherical subchondral acetabulum. (**a**) left and (**b**) right hip.

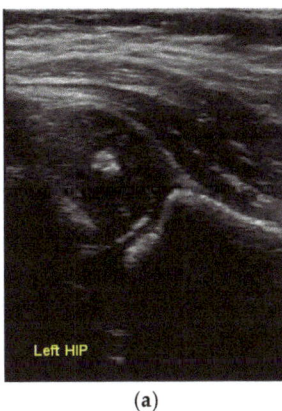 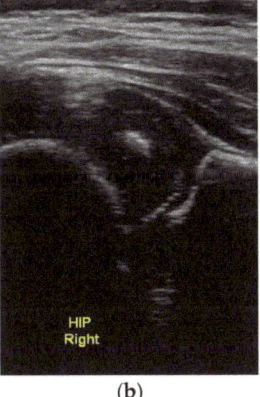

(a) (b)

Figure 3. Bilateral normal ultrasound with the presence of ossific nuclei of the femoral head, showing the normal concentric circles sign. (**a**) left and (**b**) right hip.

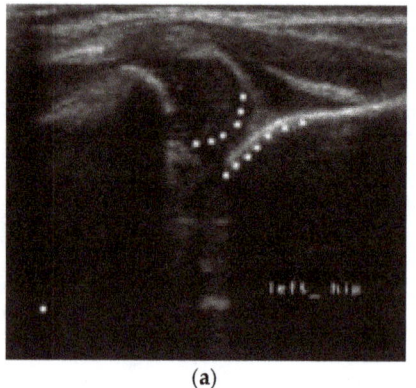 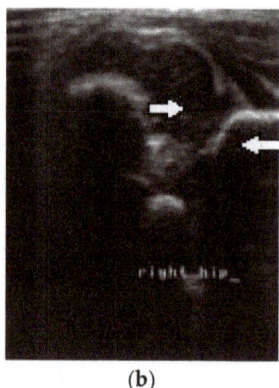

Figure 4. Bilateral DDH with disruption of the double concentric sign on the left and right side. (**a**) The acetabulum is elliptic and the head has a spherical shape (**b**) The arrows point to the femoral head and the sloping acetabulum. There is increased distance between the head and the depth of the acetabulum.

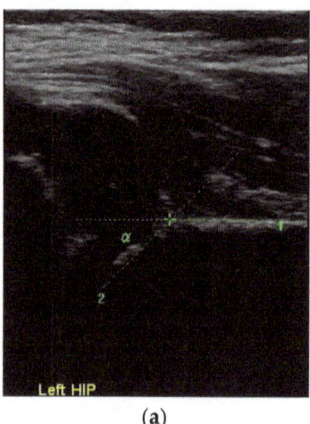 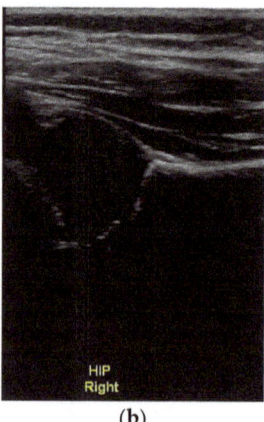

Figure 5. Image showing DDH (**a**) on the left hip, with the spherical head lying on the upper part of the elliptic shape acetabulum and (**b**) the normal right hip.

3. Results

Of the 3650 babies included in our study, 2336 (64%) were female and 1314 (36%) were male. The age at their initial examination varied, with a higher prevalence at the ages of 3–5 months.

Of the 3650 infants, 2628 (72%) were referred because of suspicious clinical signs, while the remaining 1022 (28%) were referred due to the presence of risk factors. Of these, 475 babies (13%) had been referred for both clinical signs and risk factors.

Overall, 295 babies in the group with clinical signs also had risk factors for DDH and 180 babies in the group of infants with risk factors also had clinical findings suspicious for DDH.

Risk factors for DDH included babies born in breech presentation, the presence of positive family history, and multiple pregnancies (Table 1).

Table 1. Reasons for referral to the orthopaedic unit.

			Number of Infants			Percentage %	
1.	Clinical Examination		2628			72%	
2.	Risk Factors		1022			28%	
	a.	Positive family history	a.	396	a.		30%
	b.	Breech Presentation	b.	816	b.		62%
	c.	Multiple babies	c.	105	c.		8%
3.	Combined etiology		475			13%	

Infants referred after the clinical examination involved a total of 2808 (2628 suspected infants +180 infants with clinical signs), of these 1798 (64%) babies presented with reduced abduction of the hips affecting either both hips (85%) or a unilateral hip (15%). Leg length discrepancy and pelvic tilt were the referral aetiology in 56 babies (2%), and foot abnormalities and torticollis were those in 112 babies (4%). Asymmetry of the gluteal creases was observed in 168 babies (6%) (Table 2).

Table 2. Results of clinical examination of referred infants for DDH (n = 2808).

	Number of Infants	Percentage (%)
Reduced Abduction	1798	64%
LLD and Pelvic Tilt	56	2%
Asymmetry of Creases	168	6%
Ortolani Positive	674	24%
Foot Abnormalities	112	4%

Of note, 674 infants were also referred to our clinic because of positive Ortolani and Barlow test results, including 'clicky hips'. Of these, in clinical examination, 95 children were found to be positive for the manoeuvre.

Overall, 3650 babies underwent US examination.

Using the criteria of the two concentric circles, 3522 (96.5%) babies presented normal hips. Among them, 3449 (94.5%) had an alpha angle >60° and 73 (2.0%) had an alpha angle between 50° and 60° and were classified as having immature hip. Based on the concentric circle sign, we identified contact and smooth movement of the head in the acetabulum, but these children were assigned to further evaluation, until the appearance of the ossific nucleus and normalisation of the alpha angle. In 128 infants (3.5%), there was a clear disruption of the two concentric circles and the hip was classified as subluxated or dislocated. The Graf classification was types three and four, with an alpha angle <50°. Of these, bilateral dysplasia was detected in 18 babies. The children were treated, either using a modified Pavlik or Tubingen brace when aged <3 months or with closed reduction under anaesthesia and arthrogram, if not easily reduced.

In the group of 128 children diagnosed with DDH, only eight were males. Among them, 124 children had a positive clinical sign of reduced abduction, positive Ortolani test, and apparent leg length discrepancy (LLD). The remaining four infants had a normal clinical evaluation but had been referred for breech presentation with loose broad abduction of the hips.

4. Discussion

We describe a new sign on US examination of the infantile hip. Ultrasound is an essential approach to examine hips in the first year of birth. Graf provided a clear definition for accurate assessment of the hip, emphasising the exact plane of examination with the lower limb, iliac bone, and upper part of the labrum. Measurement of the alpha angle describes the osseous part of the acetabulum. Despite considerable variability, alpha angle measurements have been described to be associated with age, sex, and side [4,7,10]. We adopted the initially defined alpha values for normal as >60°. Nonetheless, measurements of the beta angle are not always accurate. Graf divided neonatal hips into four groups and further subdivided type II into subgroups a, b, and c in order to deal with the immature group of neonatal hips. The reliability of the Graf classification has been questioned several times, as it depends on various subjective parameters, including the experience of the examiner and orientation of the US transducer, but mainly because it requires an accurate plane of examination [11–14].

Harcke et al. utilised the dynamic measurements of the neonatal hip, while Terjersen and Morin measured the coverage of the femoral head, as a percentage of the height of the femoral head is covered by the osseous part of the acetabulum [15–18]. Hosny et al. proposed a new angle for measurement, which combined the alpha and beta angles [19]. All these measurements are well established in the medical literature.

Several authors have tested the reproducibility of US tests and defined the alpha angle as the most accurately reproducible measurement. These measurements were mainly tested in neonates, while in our cohort, mainly older infants were examined. As neonates grow, it becomes easier to differentiate the immature normal hip from a dysplastic hip. Peterlein et al. described the presence of an angled or round bony roof. In our study, this was considered a normal finding when the femoral head produced the concentric circle sign with the acetabulum and had a normal alpha angle [20,21].

Rosendahl et al. described the dynamic test by dividing neonates into four groups. The authors used the term "concentricity" and the main sign during the test was evaluation of the gap between the femoral head and the acetabulum, combined with possible displacement of the labrum. They described minor or major instability by measuring the gap in the acetabular depth [8,22].

During the first week of life, hip instability with a positive Ortolani sign is common and usually improves. The strength required to perform tests of stability may overestimate the normal laxity and possibly the diagnosis of neonatal hip dysplasia, leading in overtreatment of the normal neonatal hip.

The concentric double circle sign is easily identified either in static or dynamic US examination. The periphery of the femoral head rotates but remains in contact with the acetabulum in normal hips. We did not draw circles to figure these circles as we found it easy to estimate their concentricity. However, accurate digital measurements for the sphericity of the two circles can be made during US, similar to Mose measurements of the sphericity of the femoral head in Perthes' disease.

All hips that were measured with an alpha angle >60° of Graf type I presented with a normal concentric circles sign. Hips with a normal concentric circle sign, but with an alpha angle of 50–60°, were classified as immature. They were regularly followed up to evaluate the normal development of the alpha angle in order to exclude hip dysplasia. An immature hip is expected to become normal by the second month of age, but a grey zone always exists. Hips characterized as immature may resolve spontaneously without any treatment [20,23,24].

All hipswith an alpha angle <50° indicated a clear disruption of the two concentric circles sign. In hip dislocation, the femoral head was found on the outer part of the ilium, while in subluxation, it was found on the edge of the sloping roof of the acetabulum. All these cases were further treated with orthotics using a modified Pavlik or Tubingen brace or by closed reduction under anaesthesia.

Clinical and US examination was performed simultaneously by the same paediatric orthopaedic surgeon. Usually, referrals to orthopaedic surgeons follow previously performed US examinations from trained neonatologists, radiologists, or sonographers. Ultrasonography is used to establish the diagnosis of hip dysplasia. The incidence of DDH is increased when the diagnosis is based purely on US examination [23,24].

All children with a positive Ortolani sign, when accurately performed and not mixed with a normal click, were classified as dysplastic and showed a disruption of the concentric double circle sign [25,26].

The disparity between clinical and US diagnosis in neonatal screening is well presented by Kuyng et al. [27]. They described clinical instability under the Barlow and Ortolani tests, referring to five types, including noisy hips and reported that 92% of subluxable hips were Graf I or IIa subtypes, which is a common finding in neonates with hip instability. They also reported that 73% of the dislocating or dislocated hips were Graf I or IIa subtypes on static examination. This differs from our result that all babies with a positive Ortolani finding presented with a disrupted concentric circle sign. The age of our patients and performance of the test by an experienced surgeon are possible explanations for this discrepancy.

Infants referred for minor limitation of hip abduction are generally found to be normal on US examination. Similar findings were observed in our patients. However, in infants with bilaterally dislocated hips, limited abduction may be the only important clinical sign, with the absence of instability. In these patients, US examination confirmed the clear disruption of the concentric circle sign, with the femoral head lying outside the sloping acetabulum.

The increased incidence of DDH in our patients is justified as the selected babies were referred due to positive clinical findings and risk factors but were not cases derived from a general screening test.

5. Conclusions

We present a new ultrasonographic sign that presents the femoral head and the acetabulum as two concentric circles. The sign can be reproduced both in the static and dynamic examination of the hip. It can be used in combination with alpha angle measurement to diagnose the normal development of the infant's hip. The sign is disrupted in infants with DDH. Infants defined as having immature hips according to the Graf classification should be followed up until confirmation of normal hip development is established.

Author Contributions: N.L. performed the clinical and US examinations and wrote the paper. C.C. collected data and edited the paper. P.K. collected data and edited the paper. All authors have read and agreed to the published version of the manuscript.

Funding: This research received no external funding.

Institutional Review Board Statement: No experiments were performed. All the examinations fully comply with the ethical standards of our country. The study was approved by The Institutional Review Board and the Ethic Committee of the Inter Balkan Medical Center with code no 4/15.03.22.

Informed Consent Statement: All parents were informed and agreed of the submission of their data.

Data Availability Statement: Data are available upon request from the corresponding author.

Conflicts of Interest: The authors declare no conflict of interest.

References

1. Roposch, A.; Protopapa, E.; Malaga-Shaw, O.; Gelfer, Y.; Humphries, P.; Ridout, D.; Wedge, J.H. Predicting developmental dysplasia of the hip in at-risk newborns. *BMC Musculoskelet. Disord.* **2020**, *21*, 442. [CrossRef] [PubMed]
2. Oh, E.J.; Min, J.J.; Kwon, S.-S.; Kim, S.B.; Choi, C.W.; Jung, Y.H.; Oh, K.J.; Park, J.Y.; Park, M.S. Breech Presentation in Twins as a Risk Factor for Developmental Dysplasia of the Hip. *J.Pediatr. Orthop.* **2022**, *42*, e55–e58. [CrossRef] [PubMed]
3. Harsanyi, S.; Zamborsky, R.; Krajciova, L.; Kokavec, M.; Danisovic, L. Developmental Dysplasia of the Hip: A Review of Etiopathogenesis, Risk Factors, and Genetic Aspects. *Medicina* **2020**, *56*, 153. [CrossRef] [PubMed]
4. Graf, R. Hip sonography: Background; technique and common mistakes; results; debate and politics; challenges. *Hip Int.* **2017**, *27*, 215–219. [CrossRef] [PubMed]
5. Gerscovich, E.O. A radiologist's guide to the imaging in the diagnosis and treatment of developmental dysplasia of the hip. II. Ultrasonography: Anatomy, technique, acetabular angle measurements, acetabular coverage of femoral head, acetabular cartilage thickness, three-dimensional technique, screening of newborns, study of older children. *Skelet. Radiol.* **1997**, *26*, 447–456.
6. KPrice, R.; Dove, R.; Hunter, J.B. The use of X-ray at 5 months in a selective screening programme for developmental dysplasia of the hip. *J. Child. Orthop.* **2011**, *5*, 195–200.

7. Graf, R.; Mohajer, M.; Plattner, F. Hip sonography update. Quality-management, catastrophes—Tips and tricks. *Med. Ultrason.* **2013**, *15*, 299–303. [CrossRef]
8. Rosendahl, K.; Markestad, T.; Lie, R. Ultrasound in the early diagnosis of congenital dislocation of the hip: The significance of hip stability versus acetabular morphology. *Pediatr. Radiol.* **1992**, *22*, 430–433. [CrossRef]
9. Harcke, H.T.; Grissom, L.E. Performing dynamic sonography of the infant hip. *Am. J. Roentgenol.* **1990**, *155*, 837–844. [CrossRef]
10. Schams, M.; Labruyère, R.; Zuse, A.; Walensi, M. Diagnosing developmental dysplasia of the hip using the Graf ultrasound method: Risk and protective factor analysis in 11,820 universally screened newborns. *Eur. J. Pediatr.* **2017**, *176*, 1193–1200. [CrossRef]
11. Roposch, A.A.; Graf, R.; Wright, J.G. Determining the reliability of the Graf classification for hip dysplasia. *Clin. Orthop. Relat. Res.* **2006**, *447*, 119–124. [CrossRef] [PubMed]
12. Wilkinson, A.G.; Wilkinson, S.; Elton, R.A. Values for bony acetabular roof angle and percentage femoral head cover in a selective ultrasoundneonatalhip-screening programme: Effect of age, sex and side. *J. Pediatr. Orthop. Part B* **2018**, *27*, 236–243. [CrossRef] [PubMed]
13. Kolb, A.; Benca, E.; Willegger, M.; Puchner, S.; Windhager, R.; Chiari, C. Measurement considerations on examiner-dependent factors in the ultrasound assessment of developmental dysplasia of the hip. *Int. Orthop.* **2017**, *41*, 1245–1250. [CrossRef] [PubMed]
14. Bilgili, F.; Bilgili, Ç.Ö.; Çetinkaya, E.; Polat, A.; Sungur, İ.; Saglam, Y. Reliability of computer-assisted and manual measurement methods for assessment of Graf Type 1 and Type 2 hip sonograms. *J. Ultrasound Med.* **2016**, *35*, 1269–1275. [CrossRef] [PubMed]
15. Terjesen, T. Ultrasound as the primary imaging method in the diagnosis of hip dysplasia in children aged < 2 years. *J. Pediatr. Orthop. Part B* **1996**, *5*, 123–128.
16. Clarke, N.M.; Harcke, H.T.; McHugh, P.; Lee, M.S.; Borns, P.F.; MacEwen, G.D. Real-time ultrasound in the diagnosis of congenital dislocation and dysplasia of the hip. *J. Bone Jt. Surg. Br. Vol.* **1985**, *67*, 406–412. [CrossRef]
17. Harcke, H.; Grissom, L.E. Infant hip sonography: Current concepts. In *Seminars in Ultrasound, CT and MRI*; WB Saunders: Philadelphia, AR, USA, 1994; Volume 15, pp. 256–263.
18. Morin, C.; Harcke, H.T.; MacEwen, G.D. The infant hip: Real-time US assessment of acetabular development. *Radiology* **1985**, *157*, 673–677. [CrossRef]
19. Hosny, G.; Koizumi, W.; Benson, M. Ultrasound screening of the infant's hip: Introduction of a new combined angle. *J. Pediatr. Orthop. Part B* **2002**, *11*, 204–211.
20. Peterlein, C.D.; Schüttler, K.F.; Lakemeier, S.; Timmesfeld, N.; Görg, C.; Fuchs-Winkelmann, S.; Schofer, M.D. Reproducibility of different screening classifications in ultrasonography of the newbornhip. *BMC Pediatr.* **2010**, *10*, 98. [CrossRef]
21. Falliner, A.; Schwinzer, D.; Hahne, H.J.; Hedderich, J.; Hassenpflug, J. Comparing ultrasound measurements of neonatal hips using the methods of Graf and Terjesen. *J. Bone Jt. Surgery. Br. Vol.* **2006**, *88*, 104–106. [CrossRef]
22. Rosendahl, K.; Aslaksen, A.; Lie, R.T.; Markestad, T.T. Reliability of ultrasound in the early diagnosis of developmental dysplasia of the hip. *Pediatr. Radiol.* **1995**, *25*, 219–224. [CrossRef]
23. Broadhurst, C.; Rhodes, A.M.L.; Harper, P.; Perry, D.C.; Clarke, N.M.P.; Aarvold, A. Incidence of late presentation of DDH in England. *Bone Jt. J.* **2019**, *101-B*, 281–287. [CrossRef]
24. Milligan, D.; Cosgrove, A. Monitoring of a hip surveillance programme protects infants from radiation and surgical intervention. *Bone Jt. J.* **2020**, *102-B*, 495–500. [CrossRef]
25. Marson, A.; Hunter, J.B.; Price, K.R. Value of the 'Clicky Hip' in Selective screening for developmental dysplasia of the hip. *Bone Jt. J.* **2019**, *101-B*, 635–638. [CrossRef]
26. Humphry, S.; Thompson, D.; Price, N.; Williams, P.R. Clicky hip, to refer or not to refer? *Bone Jt. J.* **2018**, *100-B*, 1249. [CrossRef]
27. Kyung, B.S.; Lee, S.H.; Jeong, W.K.; Park, S.Y. Disparity between clinical and ultrasound examinations in neonatalhip screening. *Clin. Orthop. Surg.* **2016**, *8*, 203–209. [CrossRef]

Disclaimer/Publisher's Note: The statements, opinions and data contained in all publications are solely those of the individual author(s) and contributor(s) and not of MDPI and/or the editor(s). MDPI and/or the editor(s) disclaim responsibility for any injury to people or property resulting from any ideas, methods, instructions or products referred to in the content.

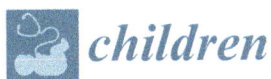

Case Report

Traumatic Hip Dislocation in Pediatric Patients: Clinical Case Series and a Narrative Review of the Literature with an Emphasis on Primary and Long-Term Complications

Eetu N. Suominen and Antti J. Saarinen *

Department of Orthopedics and Traumatology, Helsinki University Hospital, 00260 Helsinki, Finland
* Correspondence: antti.j.saarinen@helsinki.fi

Abstract: Traumatic hip dislocation is a rare injury in pediatric populations. Dislocation may be associated with low-energy trauma, such as a minor fall. Traumatic hip dislocation is associated with severe complications, such as avascular necrosis of the femoral head. Timely diagnosis and reposition decrease the rate of complications. In this study we retrospectively assessed traumatic hip dislocations in pediatric patients during a 10-year timespan in a university hospital. There were eight cases of traumatic hip dislocations. All patients had a minimum follow-up of two years and were followed with MRI scans. One patient developed avascular necrosis during the follow-up which resolved conservatively. There were no other significant complications. In conclusion, traumatic hip dislocation is a rare injury which is associated with severe complications. Patients in our case series underwent a timely reposition. The complication rate was similar to previous reports.

Keywords: hip dislocation; pediatric trauma; pediatric injury; avascular necrosis

Citation: Suominen, E.N.; Saarinen, A.J. Traumatic Hip Dislocation in Pediatric Patients: Clinical Case Series and a Narrative Review of the Literature with an Emphasis on Primary and Long-Term Complications. *Children* **2023**, *10*, 107. https://doi.org/10.3390/children10010107

Academic Editors: Axel A. Horsch, Maher A. Ghandour and Matthias Christoph M. Klotz

Received: 18 October 2022
Revised: 14 November 2022
Accepted: 16 November 2022
Published: 4 January 2023

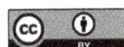

Copyright: © 2023 by the authors. Licensee MDPI, Basel, Switzerland. This article is an open access article distributed under the terms and conditions of the Creative Commons Attribution (CC BY) license (https://creativecommons.org/licenses/by/4.0/).

1. Introduction

Traumatic hip dislocation is a rare injury among the pediatric population. Patients over 10 years of age typically require a major traumatic event for dislocation [1]. However, in younger children the dislocation may occur from a minor trauma as the traumatic energy required for hip dislocation increases with age [2–4]. Posterior dislocation is the most common type of injury, making up approximately 95% of traumatic dislocations [2]. Typical characteristics of posterior dislocation are adduction, flexion, internal rotation, and shortening of the dislocated limb [5]. Associated injuries increase with age and higher energy trauma. Associated acetabular and femoral fractures are uncommon in pediatric patients.

Closed reduction under moderate conscious anesthesia can be used in adolescent patients. Reduction is usually easy to achieve, but interfering fragments originating from the hip joint structures may prevent concentric reduction. In young children, a closed reduction in an operating room with readiness to convert to open reduction is recommendable [5]. If the operating room is unavailable, closed reduction should be performed in the emergency department. The successful reduction should be confirmed using fluoroscopy [6]. Widening of the injured joint space indicates unsuccessful reduction. If a congruent and stable hip joint is not achieved using the closed reduction, an open reduction is needed. After successful reduction, immobilization with a hip spica cast is recommended for children under 10 years. Protected weight bearing for 6–8 weeks is recommended for older patients [3].

Avascular necrosis (AVN) is the feared complication of hip dislocation. The only statistically proven risk factor is delay between dislocation and reduction. If the delay is greater than 6 h, the risk of avascular necrosis is increased 20-fold [2,3,6]. Reduction may happen spontaneously, especially in young children [3]. Magnetic resonance imaging (MRI) during the primary care is warranted for patients with suspected spontaneously reduction or with signs of unsuccessful reduction to assess soft tissue entrapments not visible on radiographs [7]. As AVN may develop up to two years after the injury, follow-up clinical surveillance and control MRIs are warranted.

In this study, we describe a patient series from a tertiary university hospital during a ten-year period. We also present a narrative literature review with an emphasis on primary complications and complications during extended follow-up after traumatic hip dislocation in pediatric patients.

2. Materials and Methods

Institutional review board permission was obtained for the study. A consecutive case series of acute, traumatic hip dislocations in skeletally immature patients between 1 January 2009 and 31 December 2019 treated in the pediatric orthopedic department of Turku University Hospital, Finland were reviewed retrospectively. A retrospective cohort of patients was collected using the International Classification of Diseases (ICD) code for hip dislocation (S73) to identify the cases from the patient charts of our center. Inclusion criteria were the correct diagnosis of traumatic hip dislocation, skeletally immaturity, minimum of two years of follow-up, and adequate clinical and radiographic information. Non-traumatic dislocations were excluded from the study. No patients with traumatic dislocations were excluded.

Patient characteristics and the etiology of the injury were collected from the patient charts. Approximate time from injury to reduction was assessed. Associated injuries and successful reduction were assessed from radiographs. MRIs taken during the follow-up were evaluated. Complications were assessed during the follow-up. The mechanism of injury was defined as high energy if it was because of a motor-vehicle accident or a fall from a height of more than 3 m (10 feet). A low-energy injury was defined as a typical play activity or fall from a height of less than 3 m (10 feet) [8].

3. Results

During the study period, eight patients treated for traumatic hip dislocation were identified. Four patients were male and four female. The mean age at the time of the injury was 11.7 years (range from 4.4 to 16 years). Three patients had a dislocation after a low energy trauma. Two of these patients were aged four years, and one patient was seven years at the time of the accident. Five patients had a hip dislocation after a high energy trauma. These patients were 14 to 16 years old. Six patients had posterior and two had anterior dislocations. The detailed descriptions of the patients and accidents are presented in Table 1.

Three patients over 10-years old had associated fractures. One patient had a Hill–Sachs lesion of the femoral head with loose extra-articular osteochondral fragment at the caput–collum border. This patient had an anterior dislocation of the femoral head. Two patients had acetabulum fractures as an associated injury. In one of these patients, an MRI showed a posterocranial fracture of the acetabulum with a 7 mm lateral dislocation between acetabulum and ramus. In another patient, a caudal acetabulum fracture was observed with a 25 mm × 13 mm sized dislocated fragment. These fractures were treated conservatively. None of the patients developed complications during the follow-up. There were no recurrent dislocations.

The mean time to reduction was approximately 3 h (range from 2 to 5 h). During the follow-ups, there were no radiological or clinical evidence of growth disturbances, heterotrophic ossification, early epiphysis closure, or post-traumatic arthritis. None of the patients had abnormal neurological or vascular findings in the lower extremity. None of the patients required surgical intervention for reduction or associated injuries.

The mean duration of the follow-up was 7.9 years (range from 4.1 to 9.8 years). One patient presented with bone edema and flattening of the caput indicating AVN at 4 weeks after the injury (Patient 7 in Table 1). Time to successful reduction in this patient was five hours. The patient was treated conservatively with a 6-month weight bearing prohibition.

AVN was resolved at 6 months MRI control and the patient was asymptomatic in the clinical examination.

Table 1. Clinical characteristics and etiology of the injuries.

ID	Age at Injury (Years)	Follow-Up (Years)	Approximate Time to Reduction (Hours)	Sex	Description of the Accident	Type of Dislocation	Associated Injuries
1	15.5	12.0	3.5	Male	Motocross injury, fell after jump and landed on the hip	Anterior	Hill–Sachs lesion of the femoral head, loose extra-articular osteochondral fragment at the caput–collum border
2	15.4	10.6	2.0	Female	Fell with a moped	Posterior	
3	14.9	10.1	5.0	Male	Downhill skiing injury, fell on the hip after a jump	Posterior	
4	7.3	8.7	2.3	Female	Fell on a trampoline	Anterior	
5	16.0	6.2	unknown	Male	Downhill skiing injury, fell on the hip after a jump	Posterior	Radiograph showed 6 mm fragment next to caput. MRI showed posterocranial acetabulum fracture. 7 mm lateral dislocation between acetabulum and ramus.
6	15.8	5.9	2.0	Male	Motocross bike collided with patient	Posterior	Caudal acetabulum fracture, 25 mm × 13 mm dislocated fragment.
7	4.6	5.7	3.0	Female	Landed with the hip on abduction on a bouncing castle	Posterior	
8	4.4	4.0	3.0	Female	Sledge collision with an adult	Posterior	

4. Discussion

Several studies in recent history have studied the epidemiology, mechanism of injury, clinical presentation, diagnosis, and treatment of the traumatic hip dislocation in a pediatric population. The findings of our study are consistent with the results of the previous research. Traumatic hip dislocation in the pediatric population is an uncommon injury that requires timely diagnosis and intervention. Due to low traumatic energy or untypical etiology, pediatric hip dislocation may go unnoticed [9,10]. Special caution is needed with unconscious patients in whom the ambulatory status is unknown.

Traumatic posterior hip dislocation in children often presents with the classic lower limb deformity. The hip is in flexion, adduction, and internal rotation. The involved limb appears shorter than the contralateral limb and the femoral head can be palpated posteriorly. Radiographs should be obtained without delay after adequate pain medication. The presence of another fracture or injury can divert attention from hip dislocation and delay the diagnosis. The dislocation of the femoral head can be anterior or posterior. Similar to adult patients, the majority of hip dislocations are posterior [11]. Bilateral dislocations have been reported in the literature but are exceptional [12]. A prompt closed reduction with the patient under suitable anesthesia and analgesia is considered to be appropriate treatment. Closed reduction is usually accomplished via traction in line with the deformity. In cases in which the diagnosis of hip dislocation is delayed, some studies suggest a short period of skeletal traction after the successful reduction until pain is improved. However, the advantage of this in order to achieve easier reduction has been compromised [10].

The traumatic energy required for a traumatic hip dislocation increases with age [1,5,6]. This was also seen in our patient sample as patients younger than 10 years had minor traumatic events in contrast to adolescents, who all had high-energy trauma. When compared to adult patients, associated fractures are rare in pediatric patients after traumatic hip dislocation. Large posterior wall fractures or fractures with articular surface dislocation require internal fixation to prevent hip instability.

Radiographic assessment by anteroposterior, oblique, and lateral imaging of the pelvis is crucial before and after reduction. Plain radiographs and CT scans may not adequately show acetabulum fractures in young children due to unossified bone. In these patients an MRI is warranted [7,13,14]. MRIs also provides information on soft-tissue injuries, including labral and capsular tears along with cartilage and muscular injuries [7]. Widening of the articular space in radiographs can be caused by entrapment of soft-tissue and requires imaging with an MRI. Archer et al. reported a patient with unrecognized physeal injury in whom the attempted closed reduction resulted in a hip fracture requiring open reduction and internal fixation [5]. When any uncertainties exist regarding hip joint congruency, a CT or MRI scan should be performed to identify intra-articular bone fragments or interposed soft tissue. Concerning the additional injuries connected with traumatic hip dislocation in pediatric patients, an acetabular fracture can be underestimated with radiographs and CT scans [13].

In our patients, no severe complications occurred during the follow-up. One 4.6-year-old patient presented with AVN after a posterior dislocation after landing with the hip on abduction and flexion on a bouncing castle. Dislocation was reduced after approximately five hours from the injury with a closed reposition in the operating room after which the patient was fitted with a spica cast. AVN was discovered in a routine MRI scan at four weeks after the injury. After the imaging finding, the patient was assigned to non-weight bearing for six months. AVN resolved during the follow-up at six months and patient returned to normal activities without difficulties.

Reduction in the dislocated joint restores the normal blood flow to the femoral head. The risk of osteonecrosis is substantial and may occur in up to one-third of dislocations, depending on the severity of injury. AVN of the femoral head is the most feared and frequent serious complication related to traumatic hip dislocation. Symptoms of AVN include painless limp, pain, and restricted movement. The incidence of AVN in children younger than 18 years is reported to be 3% to 15% after an isolated hip dislocation [15,16]. AVN is caused when the arterial perforation is disturbed. Precise pathological process of the AVN remains unclear. In a cadaver study, Chung demonstrated incomplete anastomotic and transepiphyseal vessels in skeletally immature patients [17]. Undeveloped anastomotic perforation exposes the femoral head to ischemia during the dislocation [2,17]. AVN may lead to severe disability and need for a hip replacement. Evidence at present indicates an association between late hip reduction and higher rate of osteonecrosis of the femoral head in all traumatic hip dislocations [18]. Hence, all traumatic hip dislocations should be reduced as soon as possible to decrease the rate of osteonecrosis of the femoral head. When a traumatic hip dislocation is associated with femoral epiphysiolysis, the risk increases to 100% [19,20]. Because of the risk of AVN, patients should be routinely followed with MRI scans. In our study, timely reduction was achieved in all the patients and the patients were adequately followed after the dislocation.

Primary neurologic complications associated with pediatric hip dislocations are rare, presumably due to the low traumatic energy typical to these injuries. The peroneal branch of the sciatic nerve is the most likely peripheral nerve to be injured. Sciatic nerve injuries are reported in the literature with an incidence rate of approximately 5% [21]. Nerve injuries associated with traumatic hip dislocations are usually a neurapraxias and symptoms are most often transitory. The peroneal nerves are most commonly affected. Pre- and post-reductive neurovascular status should always be examined. In our patient series, no neurologic complications occurred. Other uncommon complications of the traumatic hip dislocation in pediatric patients include recurrent dislocation, heterotrophic ossification, and development of coxa magna. Recurrent dislocation may be associated with a defect in the capsule or attenuation of the hip capsule without a tear. Acute redislocation, which occurs soon after reduction, implies that the reduction was not congruent and additional investigation with a CT scan is indicated with probable open exploration [11]. Proximal femoral head displacement (epiphyseolysis) during reduction in hip dislocation has been reported in the literature [19]. The possibility of physeal fracture should be kept in mind in traumatic hip dislocation occurring in children and adolescents with an open physis.

The development of the complications in traumatic hip dislocation can be delayed several years. Older studies before follow-up with MRIs have reported avascular necrosis after three years of the injury [22]. Patients should be subjected to long-term follow-up.

Neglected or untreated traumatic hip dislocations are rare. There are few reports on neglected traumatic dislocation. Although previous studies and case reports have presented a wide variety of treatment, the optimal management remains unclear. At a time-interval between injury and reduction procedure beyond 3–4 weeks, a reductional operation should be performed [16,23]. Even if the open reduction is delayed, it may prevent deformity, and will maintain the length of the lower extremity [24]. Regarding the surgical technique, it has been proposed that the surgeon should release the adductor longus, lengthen the psoas tendon, and insert a K-wire [16]. As mentioned, the traumatic hip dislocation in children is, in majority of the patients, an isolated injury, without a concurrent acetabular fracture. Therefore, the surgical technique should be chosen so that the operation does not further compromise the articular cartilage or the vascular structures of the femoral head.

No study to date has been able to define the type of rest required or the length of time for which it should be applied and there is no evidence that this affects the long-term outcome. Early gentle range of motion and patient mobilization should be instituted. Under the age of 10 years, immobilization with a spica cast for 4 weeks, along with suitable rehabilitation is particularly important for the healing of surrounding soft tissues to make the joint become stable [1]. Yuksel et al. suggest that the non-weight bearing interval of 4 weeks and partial weight bearing after 6 weeks are appropriate periods to let the soft tissue heal [6]. According to Sahin et al., neither the type of the treatment (post-reduction traction or bed rest) nor the time from injury to full-weight bearing influenced outcomes significantly [25].

The small sample size of our patient series prevented us from performing statistical analyses. Most prior reports on traumatic hip dislocations in pediatric patients are case reports or small case series. We report a modern single center case series with extensive follow-up with routinely taken MRI scans.

5. Conclusions

Traumatic hip dislocation is a rare injury in pediatric patients and is often associated with low-energy trauma. Adequate diagnosis and repositioning prevent complications, such as avascular necrosis of the femoral head. Radiographs should be obtained when a pediatric patient is unambulatory after a traumatic event, such as a fall. A shortened leg held in adduction and internal rotation should prompt the emergency physician to consider ordering radiographs and provide analgesia for the child. Primary MRI scans might be warranted to exclude associated injuries. During follow-up, MRI scans should be routinely taken to rule out avascular necrosis. The possibility of other associated injuries should be taken into account, especially in the patients with high-energy trauma. With appropriate management, most children with traumatic hip dislocation treated promptly with closed reduction will have an excellent outcome.

Author Contributions: Conceptualization, E.N.S. and A.J.S.; methodology, E.N.S. and A.J.S.; investigation, E.N.S. and A.J.S.; resources, E.N.S. and A.J.S.; data curation, E.N.S. and A.J.S.; writing—original draft preparation, E.N.S.; writing—review and editing, A.J.S.; supervision, A.J.S.; funding acquisition, E.N.S. and A.J.S. All authors have read and agreed to the published version of the manuscript.

Funding: This research was funded by The Päivikki and Sakari Sohlberg Foundation, University of Turku, and Clinical Research Institute HUCH.

Institutional Review Board Statement: The study was conducted in accordance with the Declaration of Helsinki and approved by the Institutional Review Board of University of Turku.

Informed Consent Statement: Patient consent was waived due to the retrospective setting.

Data Availability Statement: Study data can be obtained from the corresponding author for a reasonable request.

Acknowledgments: Open Access funding provided by the University of Helsinki.

Conflicts of Interest: The authors declare no conflict of interests.

References

1. Vialle, R.; Odent, T.; Pannier, S.; Pauthier, F.; Laumonier, F.; Glorion, C. Traumatic Hip Dislocation in Childhood. *J. Pediatr. Orthop.* **2005**, *25*, 138–144. [CrossRef] [PubMed]
2. Mehlman, C.T.; Hubbard, G.W.; Crawford, A.H.; Roy, D.R.; Wall, E.J. Traumatic Hip Dislocation in Children: Long-Term Followup of 42 Patients. *Clin. Orthop. Relat. Res.* **2000**, *376*, 68–79. [CrossRef]
3. Herrera-Soto, J.A.; Price, C.T. Traumatic Hip Dislocations in Children and Adolescents: Pitfalls and Complications. *JAAOS J. Am. Acad. Orthop. Surg.* **2009**, *17*, 15–21. [CrossRef] [PubMed]
4. Offierski, C. Traumatic dislocation of the hip in children. *J. Bone Jt. Surg. Br. Vol.* **1981**, *63*, 194–197. [CrossRef]
5. Archer, J.E.; Balakumar, B.; Odeh, A.; Bache, C.E.; Dimitriou, R. Traumatic hip dislocation in the paediatric population: A case series from a specialist centre. *Injury* **2021**, *52*, 3660–3665. [CrossRef]
6. Yuksel, S.; Albay, C. Early Reduction of Pediatric Traumatic Posterior Hip Dislocation Is Much More Important Than the Treatment Procedure. *Pediatr. Emerg. Care* **2019**, *35*, e206. [CrossRef]
7. Thanacharoenpanich, S.; Bixby, S.; Breen, M.A.; Kim, Y.J. MRI Is Better Than CT Scan for Detection of Structural Pathologies After Traumatic Posterior Hip Dislocations in Children and Adolescents. *J. Pediatr. Orthop.* **2020**, *40*, 86–92. [CrossRef]
8. Musemeche, C.A.; Barthel, M.; Cosentino, C.; Reynolds, M. Pediatric falls from heights. *J. Trauma* **1991**, *31*, 1347–1349. [CrossRef]
9. Cosentino, A.; Odorizzi, G.; Schmidt, O.S. Five-years Control after a Delayed Diagnosis of a Traumatic Posterior Hip Dislocation in a 5 years Old Boy-A Case Report. *J. Orthop Case Rep.* **2021**, *11*, 47–49. [CrossRef]
10. Banskota, A.K.; Spiegel, D.A.; Shrestha, S.; Shrestha, O.P.; Rajbhandary, T. Open Reduction for Neglected Traumatic Hip Dislocation in Children and Adolescents. *J. Pediatr. Orthop.* **2007**, *27*, 187–191. [CrossRef]
11. Salisbury, R.D.; Eastwood, D.M. Traumatic Dislocation of the Hip in Children. *Clin. Orthop. Relat. Res.* **2000**, *377*, 106–111. [CrossRef]
12. Sahin, V.; Karakas, E.S.; Turk, C.Y. Bilateral traumatic hip dislocation in a child: A case report and review of the literature. *J. Trauma Acute Care Surg.* **1999**, *46*, 500–504. [CrossRef]
13. Hearty, T.; Swaroop, V.T.; Gourineni, P.; Robinson, L. Standard Radiographs and Computed Tomographic Scan Underestimating Pediatric Acetabular Fracture After Traumatic Hip Dislocation: Report of 2 Cases. *J. Orthop. Trauma* **2011**, *25*, E68–E73. [CrossRef] [PubMed]
14. Mayer, S.W.; Stewart, J.R.; Fadell, M.F.; Kestel, L.; Novais, E.N. MRI as a reliable and accurate method for assessment of posterior hip dislocation in children and adolescents without the risk of radiation exposure. *Pediatr. Radiol.* **2015**, *45*, 1355–1362. [CrossRef] [PubMed]
15. Hamilton, P.R.; Broughton, N.S. Traumatic Hip Dislocation in Childhood. *J. Pediatr. Orthop.* **1998**, *18*, 691–694. [CrossRef] [PubMed]
16. Hung, N.N. Traumatic hip dislocation in children. *J. Pediatr. Orthop. B* **2012**, *21*, 542–551. [CrossRef]
17. Chung, S.M. The arterial supply of the developing proximal end of the human femur. *J. Bone Jt. Surg. Am.* **1976**, *58*, 961–970. [CrossRef]
18. Ahmed, G.; Shiraz, S.; Riaz, M.; Ibrahim, T. Late versus early reduction in traumatic hip dislocations: A meta-analysis. *Eur. J. Orthop. Surg. Traumatol.* **2017**, *27*, 1109–1116. [CrossRef]
19. Herrera-Soto, J.A.; Price, C.T.; Reuss, B.L.; Riley, P.; Kasser, J.R.; Beaty, J.H. Proximal femoral epiphysiolysis during reduction of hip dislocation in adolescents. *J. Pediatr. Orthop.* **2006**, *26*, 371–374. [CrossRef]
20. Odent, T.; Glorion, C.; Pannier, S.; Bronfen, C.; Langlais, J.; Pouliquen, J.C. Traumatic dislocation of the hip with separation of the capital epiphysis: 5 adolescent patients with 3 9 years of follow. *Acta Orthop. Scand.* **2003**, *74*, 49–52. [CrossRef]
21. Cornwall, R.; Radomisli, T.E. Nerve Injury in Traumatic Dislocation of the Hip. *Clin. Orthop. Relat. Res.* **2000**, *377*, 84–91. [CrossRef]
22. Pearson, D.E.; Mann, R.J. Traumatic hip dislocation in children. *Clin. Orthop. Relat. Res.* **1973**, *92*, 189–194. [CrossRef] [PubMed]
23. Sulaiman, A.R.; Munajat, I.; Mohd, F.E. Outcome of traumatic hip dislocation in children. *J. Pediatr. Orthop. B* **2013**, *22*, 557–562. [CrossRef] [PubMed]
24. Kumar, S.; Jain, A.K. Neglected traumatic hip dislocation in children. *Clin. Orthop. Relat. Res.* **2005**, *431*, 9–13. [CrossRef]
25. Sahin, V.; Karakas, E.S.; Aksu, S.; Atlihan, D.; Turk, C.Y.; Halici, M. Traumatic dislocation and fracture-dislocation of the hip: A long-term follow-up study. *J. Trauma Acute Care Surg.* **2003**, *54*, 520–529.

Disclaimer/Publisher's Note: The statements, opinions and data contained in all publications are solely those of the individual author(s) and contributor(s) and not of MDPI and/or the editor(s). MDPI and/or the editor(s) disclaim responsibility for any injury to people or property resulting from any ideas, methods, instructions or products referred to in the content.

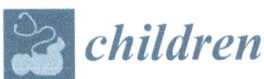

Review

Outcomes, Return to Sport, and Failures of MPFL Reconstruction Using Autografts in Children and Adolescents with Recurrent Patellofemoral Instability: A Systematic Review

Filippo Migliorini [1,2,*], Nicola Maffulli [3,4,5], Andreas Bell [2] and Marcel Betsch [6]

1. Department of Orthopaedic, Trauma, and Reconstructive Surgery, RWTH University Hospital, 52074 Aachen, Germany
2. Department of Orthopaedic and Trauma Surgery, Eifelklinik St. Brigida, 52152 Simmerath, Germany
3. Department of Medicine, Surgery and Dentistry, University of Salerno, 84081 Baronissi, Italy
4. School of Pharmacy and Bioengineering, Faculty of Medicine, Keele University, Stoke on Trent ST4 7QB, UK
5. Centre for Sports and Exercise Medicine, Barts and the London School of Medicine and Dentistry, Mile End Hospital, Queen Mary University of London, London E1 4DG, UK
6. Department of Orthopaedic and Trauma Surgery, University Hospital of Erlangen, 91054 Erlangen, Germany
* Correspondence: migliorini.md@gmail.com; Tel.: +49-0241-80-35529

Abstract: Introduction: This study systematically reviews and updates the current evidence on the outcomes of medial patellofemoral ligament (MPFL) reconstruction using autografts in children and adolescents with recurrent patellofemoral instability. The outcomes of interest were improvements in patient reported outcomes measures (PROMs), return to sport rates, and the rates of surgical failure. Methods: This systematic review was performed according to the 2020 PRISMA guidelines. The following electronic databases were accessed in October 2022: PubMed, Scopus, Web of Science. All the clinical studies which investigated the outcomes of MPFL reconstruction using autografts in children and adolescents with recurrent patellofemoral instability were accessed. Only studies which included patients younger than 18 years were considered. Techniques, case reports, guidelines, comments, editorials, letters, protocols, reviews, and meta-analyses were excluded. Studies which included patients with congenital or acute patellofemoral instability were not eligible, nor were those which focused exclusively on hyperlaxity. Results: Data from 477 patients (510 procedures) were retrieved. Of the patients, 41% (196 of 477) were women. The mean length of follow-up was 33.7 ± 28.8 months. The mean age of the patients was 14.6 ± 1.6 years. At the last follow-up, all PROMs of interest were statistically improved. The mean time to return to sport was 6.1 ± 1.1 months. Of the patients, 27% reduced their level of activity after surgical stabilization. A total of 87% of patients returned to practice sport. A total of 5% (26 of 477) and 2% (9 of 363) of patients experienced further dislocations and subluxations, respectively, during the follow-up period. Moreover, 4% (16 of 403) of patients underwent a further surgical procedure for patellofemoral instability within the follow-up period. Conclusion: MPFL reconstruction using autografts is effective in children and adolescents with recurrent patellofemoral instability.

Keywords: patellofemoral instability; recurrent; MPFL; autografts; return to sport

Citation: Migliorini, F.; Maffulli, N.; Bell, A.; Betsch, M. Outcomes, Return to Sport, and Failures of MPFL Reconstruction Using Autografts in Children and Adolescents with Recurrent Patellofemoral Instability: A Systematic Review. *Children* 2022, 9, 1892. https://doi.org/10.3390/children9121892

Academic Editors: Axel A. Horsch, Maher A. Ghandour and Matthias Christoph M. Klotz

Received: 10 November 2022
Accepted: 30 November 2022
Published: 2 December 2022

Publisher's Note: MDPI stays neutral with regard to jurisdictional claims in published maps and institutional affiliations.

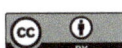

Copyright: © 2022 by the authors. Licensee MDPI, Basel, Switzerland. This article is an open access article distributed under the terms and conditions of the Creative Commons Attribution (CC BY) license (https://creativecommons.org/licenses/by/4.0/).

1. Introduction

Recurrent instability of the patella (RPI) is a multifactorial condition, which is challenging to manage particularly in skeletally immature patients [1–3]. Risk factors associated with RPI are patellar height, patellar and trochlea dysplasia, rotational and coronal malalignment, malalignment of the extensor mechanism, and injuries to the medial patellofemoral ligament (MPFL) [4,5]. The understanding of RPI has increased significantly over the last few years. RPI is a common knee injury, which occurs with an estimated incidence between 14 and 148/100,000 individuals per year, mostly in adolescents and children [6,7].

In most patients suffering their first traumatic patellar dislocation, a tear of the MPFL occurs, which is the primary stabilizer of the patella during knee flexion from 0–30° against lateral displacement [8–10]. The attachment of the MPFL to the upper third of the medial patella is quite variable in children [11–13].

Multiple techniques to surgically manage RPI in children and young adolescents have been described, with a special emphasis on MPFL reconstruction, as distal bony alignment procedures are contraindicated [14,15]. In MPFL reconstruction, a hamstring tendon graft is commonly harvested and fixed to the medial patella and femur [16]. However, fixation of the tendon graft in children and adolescents leads to a high patella fracture risk and high risk of interference with the femoral growth plate, which has led to a modification of the original technique in this population [17,18]. Given these circumstances, most MPFL reconstruction techniques described in immature patients are non-anatomical [19,20]. The clinical results are however encouraging.

MPFL reconstruction in adults has shown good clinical outcomes; however, in patients with open physes, clinical outcomes are less predictable [21–23]. Recently, many studies have been published, leading to the need of an updated review on MPFL reconstruction in children and adolescents. This study systematically reviews and updates the currently available evidence on the outcomes of autograft MPFL reconstruction in immature patients with recurrent patellofemoral instability. The outcomes of interest were improvements in patient reported outcomes measures (PROMs), return to sport rates, and the rates of surgical failure.

2. Materials and Methods

2.1. Eligibility Criteria

All the clinical studies which investigated the outcomes of MPFL reconstruction using autografts in children and adolescents affected by recurrent patellofemoral instability were accessed. Only articles in Italian, English, German, Spanish, and French were eligible. Studies with a level of evidence of I to III, according to the Oxford Centre of Evidence-Based Medicine [24], were included. Studies which included only patients younger than 18 years were considered. Guidelines, case reports, comments, letters, reviews, editorials, and protocols were not considered. Studies which performed MPFL reconstruction using synthetic or allografts were excluded. Studies which investigated patients with congenital or acute patellofemoral instability were not eligible, nor were those which focused exclusively on patients with hyperlaxity. Missing quantitative information on the endpoints of interest warranted exclusion from this investigation.

2.2. Search Strategy

This systematic review was performed according to the 2020 PRISMA guidelines [25]. The PICO algorithm was followed:

- P (pathology): recurrent patellofemoral instability;
- I (intervention): MPFL reconstruction;
- C (comparison): children and adolescents;
- O (outcomes): PROMs, return to sport rates, rates of complications.

Two authors (F.M. and A.B.) independently conducted the literature search in PubMed, Scopus, and Web of Science. The databases were accessed in October 2022. The following keywords were used with the Boolean operators AND/OR: (*patellofemoral*) AND (*instability* OR *luxation* OR *dislocation*) AND (*open physeal* OR *adolescent* OR *young* OR *children* OR *skeletally immature*) AND (*MPFL* OR *medial patellofemoral ligament*) AND (*reconstruction* OR *surgery*). Titles and abstracts resulting from the initial literature search were inspected by hand. The full texts and bibliographies of the articles of interest were accessed by hand by the same authors.

2.3. Data Extraction

Two investigators (F.M. and A.B.) independently performed data extraction. Generalities of the included studies (author, year, journal of publication, level of evidence [24], and the length of follow-up) were retrieved. Data regarding patient demographics were also collected, including mean age, gender, number of patients and knees, type of autograft. The baseline and last follow-up PROMs were retrieved using the Kujala Anterior Knee Pain Scale [26] and the Lysholm Knee Scoring Scale [27]. The rate, time, and level of the return to sport were retrieved. Data on the rates of further dislocations, subluxations, and reoperations for patellofemoral instability were also collected. The minimum clinically important difference (MCID) for the Lysholm score was 10/100 [28–30].

2.4. Statistical Analysis

Statistical analysis was conducted by the main author (F.M.) using IBM SPSS Software version 25. The arithmetic mean and standard deviation were used for representative statistics. The mean difference (MD) effect measure was used to evaluate the improvements in PROMs from the baseline to the last follow-up. Standard error (SE), t-values, and 95% confidence intervals (CI) were also evaluated. The paired t-test was performed, with values of $p < 0.05$ considered statistically significant.

3. Results

3.1. Search Result

The literature search resulted in 1239 articles. Of them, 509 were duplicates. A further 712 studies were excluded as they did not match the eligibility criteria: not matching the topic ($n = 394$), study type and design ($n = 238$), congenital or acute patellofemoral instability ($n = 42$), not using autografts ($n = 31$), language limitation ($n = 4$), and exclusive focus on hyperlaxity ($n = 3$). A further three studies were excluded as they did not report quantitative data on the outcomes of interest. The flowchart of this literature search is shown in Figure 1.

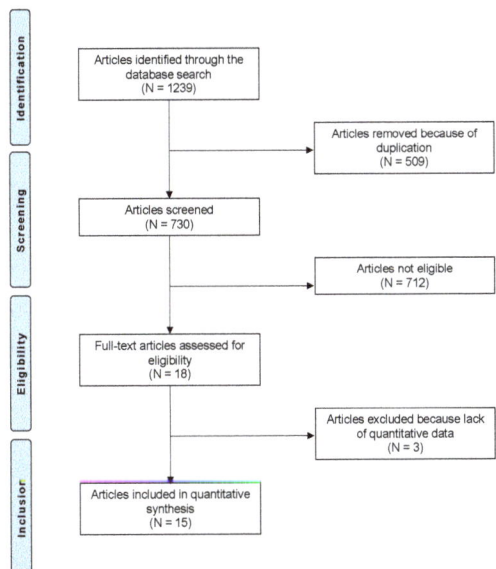

Figure 1. PRISMA flowchart of the literature search.

3.2. Demographic Data and Surgical Procedures

Data from 477 patients (510 procedures) were retrieved. Of the included patients, 41% (196 of 477) were females. The mean length of follow-up was 33.7 ± 28.8 months. The mean age of the patients was 14.6 ± 1.6 years. The demographics of the included patients are shown in Table 1.

Table 1. Baseline patient demographics (LoE: level of evidence).

Author and Year	Journal	LoE	Mean Age	Follow-Up (Months)	Women (n)	Patients (n)	Procedures (n)	Graft
Brown et al., 2008 [31]	J Knee Surg	III	11.0	14.0	1	2	2	Semitendinosus
Drez et al., 2001 [32]	Arthroscopy	IV	16.8	31.5	10	15	15	Ileotibial Band Semidendinosus, Hamstring
Fabricant et al., 2014 [33]	Knee	IV	14.9	3.0	5	27	27	Hamstring
Kumahashi et al., 2012 [34]	Arch Orthop Trauma Surg	IV	13.6	27.8	5	8	5	Semitendinosus
Lind et al., 2016 [19]	Knee Surg Sports Traumatol Arthrosc	III	12.5	39.0	9	20	20	Gracilis
Machado et al., 2017 [35]	Porto Biomed J	II	15.9	116.4	24	35	35	Gracilis
Malecki et al., 2015 [36]	Int Orthop	III	16.0	31.0	8	28	32	Adductor Magnus
Matuszewski et al., 2018 [37]	Arthroscopy	III	15.0	24.0	7	22	22	Gracilis
Nelitz et al., 2013 [38]	Am J Sports Med	IV	12.2	30.0	15	21	21	Gracilis
Nelitz et al., 2017 [39]	Knee Surg Sports Traumatol Arthrosc	III	12.8	31.5	9	25	25	Quadriceps
Parikh et al., 2013 [40]	Am J Sports Med	III	14.5	16.2	63	154	179	Gracilis
Pesenti et al., 2018 [41]	Int Orthop	IV	13.8	41.1	6	25	27	Gracilis, Semitenidnosus
Roger et al., 2019 [42]	Orthop Traumatol Surg Res	II	14.6	38.7	7	18	18	Gracilis
Saper et al., 2019 [43]	Orthop J Sport Med	IV	14.9	7.4	8	28	28	Hamstring, Not Specified
Uppstrom, et al., 2019 [44]	Knee Surg Sports Traumatol Arthrosc	IV	13.3	28.8	19	49	54	Hamstring

3.3. Clinical Outcomes

At the last follow-up, all PROMs of interest were statistically improved (Table 2).

Table 2. Results of PROMs (FU: follow-up; MD: mean difference; SE: standard error; CI: confidence interval).

Endpoint	At Baseline	At Last FU	MD	SE	95% CI	T	p
Kujala	62.0 ± 9.3	88.2 ± 8.8	26.2	0.59	25.05 to 27.35	44.69	<0.0001
Lysholm	55.3 ± 12.4	91.9 ± 3.8	36.6	0.59	35.44 to 37.77	61.63	<0.0001

3.4. Return to Sport

The mean time to return to sport was 6.1 ± 1.1 months. Of the included patients 27% had reduced their level of activity, while 87% returned to their previous level of sport.

3.5. Complications

Of the included patients, 5% (26 of 477) and 2% (9 of 363) experienced further dislocations and subluxations, respectively, during the follow-up period. Moreover, 4% (16 of 403) of patients underwent a further surgical procedure for patellofemoral instability within the follow-up period.

4. Discussion

Autograft MPFL reconstruction in children and adolescents with RPI is safe and effective, resulting in significant enhancements in clinical outcomes and low complication rates. A total of 87% of all patients were able to return to the pre-injury level of sport at approximately six months postoperatively. The rates of further patellar dislocations and subluxations were 5% and 2%, respectively. A total of 4% of all included patients underwent a further surgical procedure for RPI.

The overall quality of the 15 included studies with 477 patients was low, with the majority of the studies having a level of evidence of III to IV. This is surprising because patellar dislocations are frequent [45], and, therefore, further randomized controlled clinical trials are necessary to be able to better treat and inform patients with RPI.

The mean age of the included patients was 14.6 years, which is similar to previous studies, where they ranged from 12.5 to 14.28 years [19,46,47]. Females between the ages of 10 to 17 years are at the highest risk for patellar dislocation; however, the majority (59%) of the patients included here were males [6,48], which is in contrast to the studies of D'Ambrosi et al. and Lind et al. where they accounted for 36.5% and 45% of patients, respectively [19,46]. Of the patients, 87% returned to the same level of sport as preoperatively, while 27% had to reduce their level of sport following MPFL reconstruction. These findings confirm the results of Fisher et al., who used a quadriceps turndown technique with 94% of patients returning to a pre-injury level of sport [49]. Liu et al. found, in a retrospective study, that 94.5% of patients were able to return to sport at one year, with only 74% returning to the same level of play [50], with similar results found by Nelitz et al. [39]. RPI frequently occurs in the years near the transition to skeletal maturity; hence, most of the available literature focuses on the management of RPI in late adolescents and young adults [51]. Previously, multiple different strategies for the management of RPI have been described, including distal realignments (e.g., the Roux-Goldthwait, the Nietosvaara technique, and patellar tendon transfer), proximal realignments (e.g., MPFL reconstruction and lateral retinaculum release), or combined procedures [52–55]. The main goal of these procedures is to stabilize the patella against lateralizing forces without compromising open growth plates.

MPFL reconstruction in skeletally immature patients leads to a total rate of recurrent instability of 7%, including 5% for dislocations and 2% for subluxations. A recent review by Panni et al. found a rate of recurrent instability of 15% [47], while D'Ambrosi et al. found a recurrence rate of 5% [46]. In 2019, Wilkens et al. found a recurrence rate of patella-femoral instability of 13.8% after MPFL reconstruction, which was not different after other soft tissue procedures [56]. Overall, MPFL reconstruction in this population seems to be a safe procedure, as evidenced by the present investigation. This was confirmed by Nelitz et al. and Ladenhauf et al., who demonstrated good clinical outcomes with low postoperative dislocation rates [38,57].

In the current literature, there is some heterogeneity regarding the indications for MPFL reconstruction in children and adolescents with RPI, which must be kept in mind when analyzing the results of the present systematic review. Conservative management for first-time patella dislocations without an osteochondral injury is common; however, if after an initial trial of conservative management patients remain symptomatic or another dislocation occurs, surgical treatment should be considered. In patients with risk factors for RPI, such as trochlear and patellar dysplasia, patella alta, femoral anteversion, and increased TT-TG distances, the recurrent instability rates can be as high as 70%, and, therefore, earlier surgical intervention could be necessary [58]. There is also great heterogeneity in the current literature regarding graft fixation techniques using anchors, interference screws, or hardware free techniques [52,59], which makes it challenging to compare the outcomes of MPFL reconstruction. Further, there exist differences in terms of graft choice, e.g., autologous versus allograft, synthetic grafts, or type of graft bundle [60,61], and it must be noted that there is no agreement on the ideal graft type for this surgery.

This systematic review presents several limitations that need to be addressed. The different individual risk factors for patellofemoral instability were not considered separately. Furthermore, some in-between heterogeneities in the studies are evident. Most studies used a gracilis tendon autograft for MPFL reconstruction [19,35,37,38,40,41]. Fewer authors used the semitendinosus tendon autograft [31,32,34,41] or hamstring tendons [32,43,44]. In a previous systematic review on MPFL reconstruction in adults, the use of semitendinosus autograft achieved greater PROMs and range of motion along with a lower rate of complications compared to the gracilis tendon autograft [62]. Adductor magnus, iliotibial band, and quadriceps tendon autografts were less commonly used [32,36,39]. Most authors did not clearly state whether the type of graft bundle was a single or double bundle or whether MPFL reconstruction was combined with other realignment procedures. The lateral retinaculum release was the most commonly combined procedure [32,34,36,42–44], which was followed by tibial tuberosity transfer [36,42,43]. Chondral or meniscal procedures, tracheoplasties, and loose body removal procedures were less common [42,44]. Moreover, additional minor heterogeneities were found in the surgical fixation of autografts on the patellar side (anchor or tunnel techniques). However, given the limited and heterogeneous available data for inclusion, further subgroup analyses were not possible. As mentioned previously, there are some limitations in terms of the methodological quality of the included studies, with most studies being a retrospective cases series with a low level of evidence. Short to midterm follow-up may be sufficient for the assessment of patellar stability; however, longer follow-up is needed to reveal cases of physeal arrest or patellofemoral arthritis secondary to graft overtightening.

5. Conclusions

Autograft MPFL reconstruction in immature patients with RPI is a viable treatment option with significant clinical improvements and low complication and redislocation rates. However, further high-quality studies are needed to determine the optimal graft choice and fixation method for this challenging patient population.

Author Contributions: Conceptualization, F.M.; methodology, F.M. and A.B.; formal analysis, F.M.; writing—original draft preparation, F.M. and M.B.; writing—review and editing, N.M.; visualization, A.B. All authors have read and agreed to the published version of the manuscript.

Funding: This research received no external funding.

Institutional Review Board Statement: Not applicable.

Informed Consent Statement: Not applicable.

Data Availability Statement: Not applicable.

Conflicts of Interest: The authors declare no conflict of interest.

References

1. Malagelada, F.; Rahbek, O.; Sahirad, C.; Ramachandran, M. Results of operative 4-in-1 patella realignment in children with recurrent patella instability. *J. Orthop.* **2018**, *15*, 13–17. [CrossRef] [PubMed]
2. Hohne, S.; Gerlach, K.; Irlenbusch, L.; Schulz, M.; Kunze, C.; Finke, R. Patella Dislocation in Children and Adolescents. *Z. Orthop. Unfall.* **2017**, *155*, 169–176. [CrossRef] [PubMed]
3. Obermeyer, C.; Hoffmann, D.B.; Wachowski, M.M. Patellar dislocation in children and adolescents: Current developments in diagnostics and treatment. *Orthopade* **2019**, *48*, 868–876. [CrossRef] [PubMed]
4. Jiang, B.; Qiao, C.; Shi, Y.; Ren, Y.; Han, C.; Zhu, Y.; Na, Y. Evaluation of risk correlation between recurrence of patellar dislocation and damage to the medial patellofemoral ligament in different sites caused by primary patellar dislocation by MRI: A meta-analysis. *J. Orthop. Surg. Res.* **2020**, *15*, 461. [CrossRef] [PubMed]
5. Migliorini, F.; Oliva, F.; Maffulli, G.D.; Eschweiler, J.; Knobe, M.; Tingart, M.; Maffulli, N. Isolated medial patellofemoral ligament reconstruction for recurrent patellofemoral instability: Analysis of outcomes and risk factors. *J. Orthop. Surg. Res.* **2021**, *16*, 239. [CrossRef]
6. Fithian, D.C.; Paxton, E.W.; Stone, M.L.; Silva, P.; Davis, D.K.; Elias, D.A.; White, L.M. Epidemiology and natural history of acute patellar dislocation. *Am. J. Sports Med.* **2004**, *32*, 1114–1121. [CrossRef] [PubMed]

7. Sanders, T.L.; Pareek, A.; Hewett, T.E.; Stuart, M.J.; Dahm, D.L.; Krych, A.J. Incidence of First-Time Lateral Patellar Dislocation: A 21-Year Population-Based Study. *Sports Health* **2018**, *10*, 146–151. [CrossRef]
8. Conlan, T.; Garth, W.P., Jr.; Lemons, J.E. Evaluation of the medial soft-tissue restraints of the extensor mechanism of the knee. *J. Bone Jt. Surg. Am.* **1993**, *75*, 682–693. [CrossRef]
9. Gao, G.; Liu, P.; Xu, Y. Treatment of patellar dislocation with arthroscopic medial patellofemoral ligament reconstruction using gracilis tendon autograft and modified double-patellar tunnel technique: Minimum 5-year patient-reported outcomes. *J. Orthop. Surg. Res.* **2020**, *15*, 25. [CrossRef]
10. Krebs, C.; Tranovich, M.; Andrews, K.; Ebraheim, N. The medial patellofemoral ligament: Review of the literature. *J. Orthop.* **2018**, *15*, 596–599. [CrossRef]
11. Nomura, E.; Inoue, M.; Osada, N. Anatomical analysis of the medial patellofemoral ligament of the knee, especially the femoral attachment. *Knee Surg. Sports Traumatol. Arthrosc.* **2005**, *13*, 510–515. [CrossRef] [PubMed]
12. Smirk, C.; Morris, H. The anatomy and reconstruction of the medial patellofemoral ligament. *Knee* **2003**, *10*, 221–227. [CrossRef] [PubMed]
13. Shea, K.G.; Polousky, J.D.; Jacobs, J.C., Jr.; Ganley, T.J.; Aoki, S.K.; Grimm, N.L.; Parikh, S.N. The patellar insertion of the medial patellofemoral ligament in children: A cadaveric study. *J. Pediatr. Orthop.* **2015**, *35*, e31–e35. [CrossRef] [PubMed]
14. Marin Fermin, T.; Migliorini, F.; Kalifis, G.; Zikria, B.A.; D'Hooghe, P.; Al-Khelaifi, K.; Papakostas, E.T.; Maffulli, N. Hardware-free MPFL reconstruction in patients with recurrent patellofemoral instability is safe and effective. *J. Orthop. Surg. Res.* **2022**, *17*, 121. [CrossRef] [PubMed]
15. Letts, R.M.; Davidson, D.; Beaule, P. Semitendinosus tenodesis for repair of recurrent dislocation of the patella in children. *J. Pediatr. Orthop.* **1999**, *19*, 742–747. [CrossRef] [PubMed]
16. Wang, Q.; Huang, W.; Cai, D.; Huang, H. Biomechanical comparison of single- and double-bundle medial patellofemoral ligament reconstruction. *J. Orthop. Surg. Res.* **2017**, *12*, 29. [CrossRef] [PubMed]
17. Nelitz, M.; Williams, S.R. Anatomic reconstruction of the medial patellofemoral ligament in children and adolescents using a pedicled quadriceps tendon graft. *Arthrosc. Tech.* **2014**, *3*, e303–e308. [CrossRef] [PubMed]
18. Schiphouwer, L.; Rood, A.; Tigchelaar, S.; Koeter, S. Complications of medial patellofemoral ligament reconstruction using two transverse patellar tunnels. *Knee Surg. Sports Traumatol. Arthrosc.* **2017**, *25*, 245–250. [CrossRef]
19. Lind, M.; Enderlein, D.; Nielsen, T.; Christiansen, S.E.; Fauno, P. Clinical outcome after reconstruction of the medial patellofemoral ligament in paediatric patients with recurrent patella instability. *Knee Surg. Sports Traumatol. Arthrosc.* **2016**, *24*, 666–671. [CrossRef]
20. Shea, K.G.; Polousky, J.D.; Jacobs, J.C., Jr.; Ganley, T.J.; Aoki, S.K.; Grimm, N.L.; Parikh, S.N. The relationship of the femoral physis and the medial patellofemoral ligament in children: A cadaveric study. *J. Pediatr. Orthop.* **2014**, *34*, 808–813. [CrossRef]
21. Buchanan, G.; Torres, L.; Czarkowski, B.; Giangarra, C.E. Current Concepts in the Treatment of Gross Patellofemoral Instability. *Int. J. Sports Phys. Ther.* **2016**, *11*, 867–876. [PubMed]
22. Lippacher, S.; Dreyhaupt, J.; Williams, S.R.; Reichel, H.; Nelitz, M. Reconstruction of the Medial Patellofemoral Ligament: Clinical Outcomes and Return to Sports. *Am. J. Sports Med.* **2014**, *42*, 1661–1668. [CrossRef] [PubMed]
23. Schneider, D.K.; Grawe, B.; Magnussen, R.A.; Ceasar, A.; Parikh, S.N.; Wall, E.J.; Colosimo, A.J.; Kaeding, C.C.; Myer, G.D. Outcomes After Isolated Medial Patellofemoral Ligament Reconstruction for the Treatment of Recurrent Lateral Patellar Dislocations: A Systematic Review and Meta-analysis. *Am. J. Sports Med.* **2016**, *44*, 2993–3005. [CrossRef] [PubMed]
24. Howick, J.C.I.; Glasziou, P.; Greenhalgh, T.; Carl Heneghan Liberati, A.; Moschetti, I.; Phillips, B.; Thornton, H.; Goddard, O.; Hodgkinson, M. The 2011 Oxford CEBM Levels of Evidence. Oxford Centre for Evidence-Based Medicine. 2011. Available online: https://www.cebm.net/index.aspx?o=5653 (accessed on 1 January 2021).
25. Page, M.J.; McKenzie, J.E.; Bossuyt, P.M.; Boutron, I.; Hoffmann, T.C.; Mulrow, C.D.; Shamseer, L.; Tetzlaff, J.M.; Akl, E.A.; Brennan, S.E.; et al. The PRISMA 2020 statement: An updated guideline for reporting systematic reviews. *BMJ* **2021**, *372*, n71. [CrossRef] [PubMed]
26. Kujala, U.M.; Jaakkola, L.H.; Koskinen, S.K.; Taimela, S.; Hurme, M.; Nelimarkka, O. Scoring of patellofemoral disorders. *Arthroscopy* **1993**, *9*, 159–163. [CrossRef]
27. Lysholm, J.; Gillquist, J. Evaluation of knee ligament surgery results with special emphasis on use of a scoring scale. *Am. J. Sports Med.* **1982**, *10*, 150–154. [CrossRef]
28. Mostafaee, N.; Negahban, H.; Shaterzadeh Yazdi, M.J.; Goharpey, S.; Mehravar, M.; Pirayeh, N. Responsiveness of a Persian version of Knee Injury and Osteoarthritis Outcome Score and Tegner activity scale in athletes with anterior cruciate ligament reconstruction following physiotherapy treatment. *Physiother. Theory Pract.* **2020**, *36*, 1019–1026 [CrossRef]
29. Jones, K.J.; Kelley, B.V.; Arshi, A.; McAllister, D.R.; Fabricant, P.D. Comparative Effectiveness of Cartilage Repair With Respect to the Minimal Clinically Important Difference. *Am. J. Sports Med.* **2019**, *47*, 3284–3293. [CrossRef]
30. Agarwalla, A.; Liu, J.N.; Garcia, G.H.; Gowd, A.K.; Puzzitiello, R.N.; Yanke, A.B.; Cole, B.J. Return to Sport following Isolated Lateral Opening Wedge Distal Femoral Osteotomy. *Cartilage* **2021**, *13*, 846S–852S. [CrossRef]
31. Brown, G.D.; Ahmad, C.S. Combined medial patellofemoral ligament and medial patellotibial ligament reconstruction in skeletally immature patients. *J. Knee Surg.* **2008**, *21*, 328–332. [CrossRef]
32. Drez, D., Jr.; Edwards, T.B.; Williams, C.S. Results of medial patellofemoral ligament reconstruction in the treatment of patellar dislocation. *Arthroscopy* **2001**, *17*, 298–306. [CrossRef] [PubMed]

33. Fabricant, P.D.; Ladenhauf, H.N.; Salvati, E.A.; Green, D.W. Medial patellofemoral ligament (MPFL) reconstruction improves radiographic measures of patella alta in children. *Knee* **2014**, *21*, 1180–1184. [CrossRef] [PubMed]
34. Kumahashi, N.; Kuwata, S.; Tadenuma, T.; Kadowaki, M.; Uchio, Y. A "sandwich" method of reconstruction of the medial patellofemoral ligament using a titanium interference screw for patellar instability in skeletally immature patients. *Arch. Orthop. Trauma Surg.* **2012**, *132*, 1077–1083. [CrossRef] [PubMed]
35. Machado, S.A.F.; Pinto, R.A.P.; Antunes, A.J.A.M.; de Oliveira, P.A.R. Patellofemoral instability in skeletally immature patients. *Porto Biomed. J.* **2017**, *2*, 120–123. [CrossRef] [PubMed]
36. Malecki, K.; Fabis, J.; Flont, P.; Niedzielski, K.R. The results of adductor magnus tenodesis in adolescents with recurrent patellar dislocation. *Biomed. Res. Int.* **2015**, *2015*, 456858. [CrossRef]
37. Matuszewski, L.; Trams, M.; Ciszewski, A.; Wilczynski, M.; Trams, E.; Jakubowski, P.; Matuszewska, A.; John, K. Medial patellofemoral ligament reconstruction in children A comparative randomized short-term study of fascia lata allograft and gracilis tendon autograft reconstruction. *Medicine* **2018**, *97*, e13605. [CrossRef]
38. Nelitz, M.; Dreyhaupt, J.; Reichel, H.; Woelfle, J.; Lippacher, S. Anatomic reconstruction of the medial patellofemoral ligament in children and adolescents with open growth plates: Surgical technique and clinical outcome. *Am. J. Sports Med.* **2013**, *41*, 58–63. [CrossRef]
39. Nelitz, M.; Dreyhaupt, J.; Williams, S.R.M. Anatomic reconstruction of the medial patellofemoral ligament in children and adolescents using a pedicled quadriceps tendon graft shows favourable results at a minimum of 2-year follow-up. *Knee Surg. Sports Traumatol. Arthrosc.* **2018**, *26*, 1210–1215. [CrossRef]
40. Parikh, S.N.; Nathan, S.T.; Wall, E.J.; Eismann, E.A. Complications of medial patellofemoral ligament reconstruction in young patients. *Am. J. Sports Med.* **2013**, *41*, 1030–1038. [CrossRef]
41. Pesenti, S.; Ollivier, M.; Escudier, J.C.; Cermolacce, M.; Baud, A.; Launay, F.; Jouve, J.L.; Choufani, E. Medial patellofemoral ligament reconstruction in children: Do osseous abnormalities matter? *Int. Orthop.* **2018**, *42*, 1357–1362. [CrossRef]
42. Rogera, J.; Visteb, A.; Cievet-Bonfilsa, M.; Pracrosc, J.P.; Rauxa, S.; Chotel, F. Axial patellar engagement index and patellar tilt after medial patello-femoral ligament reconstruction in children and adolescents. *Orthop. Traumatol Surg. Res.* **2019**, *105*, 133–138. [CrossRef] [PubMed]
43. Saper, M.G.; Fantozzi, P.; Bompadre, V.; Racicot, M.; Schmale, G.A. Return-to-Sport Testing After Medial Patellofemoral Ligament Reconstruction in Adolescent Athletes. *Orthop. J. Sports Med.* **2019**, *7*, 2325967119828953. [CrossRef] [PubMed]
44. Uppstrom, T.J.; Price, M.; Black, S.; Gausden, E.; Haskel, J.; Green, D.W. Medial patellofemoral ligament (MPFL) reconstruction technique using an epiphyseal femoral socket with fluoroscopic guidance helps avoid physeal injury in skeletally immature patients. *Knee Surg. Sports Traumatol. Arthrosc.* **2019**, *27*, 3536–3542. [CrossRef] [PubMed]
45. Panni, A.S.; Vasso, M.; Cerciello, S. Acute patellar dislocation. What to do? *Knee Surg. Sports Traumatol. Arthrosc.* **2013**, *21*, 275–278. [CrossRef]
46. D'Ambrosi, R.; Corona, K.; Capitani, P.; Coccioli, G.; Ursino, N.; Peretti, G.M. Complications and Recurrence of Patellar Instability after Medial Patellofemoral Ligament Reconstruction in Children and Adolescents: A Systematic Review. *Children* **2021**, *8*, 434. [CrossRef]
47. Shamrock, A.G.; Day, M.A.; Duchman, K.R.; Glass, N.; Westermann, R.W. Medial Patellofemoral Ligament Reconstruction in Skeletally Immature Patients: A Systematic Review and Meta-analysis. *Orthop. J. Sports Med.* **2019**, *7*, 2325967119855023. [CrossRef]
48. Parikh, S.N.; Lykissas, M.G.; Gkiatas, I. Predicting Risk of Recurrent Patellar Dislocation. *Curr. Rev. Musculoskelet. Med.* **2018**, *11*, 253–260. [CrossRef]
49. Fisher, M.; Singh, S.; Samora, W.P., 3rd; Beran, M.C.; Klingele, K.E. Outcomes of MPFL Reconstruction Utilizing a Quadriceps Turndown Technique in the Adolescent/Pediatric Population. *J. Pediatr. Orthop.* **2021**, *41*, e494–e498. [CrossRef]
50. Liu, J.N.; Brady, J.M.; Kalbian, I.L.; Strickland, S.M.; Ryan, C.B.; Nguyen, J.T.; Shubin Stein, B.E. Clinical Outcomes After Isolated Medial Patellofemoral Ligament Reconstruction for Patellar Instability Among Patients With Trochlear Dysplasia. *Am. J. Sports Med.* **2018**, *46*, 883–889. [CrossRef]
51. Liu, J.N.; Steinhaus, M.E.; Kalbian, I.L.; Post, W.R.; Green, D.W.; Strickland, S.M.; Shubin Stein, B.E. Patellar Instability Management: A Survey of the International Patellofemoral Study Group. *Am. J. Sports Med.* **2018**, *46*, 3299–3306. [CrossRef]
52. Schlichte, L.M.; Sidharthan, S.; Green, D.W.; Parikh, S.N. Pediatric Management of Recurrent Patellar Instability. *Sports Med. Arthrosc. Rev.* **2019**, *27*, 171–180. [CrossRef] [PubMed]
53. Vellios, E.E.; Trivellas, M.; Arshi, A.; Beck, J.J. Recurrent Patellofemoral Instability in the Pediatric Patient: Management and Pitfalls. *Curr. Rev. Musculoskelet. Med.* **2020**, *13*, 58–68. [CrossRef] [PubMed]
54. Migliorini, F.; Luring, C.; Eschweiler, J.; Baroncini, A.; Driessen, A.; Spiezia, F.; Tingart, M.; Maffulli, N. Isolated Arthroscopic Lateral Retinacular Release for Lateral Patellar Compression Syndrome. *Life* **2021**, *11*, 295. [CrossRef] [PubMed]
55. Migliorini, F.; Maffulli, N.; Eschweiler, J.; Quack, V.; Tingart, M.; Driessen, A. Lateral retinacular release combined with MPFL reconstruction for patellofemoral instability: A systematic review. *Arch. Orthop. Trauma Surg.* **2021**, *141*, 283–292. [CrossRef]
56. Wilkens, O.E.; Hannink, G.; van de Groes, S.A.W. Recurrent patellofemoral instability rates after MPFL reconstruction techniques are in the range of instability rates after other soft tissue realignment techniques. *Knee Surg. Sports Traumatol. Arthrosc.* **2020**, *28*, 1919–1931. [CrossRef] [PubMed]

57. Ladenhauf, H.N.; Berkes, M.B.; Green, D.W. Medial patellofemoral ligament reconstruction using hamstring autograft in children and adolescents. *Arthrosc. Tech.* **2013**, *2*, e151–e154. [CrossRef]
58. Shubin Stein, B.E.; Gruber, S.; Brady, J.M. MPFL in First-Time Dislocators. *Curr. Rev. Musculoskelet. Med.* **2018**, *11*, 182–187. [CrossRef]
59. Migliorini, F.; Baroncini, A.; Eschweiler, J.; Tingart, M.; Maffulli, N. Interference screws vs. suture anchors for isolated medial patellofemoral ligament femoral fixation: A systematic review. *J. Sport Health. Sci.* **2022**, *11*, 123–129. [CrossRef]
60. Migliorini, F.; Eschweiler, J.; Spiezia, F.; Knobe, M.; Hildebrand, F.; Maffulli, N. Synthetic graft for medial patellofemoral ligament reconstruction: A systematic review. *J. Orthop. Traumatol.* **2022**, *23*, 41. [CrossRef]
61. Migliorini, F.; Trivellas, A.; Eschweiler, J.; Knobe, M.; Tingart, M.; Maffulli, N. Comparable outcome for autografts and allografts in primary medial patellofemoral ligament reconstruction for patellofemoral instability: Systematic review and meta-analysis. *Knee Surg. Sports Traumatol. Arthrosc.* **2022**, *30*, 1282–1291. [CrossRef]
62. Migliorini, F.; Trivellas, A.; Driessen, A.; Quack, V.; Tingart, M.; Eschweiler, J. Graft choice for isolated MPFL reconstruction: Gracilis versus semitendinosus. *Eur. J. Orthop. Surg. Traumatol.* **2020**, *30*, 763–770. [CrossRef] [PubMed]

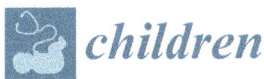

Article

Multiplier Method for Predicting the Sitting Height Growth at Maturity: A Database Analysis

Julio J. Jauregui [1], Larysa P. Hlukha [2], Philip K. McClure [2], Dror Paley [3], Mordchai B. Shualy [4], Maya B. Goldberg [4] and John E. Herzenberg [2,*]

1. Department of Orthopaedics, University of Maryland Medical Center, 110 S. Paca Street, 6th Floor, Suite 300, Baltimore, MD 21201, USA
2. International Center for Limb Lengthening, Rubin Institute for Advanced Orthopedics, Sinai Hospital of Baltimore, 2401 W. Belvedere Ave, Baltimore, MD 21215, USA
3. Paley Orthopedic and Spine Institute, 901 45th St. Kimmel Building, West Palm Beach, FL 33407, USA
4. Beth Tfiloh Dahan Community School, 3300 Old Court Rd, Pikesville, MD 21208, USA
* Correspondence: jherzenb@lifebridgehealth.org; Tel.: +1-410-601-2663

Abstract: This study aims to develop multipliers for the spine and sitting height to predict sitting height at maturity. With the aid of longitudinal and cross-sectional clinical databases, we divided the total sitting height, cervical, thoracic, and lumbar lengths at skeletal maturity by these same four factors at each age for each percentile given. A series of comparisons were then carried out between the multipliers as well as the percentiles and the varied racial and ethnic groups within them. Regarding sitting height, there was little variability and correlated with the multipliers calculated for the thoracic and lumbar spine. The multiplier method has demonstrated accuracy that is not influenced by generation, percentile, race, and ethnicity. This multiplier can be used to anticipate mature sitting height, the heights of the thoracic, cervical, and lumbar spine, as well as the lack of spinal growth after spinal fusion surgery in skeletally immature individuals.

Keywords: lumbar spine; skeletal maturity height; spine growth prediction; thoracic spine

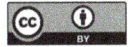

1. Introduction

Volumetric growth and ossification of the spine is a remarkably long and slow pro-cess that starts around the third month of prenatal life and continues until the second decade of life. Spine deformity, especially in early life, can negatively affect a growing spine as asymmetric forces act upon the vertebral column's growth plates. Spinal growth involves more than 130 growth plates that work in synchronicity. Because sitting height is a major component of spinal growth it provides a good parameter to observe and evaluate the progression of spinal growth [1].

Knowledge of spinal growth is of interest to spinal surgeons due to the nature of treating spine-related disorders where the growth ratios between remaining and elapsed growth are important parameters for surgical planning. Paley et al. [2] devised the multiplier method, a method of limb-length discrepancy and growth prediction. This method uses simple growth coefficients (also known as multipliers) to provide accurate predictions of limb length at maturity [3,4]. Spine growth, however, is a dynamic process and does not progress linearly; rather, it consists of periods of acceleration and subsequent de-celeration [1]. Hence, the multipliers do not isolate the growth spurt that occurs during adolescence and the growth that remains is a deciding factor for the intensifying of spinal deformities such as congenital scoliosis, kyphoscoliosis, and angular thoracolumbar kyphosis in patients with achondroplasia.

Sitting height consists of pelvic height, spine height, and skull height, and therefore serves as a capable tool for predicting spinal growth at maturity [5–7]. The known published data assessing spinal growth based on sitting-height measurements either focuses mostly on one social class or ethnic group or does not stratify by age or sex. We intended to consolidate the databases that assess sitting height and develop multipliers that predict sitting height to aid in spine deformity correction.

2. Materials and Methods

We calculated and compared the multipliers for different percentiles of 16 databases with sitting-height measurement data [1,5–18]. Fredriks et al. provided the most comprehensive assessment of spinal growth for each percentile group at each age [9]. At each age and percentile group, we divided the sitting height at skeletal maturity (Lm) by the corre-sponding sitting height at each given age (L): (M = Lm/L). We compared these multipliers (M) for each percentile group at each age. In addition, we calculated multipliers from two radiographic databases that contained measurements of the lumbar, thoracic, and cervical spine segments. These were largely obtained from standing or sitting radiographs. The databases provided measurements for a range of ages and included measurements ob-tained until subjects achieved skeletal maturity.

All data were tabulated using spreadsheet software (Excel; Microsoft, Redmond, WA, USA) with the aid of a statistical program (SPSS; IBM, Armonk, NY, USA). A series of polynomial regression analyses were used to evaluate the correlation between mean values in each of the databases using Fredriks et al.'s data as the "gold standard" database due to its inclusion of important variables such as age, ethnicity, and congenital variations. The mean sitting height that was reported for each age and stratified by sex in each of the databases was compared with the mean sitting height and the previously described SDs.

3. Results

We found that in Fredriks et al.'s database [9], the multipliers for each SD (−2.5 SD, −1 SD, 0 SD, +1 SD, +2.5 SD) at each given age for both males and females (mean variability ±0.065; maximum variability ±0.372) were similar. We also found that the variability between the multipliers was highest at birth, and generally decreased as age increased (Figures 1 and 2).

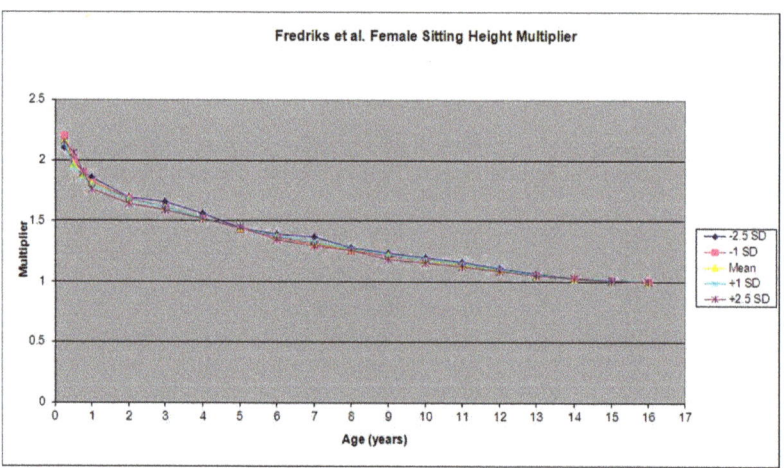

Figure 1. Mean and standard deviation for the female sitting height multiplier were calculated using data from Fredriks et al. [9].

We then compared the mean multipliers of sitting height to the multipliers for the cervical, thoracic, and lumbar segments of the spine. The multipliers of the thoracic and lumbar segments were nearly identical to those of sitting height (mean variability ±0.012; max variability ±0.043). The cervical multipliers, however, were substantially higher than those calculated from sitting height. The cervical multipliers are virtually identical to upper-extremity multipliers (mean variability ±0.0489; max variability ±0.060) [2]. See Figure 3 for a detailed comparison of all multipliers.

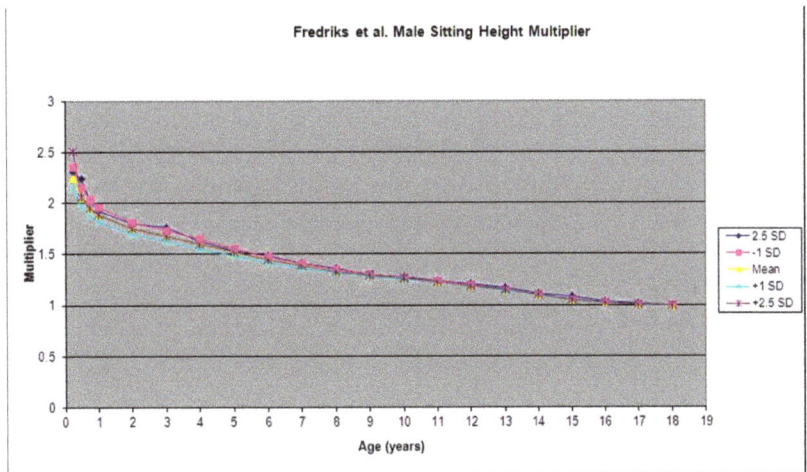

Figure 2. Mean and standard deviation for the male sitting height multiplier were calculated using data from Fredriks et al. [9].

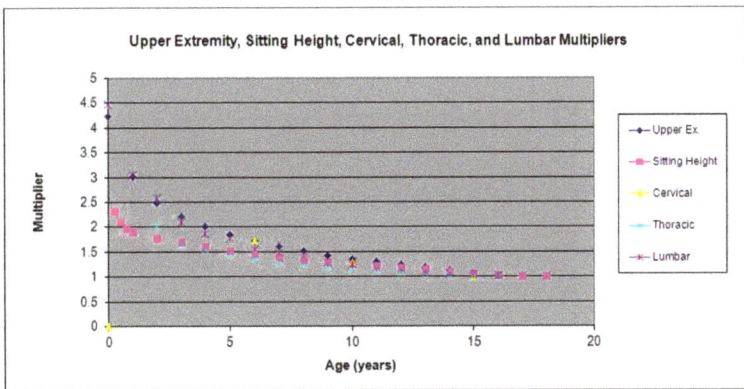

Figure 3. Upper extremity, sitting height, cervical, thoracic, and lumbar multipliers.

To diversify our data and ensure accuracy, we incorporated sitting heights from various continents and countries into our research. Zivicnjak et al. [13] published a cross-sectional study documenting the growth of 5155 (2591 female and 2564 male) Croatian children. The subjects were selected from various schools and kindergartens within the town of Zagreb to represent the entire socioeconomic spectrum. The multipliers calculated from Zivicnjak et al.'s data were virtually identical to those calculated by Fredriks et al. [9]. Pathmanathan and Prakash [14] also conducted a cross-sectional survey of northwestern Indian children. They measured the sitting height, leg length, and weight in 668 children (327 females and 341 males) between ages 6 and 16. Of the 668 children, 80% were measured more than once yearly. The multipliers calculated from this study correlated closely with those of Fredriks et al.

Our predicted multiplier method requires only a single measurement of sitting height and a simple arithmetic operation (Figure 4) to predict sitting height at skeletal maturity (Tables 1–3).

$$\text{Sitting Height (Spinal) Multiplier}$$

$$M = \frac{S_{maturity}}{S_{each\ age}}$$

$$S_{maturity} = M \times S_{current\ age}$$

Figure 4. Equation for spinal sitting height multiplier. M, age-specific multiplier; S, age-specific sitting height.

Table 1. Sitting height multiplier for 0 to 3 years of age.

Age (Years + Months)	Boys	Girls	Age (Years + Months)	Boys	Girls
0 + 1	-	-	3 + 1	1.688	1.611
0 + 2	-	-	3 + 2	1.681	1.603
0 + 3	2.315	2.153	3 + 3	1.673	1.596
0 + 4	2.165	2.052	3 + 4	1.666	1.589
0 + 5	2.131	2.024	3 + 5	1.658	1.581
0 + 6	2.096	1.995	3 + 6	1.651	1.574
0 + 7	2.04	1.944	3 + 7	1.643	1.567
0 + 8	2.006	1.916	3 + 8	1.635	1.559
0 + 9	1.971	1.887	3 + 9	1.628	1.552
0 + 10	1.968	1.839	3 + 10	1.62	1.545
0 + 11	1.934	1.839	3 + 11	1.613	1.537
1	**1.899**	**1.81**	**4**	**1.605**	**1.53**
1 + 1	1.888	1.799	4 + 1	1.598	1.523
1 + 2	1.877	1.788	4 + 2	1.591	1.516
1 + 3	1.865	1.777	4 + 3	1.585	1.508
1 + 4	1.854	1.765	4 + 4	1.578	1.501
1 + 5	1.843	1.754	4 + 5	1.571	1.494
1 + 6	1.832	1.743	4 + 6	1.564	1.487
1 + 7	1.82	1.732	4 + 7	1.557	1.479
1 + 8	1.809	1.721	4 + 8	1.55	1.472
1 + 9	1.798	1.71	4 + 9	1.544	1.465
1 + 10	1.787	1.698	4 + 10	1.537	1.458
1 + 11	1.775	1.687	4 + 11	1.53	1.45
2	**1.764**	**1.676**	**5**	**1.523**	**1.443**
2 + 1	1.758	1.671	5 + 1	1.517	1.437
2 + 2	1.753	1.666	5 + 2	1.512	1.431
2 + 3	1.747	1.662	5 + 3	1.506	1.425
2 + 4	1.741	1.657	5 + 4	1.5	1.419
2 + 5	1.736	1.652	5 + 5	1.494	1.413
2 + 6	1.73	1.647	5 + 6	1.489	1.408
2 + 7	1.724	1.642	5 + 7	1.483	1.402
2 + 8	1.719	1.637	5 + 8	1.477	1.396
2 + 9	1.713	1.633	5 + 9	1.471	1.39
2 + 10	1.707	1.628	5 + 10	1.466	1.384
2 + 11	1.702	1.623	5 + 11	1.46	1.378
3	**1.696**	**1.618**	**6**	**1.454**	**1.372**

Table 2. Sitting height multiplier for 6+ to 9 years of age.

Age (Years + Months)	Boys	Girls	Age (Years + Months)	Boys	Girls
6 + 1	1.449	1.368	9 + 1	1.291	1.212
6 + 2	1.443	1.364	9 + 2	1.288	1.209
6 + 3	1.438	1.36	9 + 3	1.286	1.206
6 + 4	1.432	1.356	9 + 4	1.283	1.203
6 + 5	1.427	1.352	9 + 5	1.281	1.2
6 + 6	1.422	1.348	9 + 6	1.278	1.197
6 + 7	1.416	1.344	9 + 7	1.276	1.193
6 + 8	1.411	1.34	9 + 8	1.273	1.19
6 + 9	1.405	1.336	9 + 9	1.271	1.187
6 + 10	1.4	1.332	9 + 10	1.268	1.184
6 + 11	1.394	1.328	9 + 11	1.266	1.181
7	1.389	1.324	10	1.263	1.178
7 + 1	1.385	1.319	10 + 1	1.26	1.175
7 + 2	1.381	1.315	10 + 2	1.258	1.172
7 + 3	1.376	1.31	10 + 3	1.255	1.169
7 + 4	1.372	1.305	10 + 4	1.252	1.166
7 + 5	1.368	1.3	10 + 5	1.249	1.163
7 + 6	1.364	1.296	10 + 6	1.247	1.161
7 + 7	1.359	1.291	10 + 7	1.244	1.158
7 + 8	1.355	1.286	10 + 8	1.241	1.155
7 + 9	1.351	1.281	10 + 9	1.238	1.152
7 + 10	1.347	1.277	10 + 10	1.236	1.149
7 + 11	1.342	1.272	10 + 11	1.233	1.146
8	1.338	1.267	11	1.23	1.143
8 + 1	1.334	1.263	11 + 1	1.227	1.14
8 + 2	1.331	1.258	11 + 2	1.224	1.136
8 + 3	1.327	1.254	11 + 3	1.221	1.133
8 + 4	1.323	1.25	11 + 4	1.217	1.129
8 + 5	1.319	1.245	11 + 5	1.214	1.126
8 + 6	1.316	1.241	11 + 6	1.211	1.122
8 + 7	1.312	1.237	11 + 7	1.208	1.119
8 + 8	1.308	1.232	11 + 8	1.205	1.115
8 + 9	1.304	1.228	11 + 9	1.202	1.112
8 + 10	1.301	1.224	11 + 10	1.198	1.108
8 + 11	1.297	1.219	11 + 11	1.195	1.105
9	1.293	1.215	12	1.192	1.101

Table 3. Sitting height Multiplier for 12+ to 15 years of age.

Age (Years + Months)	Boys	Girls	Age (Years + Months)	Boys	Girls
12 + 1	1.189	1.098	15 + 1	1.056	1.011
12 + 2	1.185	1.094	15 + 2	1.054	1.01
12 + 3	1.182	1.091	15 + 3	1.051	1.009
12 + 4	1.178	1.088	15 + 4	1.048	1.008
12 + 5	1.175	1.084	15 + 5	1.045	1.007
12 + 6	1.171	1.081	15 + 6	1.043	1.006
12 + 7	1.168	1.078	15 + 7	1.04	1.005
12 + 8	1.164	1.074	15 + 8	1.037	1.004
12 + 9	1.161	1.071	15 + 9	1.034	1.003
12 + 10	1.157	1.068	15 + 10	1.032	1.002
12 + 11	1.154	1.064	15 + 11	1.029	1.001

Table 3. Cont.

Age (Years + Months)	Boys	Girls	Age (Years + Months)	Boys	Girls
13	1.15	1.061	16	1.026	1
13 + 1	1.146	1.058	16 + 1	1.025	
13 + 2	1.142	1.056	16 + 2	1.023	
13 + 3	1.138	1.053	16 + 3	1.022	
13 + 4	1.133	1.051	16 + 4	1.021	
13 + 5	1.129	1.048	16 + 5	1.019	
13 + 6	1.125	1.046	16 + 6	1.018	
13 + 7	1.121	1.043	16 + 7	1.017	
13 + 8	1.117	1.04	16 + 8	1.015	
13 + 9	1.113	1.038	16 + 9	1.014	
13 + 10	1.108	1.035	16 + 10	1.013	
13 + 11	1.104	1.033	16 + 11	1.011	
14	1.1	1.03	17	1.01	
14 + 1	1.097	1.029	17 + 1	1.009	
14 + 2	1.093	1.027	17 + 2	1.008	
14 + 3	1.09	1.026	17 + 3	1.008	
14 + 4	1.086	1.024	17 + 4	1.007	
14 + 5	1.083	1.023	17 + 5	1.006	
14 + 6	1.08	1.021	17 + 6	1.005	
14 + 7	1.076	1.02	17 + 7	1.004	
14 + 8	1.073	1.018	17 + 8	1.003	
14 + 9	1.069	1.017	17 + 9	1.003	
14 + 10	1.066	1.015	17 + 10	1.002	
14 + 11	1.062	1.014	17 + 11	1.001	
15	1.059	1.012	18	1	

4. Discussion

The prediction of adolescent sitting height is germane to pediatricians and spinal surgeons. Other methods of growth prediction require both the determination of the subject's growth percentile and the use of a graph, all of which we have now consolidated into one simple formula (Figure 4).

Aldegheri and Agostini [19] produced a study compiled from previously published information on sitting height, but the ethnicity or race of subjects is not included. Only the means of sitting height are included without any SDs. Although the female multipliers generated show little variation from those generated from Frederik et al.'s data, the deviation between the male multipliers is considerably greater. While we are unsure of the exact reasons for the disparity between the Aldegheri and Fredriks et al. studies until age seven, we believe it has to do with the small sample size.

This work has limitations. Even though the sitting-height multiplier is meant to be universal, and we found consistency throughout all studied populations after comparing growth in many different studies, we believe that ultimately the physician should determine if each patient is following the growth curves presented by the multiplier. We also believe that whenever assessing spinal growth alterations and pathologies requiring spinal fusion or epiphysiodesis, the spinal growth will not necessarily follow the expected growth. Spinal growth can involve vertebrae changes as well as changes to the vertebral disk height. This may have implications for changes in the sitting height after maturity [18].

Longitudinal studies have demonstrated growth patterns more accurately than cross-sectional studies, as they have traced the growth of individuals over an elapsed period. However, there are far fewer longitudinal studies available due to the high cost and time limitations to perform such studies. A territory-wide cross-sectional study by Leung et al. [10] evaluated the sitting height of 25,000 Chinese children of higher socioeconomic status from birth through 18 years of age. Similarly, Lin et al. [11] assessed the sitting heights of Han children (the main ethnic group in China) and 27 minority groups. In total, 409,941 Han children and 70,298 minority children between the ages of 7 and 18 were measured. The authors reported that the sitting heights recorded from the Han cohort were generally higher than those recorded from the minority groups. However, when comparing the multipliers of Leung et al. [10] and both groups of Lin et al. [11] to the mul-tipliers generated from Fredriks et al. [9] data, a minimal difference is observed.

Lee et al. [12] published a longitudinal study observing 1,139 healthy Taipei schoolchildren ranging from 8 to 18 years of age. In addition to sitting height, they also documented arm span, skinfold thickness, and body mass index from 1994 through 1997. Alt-hough it has been suggested that longitudinal studies hold more accuracy than cross-sectional, the Lee et al. [12] multipliers held little variability to those of Fredriks et al. [9].

The multiplier method also can determine the appropriate timing of arthrodesis, as well as to predict the amount of height lost because of a specific spine operation. Each vertebra in the lumbar and thoracic spine make approximately equal growth contributions—i.e., any single vertebra in the lumbar spine contributes approximately one-fifth of the total growth of the lumbar spine, and any single vertebra in the thoracic spine contrib-utes approximately one-twelfth of the total growth of the thoracic spine [15,20]. Therefore, to predict the height of a single lumbar vertebra at maturity (Llv), multiply the current length of the lumbar spine (Lls) by the multiplier for the current age (M) and divide the result by five ([LlsM]/5 = Llv). Similarly, to predict the height of a single thoracic vertebra at maturity (Ltv), multiply the current length of the lumbar spine (Lts) by the multiplier for the current age (M) and divide the result by twelve ((LtsM)/12 = Ltv) (Figure 5).

Spinal Fusion

To predict height of single lumbar vertebra:

$$L_{vl} = (L_{sl} \times M) / 5$$

To predict height of single thoracic vertebra:

$$L_{vt} = (L_{st} \times M) / 12$$

To predict growth remaining:

$$L(M-1) \text{ or } S(M-1) = \text{growth remaining}$$

Figure 5. Equation for predicting height of the single lumbar and thoracic vertebrae and remaining growth. L, age-specific length; Lsl, age-specific length of lumbar spine; Lst, age-specific length of thoracic spine; Lvl, length of single lumbar vertebra at maturity; Lvt, length of single thoracic vertebra at maturity; M, age-specific multiplier; S, age-specific sitting height.

To calculate the growth lost as the result of arthrodesis, one must first calculate the growth remaining in the affected area of the spine. Growth remaining (G) is equal to the length of the relevant section of the spine at maturity minus the current length of the rele-vant section (M[L-1] = G). Thus, to calculate the growth lost as a result of arthrodesis (Ge), multiply the growth remaining for a single vertebra in the relevant segment of the spine ([(Lls(M-1)]/5 for lumbar vertebrae); ([Lts(M-1)]/12 for thoracic vertebrae) by the number of vertebrae fused (Vf) (Figure 5).

The prediction of sitting height is an important factor in the planning of limb lengthening for achondroplastic dwarfism [3]. As demonstrated by Paley et al., there is a close correlation between the sitting heights of these patients and normal subjects [3,16,20–22]. Hence, our sitting height multiplier also can be employed for achondroplastic patients [3]. In normal adults, sitting height comprises 53% of the total standing height at skeletal maturity [23–25]. Therefore, when lower extremity lengthening is planned in achondroplastic patients, the goal is to obtain a length in the lower extremity of 88.6% (47/53) of the pre-dicted sitting height, to achieve Vitruvian proportions.

Paley et al. have shown that the multipliers are independent of percentile groupings, height, generation, socioeconomic class, ethnicity, and race, and this independence has been clinically validated [2,4,17]. Such a relationship could be considered a mathematical property of human growth and development. The relative size and curve of the various multipliers are indicators of normal proportion; the lower extremity, having the highest multiplier, increases the most proportionally, from 35% of the height at birth to 47% of the height at skeletal maturity [20]. Sitting height, on the other hand, has a lower multiplier, decreasing proportionally from 65% of the height at birth to 53% at skeletal maturity.

5. Conclusions

Most known current data that has attempted to accurately predict spinal growth at maturity focuses on either specific ethnic groups or concentrates on a particular patient population—such those with congenital scoliosis or achondroplasia. We evaluated available databases on sitting height and multipliers for spinal growth and consolidated them to develop a multiplier for predicting sitting height growth at maturity. This method can also aid in calculating growth modification resulting from arthrodesis as well as facilitaing planning for limb lengthening procedures with challenging diagnoses such as achondroplasic dwarfism.

Author Contributions: Conceptualization, J.E.H.; methodology, J.J.J.; formal analysis, J.J.J.; resources, D.P.; data curation, L.P.H., M.B.S., M.B.G.; writing—original draft preparation, J.J.J.; writing—review and editing, L.P.H., P.K.M.; supervision, D.P., J.E.H. All authors have read and agreed to the published version of the manuscript.

Funding: This research received no external funding.

Institutional Review Board Statement: Not applicable.

Informed Consent Statement: Not applicable.

Data Availability Statement: The data presented in this study are available upon request from the corresponding author.

Acknowledgments: The authors thank Robert P. Farley, BS for assistance with the manuscript.

Conflicts of Interest: P.K.M. is a consultant for DePuy Synthes Companies, Novadip, NuVasive Specialized Orthopedics, Orthofix, and Smith & Nephew. J.E.H. is a consultant for NuVasive Specialized Orthopedics, Orthofix, OrthoPediatrics, and Smith & Nephew. The following organizations supported the institution of L.P.H., P.K.M. and J.E.H.: DePuy Synthes, NuVasive Specialized Orthopedics, Orthofix, OrthoPediatrics, Paragon 28, Pega Medical, Smith & Nephew, Stryker, Turner Imaging Systems, and WishBone Medical. J.J.J. and D.P. do not have any conflicts to report. The funders had no role in the design of the study; in the collection, analyses, or interpretation of data; in the writing of the manuscript; or in the decision to publish the results.

References

1. Cheung, J.P.Y.; Luk, K.D. Managing the pediatric spine: Growth assessment. *Asian Spine J.* **2017**, *11*, 804–816. [CrossRef] [PubMed]
2. Paley, D.; Gelman, A.; Shualy, M.B.; Herzenberg, J.E. Multiplier method for limb-length prediction in the upper extremity. *J. Hand Surg. Am.* **2008**, *33*, 385–391. [CrossRef] [PubMed]
3. Paley, D.; Matz, A.L.; Kurland, D.B.; Lamm, B.M.; Herzenberg, J.E. Multiplier method for prediction of adult height in patients with achondroplasia. *J. Pediatr. Orthop.* **2005**, *25*, 539–542. [CrossRef] [PubMed]
4. Paley, J.; Talor, J.; Levin, A.; Bhave, A.; Paley, D.; Herzenberg, J.E. The multiplier method for prediction of adult height. *J. Pediatr. Orthop.* **2004**, *24*, 732–737. [CrossRef]
5. Bundak, R.; Bas, F.; Furman, A.; Günöz, H.; Darendeliler, F.; Saka, N.; Poyrazoğlu, S.; Neyzi, O. Sitting height and sitting height/height ratio references for Turkish children. *Eur. J. Pediatr.* **2014**, *173*, 861–869. [CrossRef]
6. Abou-Hussein, S.; Abela, M.; Savona-Ventura, C. Body mass index adjustment for sitting height for better assessment of obesity risks in Maltese women. *Int. J. Risk Saf. Med.* **2011**, *23*, 241–248. [CrossRef]
7. Woynarowska, B.; Palczewska, I.; Oblacińska, A. WHO child growth standards for children 0–5 years. Percentile charts of length/height, weight, body mass index and head circumference. *Med. Wieku Rozw.* **2012**, *16*, 232–239. (In Polish)

8. Tulsi, R.S. Growth of the human vertebral column. An osteological study. *Acta Anat.* **1971**, *79*, 570–580. [CrossRef]
9. Fredriks, A.M.; van Buuren, S.; van Heel, W.J.; Dijkman-Neerincx, R.H.; Verloove-Vanhorick, S.P.; Wit, J.M. Nationwide age references for sitting height, leg length, and sitting height/height ratio, and their diagnostic value for disproportionate growth disorders. *Arch. Dis. Child.* **2005**, *90*, 807–812. [CrossRef]
10. Leung, S.S.; Lau, J.T.; Xu, Y.Y.; Tse, L.Y.; Huen, K.F.; Wong, G.W.; Law, W.Y.; Yeung, V.T.; Yeung, W.K.; Leung, N.K. Secular changes in standing height, sitting height and sexual maturation of Chinese—The Hong Kong Growth Study, 1993. *Ann. Hum. Biol.* **1996**, *23*, 297–306. [CrossRef]
11. Lin, W.S.; Zhu, F.C.; Chen, A.C.; Xin, W.H.; Su, Z.; Li, J.Y.; Ye, G.S. Physical growth of Chinese school children 7–18 years, in 1985. *Ann. Hum. Biol.* **1992**, *19*, 41–55. [CrossRef] [PubMed]
12. Lee, T.S.; Chao, T.; Tang, R.B.; Hsieh, C.C.; Chen, S.J.; Ho, L.T. A longitudinal study of growth patterns in schoolchildren in one Taipei District. II: Sitting height, arm span, body mass index and skinfold thickness. *J. Chin. Med. Assoc.* **2005**, *68*, 16–20. [CrossRef]
13. Zivicnjak, M.; Narancić, N.S.; Szirovicza, L.; Franke, D.; Hrenović, J.; Bisof, V. Gender-specific growth patterns for stature, sitting height and limbs length in Croatian children and youth (3 to 18 years of age). *Coll. Antropol.* **2003**, *27*, 321–334. [PubMed]
14. Pathmanathan, G.; Prakash, S. Growth of sitting height, subischial leg length and weight in well-off northwestern Indian children. *Ann. Hum. Biol.* **1994**, *21*, 325–334. [CrossRef] [PubMed]
15. Alhadlaq, A.M.; Al-Shayea, E.I. New method for evaluation of cervical vertebral maturation based on angular measurements. *Saudi Med. J.* **2013**, *34*, 388–394. [PubMed]
16. Marík, I.; Zemková, D.; Kubát, R.; Rygl, M.; Friedlová, J. Prediction of body height and shortening of the lower part of the body in adults with achondroplasia. *Acta Chir. Orthop. Traumatol. Cech* **1989**, *56*, 507–515. (In Czech) [PubMed]
17. Rosario, A.S.; Schienkiewitz, A.; Neuhauser, H. German height references for children aged 0 to under 18 years compared to WHO and CDC growth charts. *Ann. Hum. Biol.* **2011**, *38*, 121–130. [CrossRef]
18. Howell, F.R.; Mahood, J.K.; Dickson, R.A. Growth beyond skeletal maturity. *Spine* **1992**, *17*, 437–440. [CrossRef]
19. Aldegheri, R.; Agostini, S. A chart of anthropometric values. *J. Bone Joint Surg.* **1993**, *75*, 86–88. [CrossRef]
20. Raimondi, A.J.; Di Rocco, C. Principles of Pediatric Neurosurgery. In *The Pediatric Spine, Development and Dyscratic State*; Raimondi, A.J., Choux, M., Di Rocco, C., Eds.; Springer: New York, NY, USA, 1989; pp. 39–83.
21. Shchurov, V.A.; Kudrin, B.I.; Gerasimov, S.A. Anthropometric approach to basing the surgical correction of body length and proportions in achondroplasia patients. *Ortop. Travmatol. Protez* **1981**, *9*, 30–33. (In Russian)
22. Hunter, A.G.; Hecht, J.T.; Scott, C.I., Jr. Standard weight for height curves in achondroplasia. *Am. J. Med. Genet.* **1996**, *62*, 255–261. [CrossRef]
23. Mather, G. Head-body ratio as a visual cue for stature in people and sculptural art. *Perception* **2010**, *39*, 1390–1395. [CrossRef] [PubMed]
24. Le Floch-Prigent, P. The Vitruvian Man: An anatomical drawing for proportions by Leonardo Da Vinci. *Morphologie* **2008**, *92*, 204–209. (In French) [CrossRef] [PubMed]
25. Creed, J.C. Leonardo da Vinci, Vitruvian Man. *JAMA* **1986**, *256*, 1541. [CrossRef] [PubMed]

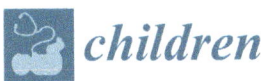

Article

The Extension of Surgery Predicts Acute Postoperative Pain, While Persistent Postoperative Pain Is Related to the Spinal Pathology in Adolescents Undergoing Posterior Spinal Fusion

Tommi Yrjälä [1], Ilkka Helenius [2,*], Tiia Rissanen [3], Matti Ahonen [4], Markku Taittonen [1] and Linda Helenius [1]

[1] Department of Anesthesia and Intensive Care, University of Turku and Turku University Hospital, 20521 Turku, Finland
[2] Department of Orthopedics and Traumatology, University of Helsinki and Helsinki University Hospital, 00029 Helsinki, Finland
[3] Department of Biostatistics, University of Turku, 20500 Turku, Finland
[4] Department of Pediatric Surgery, Orthopedics and Traumatology, University of Helsinki and Helsinki University Hospital, 00029 Helsinki, Finland
* Correspondence: ilkka.helenius@helsinki.fi

Abstract: Persistent pain after posterior spinal fusion affects 12 to 42% of patients with adolescent idiopathic scoliosis. The incidence of persistent pain among surgically treated children with Scheuermann kyphosis and spondylolisthesis is not known. The aim of our study was to determine the predictors and incidence of acute and chronic postoperative pain in adolescents undergoing posterior spinal fusion surgery. The study was a retrospective analysis of a prospectively collected pediatric spine register data. The study included 213 consecutive patients (158 AIS, 19 Scheuermann kyphosis, and 36 spondylolisthesis), aged 10–21 years undergoing posterior spinal fusion at a university hospital between March 2010 and March 2020. The mean (SD) daily postoperative opioid consumption per kilogram was significantly lower in the spondylolisthesis patients 0.36 mg/kg/day (0.17) compared to adolescent idiopathic scoliosis 0.51 mg/kg/day (0.25), and Scheuermann kyphosis 0.52 mg/kg/day (0.25) patients after surgery ($p = 0.0004$). Number of levels fused correlated with the daily opioid consumption ($r_s = 0.20$, $p = 0.0082$). The SRS-24 pain domain scores showed a statistically significant improvement from preoperative levels to two-year follow-up in all three groups ($p \leq 0.03$ for all comparisons). The spondylolisthesis patients had the lowest SRS pain domain scores (mean 4.04, SD 0.94), reporting more pain two years after surgery, in comparison to AIS (mean 4.31, SD 0.60) ($p = 0.043$) and SK (mean 4.43, SD 0.48) patients ($p = 0.049$). Persistent postoperative pain in adolescents undergoing posterior spinal fusion is related to disease pathology while higher acute postoperative pain is associated with a more extensive surgery. Spondylolisthesis patients report more chronic pain after surgery compared to AIS and SK patients.

Keywords: adolescent idiopathic scoliosis; Scheuermann kyphosis; spondylolisthesis; posterior spinal fusion; postsurgical pain

1. Introduction

Adolescent idiopathic scoliosis (AIS), Scheuermann kyphosis (SK), and spondylolisthesis are the most common indications for instrumented posterior spinal fusion (PSF) in adolescents. The primary goal of the surgical treatment for AIS and SK is to prevent progression of the deformity [1–3]. In spondylolisthesis, the aim is mainly to relieve pain and additionally to prevent progression or reduce sagittal deformity in high-grade slips [1]. The extension of the procedure varies between AIS, SK, and spondylolisthesis patients. Spinal deformity correction requires a long posterior instrumentation, while spondylolisthesis is treated with a single or two-level lumbar fusion [1]. Previous studies have suggested that PSF reduces pain in patients with AIS and spondylolisthesis, while pain outcomes after surgery for SK remain unclear [3–7].

Postoperative pain with nociceptive, neuropathic, and inflammatory components are induced from major tissue trauma after the surgical procedure [8]. Nociceptors of skin, muscles, fascia, ligaments, vertebrae, and facet joint capsules elicit the sensation of pain. Spinal surgery involves manipulation of the spine, spinal cord, and the nerve roots. These components may also suffer from inadequate perfusion and hypoxia, which may cause neuropathic pain after surgery. Tissue injury induces an inflammatory response. Damaged cells release pro-inflammatory agents such as bradykinin, histamine, cytokines, and prostanoids. Some of these inflammatory mediators act on the modulation of pain in dorsal root ganglia and directly on nociceptors.

Persistent postoperative pain is defined as a pain on the surgical site lasting over three months after surgery, well beyond the healing process [9]. Persistent postsurgical pain is associated with increased functional disability, psychological distress, and economic costs [10]. The data from AIS patients show an incidence of postoperative persistent pain between 12 to 42% [5,11–13]. However, the literature regarding the persistent postsurgical pain in SK and spondylolisthesis patients is inadequate.

The aim of our research was to determine the incidence and the predictors of acute and chronic postoperative pain in adolescents undergoing PSF. We hypothesized that acute pain is associated with the extension of surgery and that chronic postsurgical pain is more dependent on the disease pathology.

2. Materials and Methods

The study was approved by the Ethics Committee, Hospital District of Southwest Finland (ETMK 95/180/2011 and ETMK 38/1800/2015). Informed consent was obtained from all subjects involved in the study and from their parents if under 18 years old.

2.1. Study Design

The study was a retrospective analysis of a prospectively collected pediatric spine register assessing risk factors for acute and persistent pain in adolescents after instrumented PSF surgery. We reviewed 221 patients (166 AIS, 19 SK, and 36 spondylolistheses) entered consecutively into this register between March 2010 and March 2020. The date of last follow-up was 5 October 2022. This spine register is a database of children and adolescents undergoing spinal fusion surgery for AIS, SK, or spondylolisthesis at our university hospital. Eight patients were excluded from further analyses, and all of these were from the AIS group: two patients' postoperative opioid usage was not adequately documented; two patients needed early re-operation for a neurologic deficit; one patient had a combined anteroposterior approach; one patient had chronic renal insufficiency; one patient had a concomitant neurological condition, and one patient was operated for both AIS and spondylolisthesis, leaving 213 patients for further analyses. The same skilled orthopedic spine surgeon performed surgeries on all the patients. Pain was analyzed using Scoliosis Research Society-24 (SRS-24) outcome questionnaire. The data on opioid consumption was obtained from patient records.

The anesthetic management of the AIS, SK and spondylolisthesis patients was standardized. The total intravenous anesthesia protocol has been used unchanged since 2009 in our university hospital. Anesthesia was maintained with target-controlled infusions of propofol and remifentanil titrated to maintain the bispectral index (BIS) within predetermined limits. As all patients received similar weight-based remifentanil infusions intraoperatively, this was not included in the amount of postoperative opioid reported. Muscle relaxant was not used in any of the patients at any time. Dexmedetomidine-infusion (1 µg/kg/h) was used for supplemental hypnosis and analgesia in all patients. Mean arterial pressure was maintained between 65–75 mmHg with noradrenaline infusion if needed. Normothermia was maintained. Neurophysiological measurements were done every 20 min and at certain time points. None of the patients needed postoperative ventilation.

The majority (71%, 151/213) of the AIS, SK and spondylolisthesis patients received patient-controlled analgesia (PCA) with oxycodone for the first 48 postoperative hours. The typical oxycodone PCA contained an on-demand oxycodone-bolus of 0.03 mg/kg/dose at a maximum of three doses per hour, with no basal infusion. The patients without PCA (n = 62), received intravenous and oral oxycodone as needed. The patients' oral oxycodone dosages were converted to equivalent intravenous doses (0.6 * per dose) [14]. Postoperative opioid use included all opioids received postoperatively in the postoperative anesthesia care unit (PACU), pediatric intensive care unit (PICU), and postoperative ward during the hospital stay. All patients received oral paracetamol at 15–20 mg/kg three times per day. Epidural analgesia was not used by any of the patients. A numerical rating scale (NRS) was used to evaluate pain.

Perioperative variables collected included gender, age, height, weight, body mass index (BMI), fusion levels, surgical time, intraoperative blood loss, number of levels fused, length of hospital stay, opioid amount on first 48 h after operation, total opioid consumption during hospital stay, SRS-24 questionnaire preoperatively, six months postoperatively, and two years postoperatively.

The patients were mobilized according to our established process. The urinary catheter was removed on day 2 after surgery. The patients were requested to stand up and take a few steps on the first postoperative day. On the second postoperative day the patients were supported to walk around on the ward.

2.2. Scoliosis Research Society Outcome Questionnaire

The SRS-24 is a disease-specific health-related quality of life questionnaire, which is developed for scoliosis patients. The SRS-24 questionnaire is also used for other spinal surgery patients. Patients filled out the SRS-24 questionnaire preoperatively, and six and 24 months postoperatively. The SRS-24 questionnaire has seven domains: pain, general self-image, general function, general activity, postoperative self-image, postoperative function, and patient satisfaction. The scores in each field range from 1.0 to 5.0, with higher scores pointing out better patient outcomes. A score under 4 in the pain domain was considered clinically relevant and indicated moderate to severe pain [3]. The maximum score of this questionnaire is 120. The questions from 16 to 24 are related to the treatment and can therefore only be filled out after surgery. The first SRS-24 question, which asks patients to rate their pain on a scale of 1 to 9, was analyzed separately, 1 indicating no pain and 9 considered to be severe pain. A pain score over 4 was considered as moderate to severe pain.

2.3. Surgical Technique

All AIS and SK patients were operated on using a posterior-only approach and had spinal cord monitoring. Bilateral segmental pedicle screw instrumentation (MESA 5.5, Stryker spine, Leesburg, VA, USA, 6.35CD Legacy or Solera 6.0, Medtronics Spinal and Biologics, Memphis, TN, USA) were used to correct the spinal deformity. Pedicle screws were inserted using a free-hand approach. Apical posterior column osteotomies were performed in all SK patients and in 46 (29.1%) of the AIS patients to facilitate deformity correction. Selection of fusion levels was according to the Lenke classification and last substantially touched vertebra for AIS [15] and stable sagittal vertebra for SK in the lumbar spine and T2 or T3 as the upper instrumented vertebra [16].

All spondylolisthesis patients had pedicle screw instrumentation with intercorporeal fusion using a TLIF cage (Crescent, Medtronic) with an autologous bone graft from the decompression. Neural elements were widely decompressed for nerve roots (L5, S1) and cauda equinae. Patients with low-grade spondylolisthesis had pedicle screws inserted into L5 and S1 to reduce the spondylolisthesis and patients with high-grade spondylolisthesis underwent instrumentation from L4 to S1 with pelvic instrumentation (iliac or S2 alar iliac screws).

2.4. Statistical Methods

Associations between the opioid consumption and variables (study group, gender, surgery time, intraoperative blood loss and preoperative pain) were summarized with descriptive statistics and studied one by one with the Spearman correlation (for continuous variables) and the Kruskal-Wallis test (for categorical variables). Associations between chronic pain and explanatory variables (study group, gender, surgery time, intraoperative blood loss and preoperative pain) were studied with the Spearman correlation and the Kruskal-Wallis test (three groups). Study group effects with surgical outcomes (surgery time, intraoperative blood loss and length of hospital stay) were studied with the Kruskal-Wallis test and the Dwass-Steel-Critchlow-Fligner pairwise test. Differences between study groups in the SRS-24 preoperative and two-year postoperative scores, the SRS-24 pain preoperative and two-year postoperative scores and the SRS-24 self-image and two-year postoperative scores were studied with a mixed model for repeated measures. Differences between study groups in the SRS-24 function and activity domain scores were analyzed with the Kruskal-Wallis test.

The normality of variables was assessed visually and using the Shapiro-Wilk test. In all tests, the statistical significance level was set at 0.05 (two-tailed). The analyses were carried out using the SAS system, version 9.4 for Windows (SAS Institute Inc., Cary, NC, USA).

3. Results

A total of 213 consecutive adolescents (146 females (69%) and 67 males (31%)) with a mean age of 15.6 years (range 10–21 years) at the time of surgery were included in this study. The cohort consisted of 158 (74.2%) AIS patients, 19 (8.9%) patients with Scheuermann kyphosis and 36 (16.9%) spondylolisthesis patients. The majority of the AIS (114 (72.2%)) and spondylolisthesis (29 (80.6%)) patients were females as opposed to the SK patients, with only 15.8% (3) females. Twenty-three (10.8%) of these patients were under the age of 13 years at the time of surgery.

3.1. Surgical Outcome

There were significant differences in surgery time, intraoperative blood loss, number of levels fused, and length of hospital stay between the study groups. The Scheuermann patients had the greatest intraoperative blood loss compared to the other patient groups. The spondylolisthesis patients had the longest surgical time and the shortest hospital stay (Table 1).

Table 1. Demographic characteristics.

Variables	AIS (n = 158)	SK (n = 19)	Spondylolisthesis (n = 36)	p Value
Sex (male:female)	44:114	3:16	7:29	<0.001
Age (years)	15.6 (2.2)	16.7 (1.3)	14.7 (1.9)	0.002
Weight (kg)	58.3 (13.5)	80.6 (27.8)	57.2 (12.5)	<0.001
BMI (kg/m^2)	20.9 (3.9)	25.7 (7.5)	21.3 (3.7)	0.018
Surgical time (h)	2.95 (0.75)	3.45 (0.53)	3.49 (1.00)	<0.001
Intraoperative blood loos (mL)	529 (350)	616 (200)	344 (203)	<0.001
Number of levels fused (n)	10.8 (1.2)	12.9 (0.5)	2.6 (0.5)	<0.001
Daily oxycodone dose/kg during hospital stay (mg/kg/day)	0.51 (0.25)	0.52 (0.25)	0.36 (0.17)	<0.001
Major curve				
Preop	52 (8.5)	79 (5.6)		
Postop	13 (4.6)	48 (8.4)		
Length of hospital stay (day)	7.2 (1.6)	7.8 (1.6)	6.2 (2.1)	<0.001

Data presented as mean and standard deviation or number and percentage.

3.2. Preoperative Pain and SRS-24 Scores

Preoperative mean (SD) SRS-24 pain scores were significantly lower in the spondylolisthesis patients, meaning more pain, 3.24 (0.9) compared to AIS 3.96 (0.7) and SK 4.02

(0.6) patients, $p < 0.001$ in both comparisons (Table 2). Seventy-six percent (25/33 patients) of the spondylolisthesis patients had a preoperative SRS pain score under 4, as compared to 42% (62/146 patients) in the AIS group and 28% (5/18 patients) in the SK group. Preoperatively 17% (25 of 146) of the AIS patients, 17% (3 of 18) of SK, and 52% (17 of 33) of the spondylolisthesis patients reported moderate to severe pain on question 1 of the SRS-24 questionnaire.

Table 2. SRS-24 domain scores in the groups.

SRS-24 Domains	AIS	Scheuermann Kyphosis	Spondylolisthesis	p-Value AIS vs. SK	p-Value AIS vs. Spondylolisthesis
Pain					
preoperative	3.96 (0.72)	4.02 (0.64)	3.24 (0.86)	0.82	<0.001
6-mth FU	4.25 (0.63)	4.36 (0.49)	3.60 (0.71)	0.46	<0.001
2-year FU	4.31 (0.60)	4.43 (0.48)	4.04 (0.94)	0.46	0.04
Self-image					
preoperative	3.83 (0.70)	3.54 (0.92)	4.00 (0.67)	0.05	0.23
6-mth FU	4.05 (0.68)	3.96 (0.50)	4.19 (0.50)	0.84	0.53
2-year FU	4.14 (0.68)	4.11 (0.61)	4.21 (0.58)	0.88	0.42
Function					
preoperative	4.03 (0.47)	3.96 (0.44)	3.84 (0.54)	0.67	0.14
6-mth FU	3.95 (0.52)	4.04 (0.69)	3.95 (0.60)	0.56	0.69
2-year FU	4.13 (0.56)	4.07 (0.42)	4.10 (0.53)	0.56	0.74
Activity					
preoperative	4.45 (0.81)	4.57 (0.47)	3.52 (1.13)	0.42	<0.001
6-mth FU	3.93 (0.98)	3.84 (1.10)	3.97 (1.00)	0.37	0.38
2-year FU	4.66 (0.67)	4.44 (0.88)	4.39 (1.09)	0.13	0.24
Total score					
preoperative	4.05 (0.50)	4.02 (0.49)	3.55 (0.60)	0.69	<0.001
6-mth FU	3.84 (0.45)	3.94 (0.46)	3.88 (0.44)	0.35	0.61
2-year FU	4.05 (0.42)	4.09 (0.46)	3.93 (0.64)	0.72	0.18

Data presented in mean (SD).

Preoperative mean (SD) SRS-24 total scores were significantly higher in AIS (4.05 (0.50)) and SK (4.02 (0.49)) patients compared to spondylolisthesis patients (3.55 (0.60)), $p < 0.001$ for both comparisons. Similarly, preoperative mean (SD) SRS-24 activity scores were significantly lower in spondylolisthesis patients, meaning less activity (3.52 (1.13)) compared to AIS (4.45 (0.81)) and SK (4.57 (0.47)) patients, ($p < 0.001$ for both comparisons).

3.3. Acute Postoperative Pain

There was a statistically significant difference in the opioid consumption after surgery between the three groups. The mean (SD) daily postoperative opioid consumption was significantly lower in the spondylolisthesis patients (0.36 mg/kg/day (0.17)) compared to AIS (0.51 mg/kg/day (0.25)) and SK (0.52 mg/kg/day (0.25)) patients ($p < 0.001$). Patients' age, gender, BMI, surgery time, intraoperative blood loss or preoperative pain were not associated with increased opioid consumption postoperatively. The number of fused vertebrae correlated with the daily opioid consumption ($r_s = 0.20$, $p = 0.0082$).

The difference in the oxycodone consumption during first 48 postoperative hours did not reach statistical significance. The mean (SD) 48 h oxycodone consumption in AIS, SK and spondylolisthesis groups were 1.68 mg/kg (1.08), 1.80 mg/kg (0.78) and 1.40 mg/kg (0.75), respectively, ($p = 0.10$). There was a correlation between longer surgical time and increased 48 h opioid consumption ($r_s = 0.16$, $p = 0.020$). Patient gender, intraoperative blood loss or preoperative pain were not associated with increased 48 h oxycodone consumption after surgery.

3.4. Persistent Postoperative Pain

The SRS-24 pain domain scores showed a statistically significant improvement from preoperative levels to two-year follow-up in all three groups. This domain increased from a mean of 3.96 to 4.31 in the AIS patients ($p < 0.001$), 3.24 to 4.04 in the spondylolisthesis patients ($p < 0.001$), and 4.02 to 4.43 in the SK group ($p = 0.03$), respectively. At two years postoperatively, 11% (14 of 129) of AIS, 7% (1 of 14) of SK, and 16% (4 of 25) of the spondylolisthesis patients reported moderate to severe pain on question 1 in the SRS-24 questionnaire.

The patients with spondylolisthesis had the lowest SRS pain scores (mean 4.04, SD 0.94) at two years after surgery in comparison to AIS (mean 4.31, SD 0.60) ($p = 0.043$) and SK (mean 4.43, SD 0.48) ($p = 0.049$) patients. There was no statistical difference in SRS pain scores between the AIS and SK patients ($p = 0.46$) at the two-year follow-up. Patients' age, gender, BMI, surgery time, intraoperative blood loss or preoperative pain were not associated with more persistent postoperative pain.

At the two-year follow-up, 27 (21%) of 129 AIS patients, 3 (20%) of 15 SK patients, and 9 (36%) of 25 patients in the spondylolisthesis group had a SRS pain score under 4 ($p = 0.26$). At the two-year follow-up there was a positive correlation between the scores in self-image and pain in the AIS patients ($r_s = 0.30$, $p < 0.001$). This correlation between self-image and pain was not seen in the other groups.

3.5. Subgroup Analysis of AIS Patients

In a subgroup analysis with AIS patients only, there was a correlation between preoperative pain and daily postoperative opioid consumption ($r_s = 0.29$, $p < 0.001$) and persistent pain ($p < 0.001$). Patient gender affected the opioid consumption after surgery ($p = 0.013$) but not the persistent postoperative pain. Intraoperative blood loss, surgery time or number of fused vertebras were not associated with opioid consumption after surgery nor with persistent postoperative pain.

4. Discussion

To the best of our knowledge, this is among the first studies comparing persistent postoperative pain development of surgically treated AIS, SK, and spondylolisthesis patients. In our study, the extension of surgery (levels fused) predicted acute postoperative pain and greater opioid use during hospital stay. However, diagnosis and disease pathology were stronger predictors for chronic pain.

Preoperative pain is a common risk factor for persistent pain after PSF in AIS patients [13,17–19]. This might explain why spondylolisthesis patients had a higher incidence of persistent pain after surgery than AIS and SK patients. Other risk factors for chronic pain after PSF in AIS patients according to the literature are child anxiety [11,18,19], longer operative time [11,20], and self-image [4]. The development of chronic postoperative pain seems to be multifactorial [8]. There is paucity in literature regarding chronic postsurgical pain after deformity correction in spondylolisthesis and SK patients. Multimodal analgesia is an important component in reducing chronic pain, but the optimal treatment protocol for adolescent spinal surgery is still not established [12,21]. Studies have shown that acute postsurgical pain predicts chronic pain in adolescents [11,22]. However, in the study conducted by Li et al. [23], it was found that opioid consumption during the acute postoperative period did not significantly predict pain six months after surgery. In our study, the mean daily postoperative opioid consumption was significantly lower in the spondylolisthesis patients compared to AIS and SK patients. Spondylolisthesis patients had more persistent pain compared to AIS and SK patients. In the subgroup analysis with AIS patients, the opioid consumption during immediate postoperative period did not predict pain six months or two years after surgery. Patients with spondylolisthesis had the lowest preoperative SRS-24 activity scores, meaning less activity compared to AIS and SK patients. They also had more preoperative pain compared to AIS and SK patients, which could lead to lower activity scores. Secondly, the conservative treatment of spondylolisthesis patients includes restriction of physical activity. Lower pain and activity scores resulted in lower preoperative SRS-24 total scores, reflecting a lower health-related quality of life in the spondylolisthesis patients compared to AIS and SK patients.

The indications for PSF differ in patients with AIS, SK, and spondylolisthesis [1,24]. Patients with AIS and SK undergo surgery for spinal deformity and spondylolisthesis patients mainly for low back and/or radicular pain. Surgical techniques also differ in nature. Multiple levels of spinal fusion are required to address deformity, while one or two-level spinal fusion with or without pelvic instrumentation is adequate to reduce or stabilize spondylolisthesis. Ideally, AIS and SK patients undergo surgery without nerve root manipulation. Wide nerve root decompression and retraction is needed in patients with spondylolisthesis. Additionally, reduction of high-grade spondylolisthesis improves possibilities of spinal union, but increases tension on L5 nerve roots [25]. Our study indicates that the extent of intraoperative tissue injury (multiple spinal fusion levels) explains relatively well immediate postoperative pain and opioid requirement after surgery. In contrast, preoperative pain and perioperative nerve root manipulation may be associated with more long-term pain, as observed in patients with spondylolisthesis.

Carreon et al. [26] determined the minimum clinically important difference (MCID) in Scoliosis Research Society-22 appearance, activity, and pain domains after surgical correction of AIS. The MCID in pain domain was 0.20. In our study, the surgical treatment of spinal deformity reduced pain after two years in all three groups of patients, and in every patient group the improvement was greater than 0.20. The greatest improvement in pain domain scores was seen in the spondylolisthesis patients. However, spondylolisthesis patients had still more chronic pain after surgery compared to AIS and SK patients.

Limitations and Strengths

This study represents a retrospective analysis of a prospectively collected pediatric spine register with 213 consecutive adolescents with almost complete preoperative and two-year health-related quality of life data. AIS is the most common indication for spinal fusion in the adolescent age group, while the need for surgery of pediatric spondylolisthesis and Scheuermann kyphosis is much more limited. This resulted in a noticeably larger group of patients in the AIS as compared to SK and spondylolisthesis groups. Therefore, one limitation is the relatively small number of spondylolisthesis and Scheuermann kyphosis patients in the register that included 158 AIS patients but only 19 SK and 36 spondylolisthesis patients. Perioperative pain management was standardized. Health-related quality of life and pain were evaluated using the SRS-24 questionnaire, which is a validated outcome tool for adolescents undergoing instrumented posterior spinal fusion. Surgical management was standardized and included a selection of fusion levels according to the Lenke classification and last substantially touched vertebra for AIS [15], stable sagittal vertebral body for Scheuermann kyphosis [16], and one-level fusion for low-grade and two-level fusions for high-grade spondylolisthesis. All the patients were operated on by the same experienced orthopedic spine surgeon. Postoperative pain management included either oxycodone PCA or intravenous and oral oxycodone during the first 48 h postoperatively.

5. Conclusions

Instrumented posterior spinal fusion significantly reduced pain two years after surgery in AIS, SK, and spondylolisthesis patients. A larger number of levels fused was associated with a higher postoperative opioid consumption, as patients with AIS and SK required significantly more opioids than the patients with spondylolisthesis. In contrast, spondylolisthesis patients had more persistent pain two years after surgery compared to AIS and SK patients, suggesting that spinal pathology is more predictive of long-term pain.

Author Contributions: Conceptualization, T.Y., I.H., M.A., M.T. and L.H.; Data curation, I.H., M.T. and L.H.; Formal analysis, T.Y., I.H., T.R. and L.H.; Investigation, T.Y.; Methodology, I.H. and L.H.; Project administration, I.H.; Supervision, I.H., M.T. and L.H.; Writing—original draft, T.Y.; Writing—review & editing, T.Y., I.H., T.R., M.A., M.T. and L.H. All authors have read and agreed to the published version of the manuscript.

Funding: Scientific funding obtained from Turku and Helsinki University Hospitals (11265 and 1), Medtronic (ERP-2020-12238), Stryker Spine (S-I-027), Cerapedics, and Pediatric Research Foundation (HUCH 70295). The funding body did not play a role in the investigation or writing of the manuscript. The funds were only used for salary for research nurse and funding research leaves.

Institutional Review Board Statement: The study was conducted in accordance with the Declaration of Helsinki, and approved by the Ethics Committee, Hospital District of Southwest Finland (ETMK 95/180/2011 and ETMK 38/1800/2015).

Informed Consent Statement: Informed consent was obtained from all subjects involved in the study and from their parents if under 18 years old.

Data Availability Statement: The data generated and analyzed during the current study are available from the corresponding author on reasonable request.

Acknowledgments: Open access funding provided by University of Helsinki.

Conflicts of Interest: Ilkka Helenius has been working as a consultant for Medtronic and K2M.

References

1. Helenius, I.; Remes, V.; Lamberg, T.; Schlenzka, D.; Poussa, M. Long-Term Health-Related Quality of Life After Surgery for Adolescent Idiopathic Scoliosis and Spondylolisthesis. *J. Bone Jt. Surg. -Ser. A* **2008**, *90*, 1231–1239. [CrossRef] [PubMed]
2. Aghdasi, B.; Bachmann, K.R.; Clark, D.; Koldenhoven, R.; Sultan, M.; George, J.; Singla, A.; Abel, M.F. Patient-reported Outcomes Following Surgical Intervention for Adolescent Idiopathic Scoliosis A Systematic Review and Meta-Analysis. *Clin. Spine Surg.* **2020**, *33*, 24–34. [CrossRef] [PubMed]
3. Djurasovic, M.; Glassman, S.D.; Sucato, D.J.; Lenke, L.G.; Crawford, C.H.; Carreon, L.Y. Improvement in Scoliosis Research Society-22R Pain Scores After Surgery for Adolescent Idiopathic Scoliosis. *Spine* **2018**, *43*, 127–132. [CrossRef]
4. Landman, Z.; Oswald, T.; Sanders, J.; Diab, M. Prevalence and Predictors of Pain in Surgical Treatment of Adolescent Idiopathic Scoliosis. *Spine* **2011**, *36*, 825–829. [CrossRef] [PubMed]
5. Helenius, L.; Diarbakerli, E.; Grauers, A.; Lastikka, M.; Oksanen, H.; Pajulo, O.; Löyttyniemi, E.; Manner, T.; Gerdhem, P.; Helenius, I. Back Pain and Quality of Life after Surgical Treatment for Adolescent Idiopathic Scoliosis at 5-Year Follow-up: Comparison with Healthy Controls and Patients with Untreated Idiopathic Scoliosis. *J. Bone Jt. Surg.* **2019**, *101*, 1460–1466. [CrossRef]
6. Green, C.; Brown, K.; Caine, H.; Dieckmann, R.J.; Rathjen, K.E. Prospective Comparison of Patient-selected Operative Versus Nonoperative Treatment of Scheuermann Kyphosis. *J. Pediatr. Orthop.* **2020**, *40*, e716–e719. [CrossRef]
7. Sieberg, C.B.; Simons, L.E.; Edelstein, M.R.; DeAngelis, M.R.; Pielech, M.; Sethna, N.; Hresko, M.T. Pain Prevalence and Trajectories Following Pediatric Spinal Fusion Surgery. *J. Pain* **2013**, *14*, 1694–1702. [CrossRef]
8. Seki, H.; Ideno, S.; Ishihara, T.; Watanabe, K.; Matsumoto, M.; Morisaki, H. Postoperative pain management in patients undergoing posterior spinal fusion for adolescent idiopathic scoliosis: A narrative review. *Scoliosis Spinal Disord.* **2018**, *13*, 17. [CrossRef] [PubMed]
9. Schug, S.A.; Lavand'Homme, P.; Barke, A.; Korwisi, B.; Rief, W.; Treede, R.D. The IASP classification of chronic pain for ICD-11: Chronic postsurgical or posttraumatic pain. *Pain* **2019**, *160*, 45–52. [CrossRef]
10. Rosenbloom, B.N.; Pagé, M.G.; Isaac, L.; Campbell, F.; Stinson, J.N.; Wright, J.G.; Katz, J. Pediatric Chronic Postsurgical Pain And Functional Disability: A Prospective Study Of Risk Factors Up To One Year After Major Surgery. *J. Pain Res.* **2019**, *12*, 3079–3098. [CrossRef] [PubMed]
11. Chidambaran, V.; Ding, L.; Moore, D.; Spruance, K.; Cudilo, E.; Pilipenko, V.; Hossain, M.; Sturm, P.; Kashikar-Zuck, S.; Martin, L.; et al. Predicting the pain continuum after adolescent idiopathic scoliosis surgery: A prospective cohort study. *Eur. J. Pain* **2017**, *21*, 1252–1265. [CrossRef] [PubMed]
12. Lee, C.S.; Merchant, S.; Chidambaran, V. Postoperative Pain Management in Pediatric Spinal Fusion Surgery for Idiopathic Scoliosis. *Pediatr. Drugs* **2020**, *22*, 575–601. [CrossRef] [PubMed]
13. Hwang, S.W.; Harms Study Group; Pendleton, C.; Samdani, A.F.; Bastrom, T.P.; Keeny, H.; Lonner, B.S.; Newton, P.O.; Pahys, J.M. Preoperative SRS pain score is the primary predictor of postoperative pain after surgery for adolescent idiopathic scoliosis: An observational retrospective study of pain outcomes from a registry of 1744 patients with a mean follow-up of 3.4 years. *Eur. Spine J.* **2020**, *29*, 754–760. [CrossRef] [PubMed]
14. Kalso, E. Oxycodone. *J. Pain Symptom Manag.* **2005**, *29*, 47–56. [CrossRef]
15. Beauchamp, E.C.; Lenke, L.G.; Cerpa, M.; Newton, P.O.; Kelly, M.P.; Blanke, K.M.; Harms Study Group Investigators. Selecting the "Touched Vertebra" as the Lowest Instrumented Vertebra in Patients with Lenke Type-1 and 2 Curves: Radiographic Results After a Minimum 5-Year Follow-up. *J. Bone Jt Surg.* **2020**, *102*, 1966–1973. [CrossRef]
16. Cho, K.J.; Lenke, L.G.; Bridwell, K.H.; Kamiya, M.; Sides, B. Selection of the optimal distal fusion level in posterior instrumentation and fusion for thoracic hyperkyphosis: The sagittal stable vertebra concept. *Spine* **2009**, *34*, 765–770. [CrossRef]
17. Bastrom, T.P.; Marks, M.C.; Yaszay, B.; Newton, P.O. Prevalence of postoperative pain in adolescent idiopathic scoliosis and the association with preoperative pain. *Spine* **2013**, *38*, 1848–1852. [CrossRef]
18. Connelly, M.; Fulmer, R.D.; Prohaska, J.; Anson, L.; Dryer, L.; Thomas, V.; Ariagno, J.E.; Price, N.; Schwend, R. Predictors of Postoperative Pain Trajectories in Adolescent Idiopathic Scoliosis. *Spine* **2014**, *39*, E174–E181. [CrossRef]
19. Bailey, K.M.; Howard, J.J.; El-Hawary, R.; Chorney, J. Pain Trajectories Following Adolescent Idiopathic Scoliosis Correction. *J. Bone Jt. Surg.* **2021**, *6*, e20.00122. [CrossRef] [PubMed]

20. Helenius, L.; Yrjälä, T.; Oksanen, H.; Pajulo, O.; Löyttyniemi, E.; Taittonen, M.; Helenius, I. Pregabalin and Persistent Postoperative Pain Following Posterior Spinal Fusion in Children and Adolescents A Randomized Clinical Trial. *J. Bone Jt. Surg.* **2021**, *103*, 2200–2206. [CrossRef] [PubMed]
21. Ricciardelli, R.M.; Walters, N.M.; Pomerantz, M.; Metcalfe, B.; Afroze, F.; Ehlers, M.; Leduc, L.; Feustel, P.; Silverman, E.; Carl, A. The efficacy of ketamine for postoperative pain control in adolescent patients undergoing spinal fusion surgery for idiopathic scoliosis. *Spine Deform.* **2020**, *8*, 433–440. [CrossRef] [PubMed]
22. Ocay, D.D.; Li, M.M.J.; Ingelmo, P.; Ouellet, J.A.; Pagé, M.G.; Ferland, C.E. Predicting Acute Postoperative Pain Trajectories and Long-Term Outcomes of Adolescents after Spinal Fusion Surgery. *Pain Res. Manag.* **2020**, *2020*, 9874739. [CrossRef] [PubMed]
23. Li, M.M.; Ocay, D.D.; Teles, A.R.; Ingelmo, P.M.; Ouellet, J.A.; Pagé, M.G.; Ferland, C.E. Acute postoperative opioid consumption trajectories and long-term outcomes in pediatric patients after spine surgery. *J. Pain Res.* **2019**, *12*, 1673–1684. [CrossRef] [PubMed]
24. Bourassa-Moreau, É.; Labelle, H.; Parent, S.; Hresko, M.T.; Sucato, D.; Lenke, L.G.; Marks, M.; Mac-Thiong, J.M. Expectations for Postoperative Improvement in Health-Related Quality of Life in Young Patients with Lumbosacral Spondylolisthesis: A Prospective Cohort Study. *Spine* **2019**, *44*, E181–E186. [CrossRef]
25. Longo, U.G.; Loppini, M.; Romeo, G.; Maffulli, N.; Denaro, V. Evidence-based surgical management of spondylolisthesis: Reduction or arthrodesis in situ. *J. Bone Jt. Surg.* **2014**, *96*, 53–58. [CrossRef]
26. Carreon, L.Y.; Sanders, J.O.; Diab, M.; Sucato, D.J.; Sturm, P.F.; Glassman, S.D. The Minimum Clinically Important Difference in SRS-22 appearance, activity and pain domains after surcigal correction of adolescent idiopathic scoliosis. *Spine* **2010**, *35*, 2079–2083. [CrossRef]

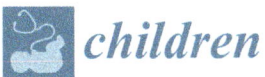

Article

Retrospective Analysis of FED Method Treatment Results in 11–17-Year-Old Children with Idiopathic Scoliosis

Sandra Trzcińska [1] and Kamil Koszela [2,*]

1. Department of Physiotherapy, College of Rehabilitation in Warsaw, 01-234 Warsaw, Poland
2. Neuroorthopedics and Neurology Clinic and Polyclinic, National Institute of Geriatrics, Rheumatology and Rehabilitation, 02-637 Warsaw, Poland
* Correspondence: kamil.aikido@interia.pl; Tel.: +48-601-441-115

Abstract: (1) Background: Idiopathic scoliosis is a major treatment problem due to its unknown origin and its three-dimensional nature. Attempts to cure it and search for new methods of physiotherapeutic treatment that would lead to its correction are one of the key issues of modern medicine. One of them is the fixation, elongation, de-rotation method (FED), used in the conservative treatment of idiopathic scoliosis. The aim of the study was evaluation of the short-term effectiveness of the FED method in the treatment of patients with idiopathic scoliosis. (2) Methods: Each patient underwent therapy based on the guidelines of the FED method. Patients were tested with the Bunnell scoliometer and the Zebris computer system. The treatment period was three weeks, after which the examinations were repeated. (3) Results: The results appeared to be statistically significant for all tested variables. (4) Conclusions: The examinations showed that the FED method had a statistically significant effect on the improvement of all parameters of posture examination, regardless of the size of the scoliotic deformation angle and bone maturity.

Keywords: scoliosis; musculoskeletal disorders; spine; conservative treatment; rehabilitation

Citation: Trzcińska, S.; Koszela, K. Retrospective Analysis of FED Method Treatment Results in 11–17-Year-Old Children with Idiopathic Scoliosis. *Children* 2022, 9, 1513. https://doi.org/10.3390/children9101513

Academic Editors: Axel A. Horsch, Maher A. Ghandour and Matthias Christoph M. Klotz

Received: 28 August 2022
Accepted: 30 September 2022
Published: 3 October 2022

Publisher's Note: MDPI stays neutral with regard to jurisdictional claims in published maps and institutional affiliations.

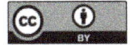

Copyright: © 2022 by the authors. Licensee MDPI, Basel, Switzerland. This article is an open access article distributed under the terms and conditions of the Creative Commons Attribution (CC BY) license (https://creativecommons.org/licenses/by/4.0/).

1. Introduction

Idiopathic scoliosis is a major treatment problem due to its unknown origin and its three-dimensional nature. Attempts to cure it and search for new methods of physiotherapeutic treatment that would lead to its correction are one of the key issues of modern medicine.

One of the less known methods used in Poland for the treatment of patients with idiopathic scoliosis is the FED method (fixation, elongation, de-rotation) established in Spain. The FED treatment method uses a device where corrective forces act on the curvature. The strength of the device is focused on stabilizing, stretching, and de-rotating the spine, under the control of an innovative computer program [1]. As a method that uses a special apparatus for the correction of scoliotic deformity, it has been of great interest to medics in recent years. However, reports that assess the effects of its application are still insufficient [2].

There are several ways to test the effectiveness of the FED method in treating patients with idiopathic scoliosis. The most popular, but harmful due to radiation exposure, is a radiological examination, which is still the standard for diagnosing scoliosis [3–5]. Scoliosis patients can get 10 to 25 spinal X-rays over several years equating to a maximum 10 to 25 mGy of cumulative exposure. Patients who were diagnosed at a younger age and received early and ongoing treatment may be subjected to up to 40 to 50 X-rays, 50 mGy in total [6]. Other non-invasive devices have been used more and more frequently to assess the effects of therapeutic activities undertaken, including the assessment and comparison of various treatments and methods. Such a test can be both a clinical examination, including a scoliometer test as a simple and reliable device for measuring the transverse plane of the spine-trunk rotation, and a more modern three-dimensional posture test, such as the Zebris system. The Zebris system is a modern and specialized apparatus that uses ultrasound, enabling non-invasive examination of the body posture by creating a three-dimensional image of the patient's figure. The system performs a computer analysis to create a report [7]. While the scoliometer is traditionally used to measure trunk rotation at the apex of the curvature, it can also be used to assess global trunk rotation, which evaluates the overall impact of therapy on the spine. A similar test assessing the overall effect of the therapy, but in the frontal plane, is the examination of scoliotic deformity with the Zebris system.

The aim of the study was to evaluate the results of the FED method in patients with idiopathic scoliosis in the short term.

2. Materials and Methods

2.1. Study Population

The study included 81 subjects, 72 girls and 9 boys, aged from 11 to 17 (mean 14.28 ± 1.63). Each of the subjects had a current radiograph, which assessed the following: Risser test, the size of the Cobb angle for individual curvatures and the type of scoliosis was marked according to the King-Moe classification. All patients had idiopathic double-curve scoliosis of type I or II, characterized by the presence of a sigmoid curve in the thoracic (type I) or in the lumbar (type II) segments greater than the other one.

Inclusion Criteria

- Current X-ray scan (not older than 1 month) covering the pelvic girdle, diagnosed double-curve idiopathic scoliosis of type I and II according to King-Moe classification, with the Cobb angle between 10 and 60 degrees of primary scoliosis;
- Age 11–17 years;
- Incomplete ossification;
- No contraindications to the therapy from other systems;
- Consent to examination procedures.
- Exclusion criteria:
- Scoliosis of other than idiopathic origin;
- Risser sign = 5–finished ossification;
- Coexisting diseases of other organs that prevent participation in the program;
- Lack of consent of the patient and the guardian to examinations and participation in the program.

2.2. Study Protocol

Each patient underwent therapy based on the guidelines of the FED method, which consisted of three basic elements: physical therapy as well as analytical and instrumental kinesiotherapy. The main component of the treatment was a special device that corrected the spine in 3 planes. With the help of a special vest, the patient was suspended in the device. Elongation was performed by a computer-controlled hoist, which, at the same time, regulated the pressure of the mobile arm correcting the apex of the scoliotic curve. Other arms stabilized the scoliotic curve at its ends. The pressure force was determined depending on the patient's ability, up to a maximum of 100 kg. The time of the procedure was 30 min, the time of corrective pressure performed by the pneumatic movable arm was 20 s, and the break was 10 s. The arm corrected the curve both in the frontal and rotational planes, owing to the possibility of its angular positioning. In order to prepare the patient for the therapy in the device, the tissues were made more flexible and blood supply improved in the places to be subjected to the therapy, so, in this study, electrostimulation of the muscles on the convex side of the curve and thermal treatment, in which warm compresses were placed in the deformation concavity, were used. Both procedures lasted 15 min. Then the patient performed exercises for about 20–30 min, individually selected in accordance with the guidelines of the FED method. The selection of exercises was based on the King-Moe classification, which divides scoliosis into 5 types in terms of the location of scoliotic curvatures. In addition, patients wore the Boston brace every day for approximately 21–22 h a day, except for FED therapy (up to 3 h) and personal care. The Boston brace was made on the basis of a plaster cast and self-report was used.

Each participant was tested with the Bunnell scoliometer and the Zebris computer system on the day before therapy began. The treatment period was 3 weeks, after which the examinations were repeated on the day the therapy completed. In the study, the scoliometer assessed both the trunk rotation angle at the apex of both scoliotic curves for the thoracic (ATR Th) and lumbar (ATR L) spine, and the total spine rotation using the SDR summing parameter, which consisted in summing the values of the rotation on both curves as positive values regardless of their direction. The computer examination assessed overall scoliotic deformation (SD) in the frontal plane. This parameter was the sum of the angles of tangents from the seventh cervical to the fifth lumbar vertebrae (C7-L5).

This study was conducted according to the guidelines of the Declaration of Helsinki, and approved by the Bioethics Committee for Scientific Research at the College of Rehabilitation in Warsaw, number 100/2022.

2.3. Data Analysis

In order to answer the research questions, statistical analyses were performed with the IBM SPSS Statistics 27 (Armonk, NY, USA). This was used to analyze basic descriptive statistics, with Shapiro–Wilk test, and Student's t-test for dependent samples, and Wilcoxon test and Spearman's rho correlation analysis. The level of significance was considered to be $\alpha = 0.05$.

3. Results

3.1. Data Analysis

Most patients (66.7%) had type II scoliosis according to the King-Moe classification. The mean Cobb angle at the thoracic level [°] was 35.91 ± 10.43, and at the lumbar level it was 33.54 ± 10.94. Detailed results are presented in Tables 1 and 2.

Table 1. Gender and type of scoliosis.

		n	%
Gender (n = 81)	Girls	72	88.90%
	Boys	9	11.10%
King-Moe Classification (n = 81)	Type I	27	33.30%
	Type II	54	66.70%

n—number.

Table 2. Age and X-ray analysis of indicators.

	n	$\bar{x}$	Min.	Max.
Age [years]	81	14.28 ± 1.63	11.00	17.00
Risser sign [score]	81	2.85 ± 0.94	1.00	4.00
Cobb angle at the thoracic level [°]	81	35.91 ± 10.43	13.00	56.00
Cobb angle at the lumbar level [°]	81	33.54 ± 10.94	10.00	59.00
King-Moe Classification Type I-Cobb angle at the lumbar level	27	40.48 ± 6.70	24.00	59.00
King-Moe Classification Type II-Cobb angle at the thoracic level	54	39.01 ± 7.69	16.00	53.00

n—number, x—mean, SD—standard deviation, Min—the lowest value, Max—the highest value.

3.2. Basic Descriptive Statistics with the Shapiro-Wilk Test

In the first step of the analysis, the distributions of quantitative variables were checked. For this purpose, basic descriptive statistics were calculated together with the Shapiro-Wilk test examining the normality of the distribution. The results of the analysis are presented in Table 3.

Table 3. Basic descriptive statistics of the studied variables together with the Shapiro-Wilk test for normality.

	$\bar{x}$	Me	Sk.	Kurt.	Min.	Max.	W	p
Before Therapy (n = 81)								
The trunk rotation angle-ATR Th [°]	11.30 ± 4.63	11.00	0.08	−0.47	1.00	22.00	0.99	0.535
The lumbar rotation angle-ATR L [°]	7.75 ± 4.90	7.00	0.50	−0.44	0.00	19.00	0.95	0.003 *
Sum of two rotations-SDR [°]	19.05 ± 5.46	18.00	0.48	−0.11	8.00	33.00	0.97	0.066
Scoliotic deformation angle-SD [°]	37.06 ± 14.21	35.00	1.10	2.51	8.30	90.60	0.94	<0.001 *
After Therapy (n = 81)								
The trunk rotation angle-ATR Th [°]	8.51 ± 4.19	8.00	0.13	−0.34	0.00	18.00	0.98	0.430
The lumbar rotation angle-ATR L [°]	5.05 ± 4.18	4.00	0.88	0.08	0.00	16.00	0.91	<0.001 *
Sum of two rotations-SDR [°]	13.56 ± 4.69	13.00	0.21	−0.57	4.00	23.00	0.98	0.114
Scoliotic deformation angle-SD [°]	24.25 ± 12.09	21.80	1.42	3.33	0.00	69.80	0.88	<0.001 *

n—number, x—mean, SD—standard deviation, Me—median, Sk—skewness, Kurt—kurtosis, Min—the lowest value, Max—the highest value, W—Shapiro-Wilk test, p—level of significance, *—statistical significance.

The results of the Shapiro-Wilk test appeared to be statistically significant for the lumbar rotation angle-ATR L [°] and for the scoliotic deformation angle-SD [°] both before and after the therapy. This meant that distributions of these variables differed from the normal distribution. However, in the case of the lumbar rotation angle-ATR L [°], the value of the skewness did not exceed the absolute value of one, which indicated that the asymmetry was insignificant. Therefore, the analyses for the trunk and lumbar rotation angles-ATR Th [°] and AR L [°], and for the sum of two rotations-SDR [°], were performed based on parametric tests. Yet, for the scoliotic deformation angle-SD [°], the skewness exceeded the value of one. A detailed analysis showed that this value of skewness resulted from the presence of two outliers (+ 3SD). Thus, for these variables, the analyses were based on non-parametric tests.

3.3. Comparison of the Value of the Trunk Rotation Angle-ATR Th [°], the Lumbar Rotation Angle-ATR L [°], the Sum of Two Rotations SDR [°] and the Angle of Scoliotic Deformation-SD [°], before and after the Therapy

In the next step, it was checked whether the applied therapy influenced values of the trunk rotation angle-ATR Th [°], the lumbar rotation angle-ATR L [°], the sum of two rotations-SDR [°] and the angle of scoliotic deformation-SD [°]. For this purpose, the Student's t-test was performed for dependent samples and, in the case of the scoliotic deformation angle, the non-parametric Wilcoxon test was performed. The analyses were performed for all patients, taking into account the division into gender and type of scoliosis, based on the King-Moe classification (Table 4).

The results appeared to be statistically significant for all tested variables. The values of individual parameters, the trunk and lumbar rotation angles, the sum of two rotations and the scoliotic deformation angle, were significantly lower after the therapy than before. Differences in measurements were observed in both girls and boys, and in subjects with scoliosis types I and II. Each of the differences between the measurements before and after the therapy was significant.

Table 4. Results of Student's *t*-test for dependent samples and Wilcoxon's test comparing individual parameters measured with a scoliometer and Zebris, before and after therapy.

	Before Therapy $\bar{x}$	After Therapy $\bar{x}$	t/Z	p	95% CI LL	UL	d Cohena/r
Total (n = 81)							
The trunk rotation angle-ATR Th [°]	11.30 ± 4.63	8.51 ± 4.19	15.23	<0.001 *	2.43	3.15	1.69
The lumbar rotation angle-ATR L [°]	7.75 ± 4.90	5.05 ± 4.18	12.55	<0.001 *	2.27	3.13	1.39
Sum of two rotations [°]	19.05 ± 5.46	13.56 ± 4.69	19.17	<0.001 *	4.92	6.06	2.13
Scoliotic deformation angle-SD [°]	37.06 ± 14.21	24.25 ± 12.09	−7.40	<0.001 *	10.63	14.99	0.58
Girls (n = 72)							
The trunk rotation angle- ATR Th [°]	11.03 ± 4.63	8.26 ± 4.18	14.01	<0.001 *	2.37	3.16	1.65
The lumbar rotation angle-ATR L [°]	7.82 ± 4.94	5.07 ± 4.25	11.68	<0.001 *	2.28	3.22	1.38
Sum of two rotations [°]	18.85 ± 5.47	13.33 ± 4.73	17.70	<0.001 *	4.89	6.13	2.09
Scoliotic deformation angle-SD [°]	37.49 ± 13.83	24.38 ± 12.61	−6.96	<0.001 *	10.83	15.38	0.58
Boys (n = 9)							
The trunk rotation angle-ATR Th [°]	13.44 ± 4.28	10.44 ± 4.00	6.00	<0.001 *	1.85	4.15	2.00
The lumbar rotation angle-ATR L [°]	7.22 ± 4.84	4.89 ± 3.82	4.95	0.001 *	1.25	3.42	1.65
Sum of two rotations [°]	20.67 ± 5.39	15.33 ± 4.12	7.54	<0.001 *	3.70	6.96	2.51
Scoliotic deformation angle-SD [°]	33.62 ± 17.46	23.16 ± 6.89	−2.67	0.008 *	1.63	19.30	0.63
Scoliosis type I (n = 27)							
The trunk rotation angle-ATR Th [°]	9.00 ± 4.09	6.33 ± 3.45	7.45	<0.001 *	1.93	3.40	1.43
The lumbar rotation angle-ATR L [°]	9.67 ± 4.84	7.07 ± 4.20	9.66	<0.001 *	2.04	3.14	1.86
Sum of two rotations [°]	18.67 ± 6.00	13.41 ± 4.94	11.73	<0.001 *	4.34	6.18	2.26
Scoliotic deformation angle-SD [°]	35.57 ± 12.26	22.32 ± 9.24	−4.45	<0.001 *	9.29	17.20	0.61
Scoliosis type II (n = 54)							
The trunk rotation angle-ATR Th [°]	12.44 ± 4.49	9.59 ± 4.13	13.55	<0.001 *	2.43	3.27	1.84
The lumbar rotation angle-ATR L [°]	6.80 ± 4.69	4.04 ± 3.82	9.34	<0.001 *	2.17	3.35	1.27
Sum of two rotations [°]	19.24 ± 5.22	13.63 ± 4.60	15.22	<0.001 *	4.87	6.35	2.07
Scoliotic deformation angle-SD [°]	37.81 ± 15.14	25.21 ± 13.26	−5.95	<0.001 *	9.90	15.29	0.57

n—number, *x*—mean, *SD*—standard deviation, *t*—*t*-test, *Z*—Wilcoxon test, *p*—level of significance, 95% CI—95% Confidence Interval, *LL*—Lower Limit, *UL*—Upper Limit, *d Cohena*—effect size for Student's *t* test for dependent samples, *r*—effect size for Wilcoxon test, *—statistical significance.

3.4. Correlations between Parameters Measured with X-ray, Scoliometer and Scolioscan

In the next step, it was verified whether the measurements made with the use of a scoliometer and Zebris computer system correlated with each other. For this purpose, Spearman's rho correlation analyses were performed. The parameters were compared before and after therapy and for all observations in general. The results are presented in Table 5.

The analysis showed six statistically significant correlations. For the measurements performed before the therapy, a significant correlation was observed only in the case of the sum of two rotations-SDR [°]. In the case of measurements performed after the therapy, statistically significant correlations concerned the trunk rotation angle-ATR Th [°] and again the sum of two rotations-SDR [°]. On the other hand, the analysis performed for all measurements in total showed that the angle of scoliotic deformation-SD [°] was significantly related to each of the results obtained with the use of the scoliometer. Parameters that were measured with the scoliometer were positively related to the scoliotic deformation angle, which was measured with the Zebris computer system. Three of the statistically significant correlations were weak and three were moderately strong.

Table 5. Correlation analysis for measurements made with a scoliometer and Zebris computer system.

Measurements Made with a Scoliometer		Scoliotic Deformation Angle-SD [°]-Measurement Made with Zebris System		
		Before Therapy ($n = 81$)	After Therapy ($n = 81$)	Total ($n = 162$)
The trunk rotation angle-ATR Th [°]	rho Spearman	0.21	0.24	0.33
	significance	0.06	0.03 *	<0.001 *
The lumbar rotation angle-ATR L [°]	rho Spearman	0.16	0.13	0.23
	significance	0.16	0.26	0.003 *
Sum of two rotations [°]	rho Spearman	0.28	0.32	0.44
	significance	0.01 *	0.004 *	<0.001 *

n—number, *—statistical significance.

3.5. Comparison of the Value of the Trunk Rotation Angle-ATR Th [°], the Lumbar Rotation Angle-ATR L [°], the Sum of Two Rotations SDR [°] and the Angle of Scoliotic Deformation-SD [°], before and after the Therapy Depending on the Dimensions of the Larger Curve

In the next step, it was verified whether, as a result of the therapy, in the groups distinguished by the dimensions of the larger curvature, the individual measured parameters changed, i.e., the trunk rotation angle-ATR Th [°], the lumbar rotation angle-ATR L [°], the sum of two rotations-SDR [°] and the angle of scoliotic deformation-SD [°]. The analyses were carried out in groups distinguished according to the value of the larger Cobb angle (at the level of the thoracic or lumbar spine). It was assumed that I° results were up to 24°, II°, 25–45°, and III°, above 45°. Due to the very small number of individuals with I° ($n = 4$), the analyses were performed only for those with II° and III°. The Student's t-test was used for dependent samples, and, in the case of the scoliotic deformation angle, the non-parametric Wilcoxon test was used (Table 6).

The results were statistically significant for all variables in every group. The values of trunk and lumbar rotation angles [°] (ATR Th and ATR L), sum of two rotations [°] and scoliotic deformation angle-SD [°] were lower after the therapy compared to those before the therapy. In both groups and for all variables, the observed differences were strong.

Table 6. Results of Student's t-test for dependent samples and Wilcoxon's test-comparison of individual parameters measured with the scoliometer and Zebris, before and after therapy, with division into groups distinguished on the basis of the value of greater Cobb angle.

	Before Therapy $\bar{x}$	After Therapy $\bar{x}$	t/Z	p	95% CI LL	95% CI UL	d Cohena/r
II°—Value of Greater Cobb Angle 25–45° ($n = 56$)							
The trunk rotation angle-ATR Th [°]	10.34 ± 4.36	7.91 ± 3.95	12.99	<0.001 *	2.05	2.80	1.74
The lumbar rotation angle-ATR L [°]	7.18 ± 4.84	4.64 ± 4.05	10.05	<0.001 *	2.03	3.04	1.34
Sum of two rotations [°]	17.52 ± 3.90	12.55 ± 3.60	16.07	<0.001 *	4.35	5.58	2.15
Scoliotic deformation angle-SD [°]	32.92 ± 10.25	20.94 ± 8.91	−6.11	<0.001 *	9.56	14.41	0.58

Table 6. Cont.

	Before Therapy $\bar{x}$	After Therapy $\bar{x}$	t/Z	p	95% CI LL	95% CI UL	d Cohena/r
III°—Value of Greater Cobb Angle > 45° (n = 21)							
The trunk rotation angle-ATR Th [°]	14.14 ± 4.41	10.24 ± 4.40	10.18	<0.001 *	3.10	4.70	2.22
The lumbar rotation angle-ATR L [°]	9.43 ± 5.08	6.43 ± 4.55	6.34	<0.001 *	2.01	3.99	1.38
Sum of two rotations [°]	23.57 ± 6.64	16.67 ± 5.79	11.48	<0.001 *	5.65	8.16	2.51
Scoliotic deformation angle-SD [°]	49.34 ± 16.89	32.85 ± 15.20	−3.88	<0.001 *	11.21	21.77	0.60

n—number, x—mean, SD—standard deviation, t—t-test, Z—Wilcoxon test, p—level of significance, 95% CI—95% Confidence Interval, LL—Lower Limit, UL—Upper Limit, d Cohena—effect size for Student's t test for dependent samples, r—effect size for Wilcoxon test, *—statistical significance.

3.6. Comparison of the Value of the Trunk Rotation Angle-ATR Th [°], the Lumbar Rotation Angle-ATR L [°], the Sum of Two Rotations SDR [°] and the Angle of Scoliotic Deformation-SD [°], before and after the Therapy Depending on the Risser Sign Grade

The results were statistically significant for all variables in every group. The values of trunk and lumbar rotation angles [°] (ATR Th and ATR L), sum of two rotations [°] and scoliotic deformation angle-SD [°] were lower after the therapy compared to those before the therapy. In both groups and for all variables, the values were lower after the therapy compared to those before the therapy independently of the Risser Sign Grade, the observed differences were strong (Table 7).

Table 7. Results of Student's t-test for dependent samples and Wilcoxon's test-comparison of individual parameters measured with the scoliometer and Zebris, before and after therapy, with division into groups distinguished on the basis of Risser Sign Grade.

	Before Therapy $\bar{x}$	After Therapy $\bar{x}$	t/Z	p	95% CI LL	95% CI UL	d Cohena/r
Risser Sign Grade 1 (n = 9)							
The trunk rotation angle-ATR Th [°]	11.89 ± 3.33	8.89 ± 4.14	4.24	0.002 *	1.37	4.63	1.41
The lumbar rotation angle-ATR L [°]	8.44 ± 5.41	6.56 ± 4.77	3.69	0.006 *	0.71	3.07	1.23
Sum of two rotations [°]	20.33 ± 7.50	15.44 ± 6.69	5.82	<0.001 *	2.95	6.83	1.94
Scoliotic deformation angle-SD [°]	48.14 ± 14.10	33.73 ± 13.38	−2.67	0.008 *	8.67	20.15	0.63
Risser Sign Grade 2 (n = 15)							
The trunk rotation angle-ATR Th [°]	12.40 ± 5.14	9.67 ± 4.78	7.12	<0.001 *	1.91	3.56	1.84
The lumbar rotation angle-ATR L [°]	7.40 ± 5.28	4.47 ± 4.24	5.12	<0.001 *	1.70	4.16	1.32
Sum of two rotations [°]	19.80 ± 5.20	14.13 ± 3.93	8.16	<0.001 *	4.18	7.16	2.11
Scoliotic deformation angle-SD [°]	39.16 ± 10.82	26.83 ± 11.69	−3.41	<0.001 *	8.13	16.53	0.62
Risser Sign Grade 3 (n = 36)							
The trunk rotation angle-ATR Th [°]	10.36 ± 4.82	7.83 ± 4.05	10.10	<0.001 *	2.02	3.04	1.68
The lumbar rotation angle-ATR L [°]	8.17 ± 5.28	5.31 ± 4.68	8.34	<0.001 *	2.16	3.56	1.39
Sum of two rotations [°]	18.53 ± 5.60	13.14 ± 4.77	12.38	<0.001 *	4.51	6.27	2.06
Scoliotic deformation angle-SD [°]	34.87 ± 15.15	21.10 ± 11.18	−5.23	<0.001 *	10.83	16.70	0.62

Table 7. Cont.

	Before Therapy $\bar{x}$	After Therapy $\bar{x}$	t/Z	p	95% CI LL	95% CI UL	d Cohena/r
Risser Sign Grade 4 (n = 21)							
The trunk rotation angle-ATR Th [°]	11.86 ± 4.37	8.67 ± 4.10	8.10	<0.001 *	2.37	4.01	1.77
The lumbar rotation angle-ATR L [°]	7.00 ± 3.86	4.38 ± 2.84	7.11	<0.001 *	1.85	3.39	1.55
Sum of two rotations [°]	18.86 ± 4.61	13.05 ± 4.12	10.24	<0.001 *	4.63	6.99	2.23
Scoliotic deformation angle-SD [°]	34.57 ± 13.06	23.73 ± 11.61	−3.13	0.002 *	4.60	17.07	0.48

n—number, x—mean, SD—standard deviation, t—t-test, Z—Wilcoxon test, p—level of significance, 95% CI—95% Confidence Interval, LL—Lower Limit, UL—Upper Limit, d Cohena—effect size for Student's t test for dependent samples, r—effect size for Wilcoxon test, *—statistical significance.

4. Discussion

The FED method is a relatively little-known method of treatment. It originated in Spain, where most of the scientific reports on its effectiveness come from [8–11]. Conducted studies have concerned mainly single cases or studies in smaller groups of patients. At the time when the method became fairly common in Poland, projects concerning larger research groups began to appear [12–14]. Today, many reports assessing its effectiveness in the treatment of patients with idiopathic scoliosis come from Poland. The number of centers using this type of treatment is constantly growing and the method has a large number of supporters. The reports that appear, especially in recent years, prove its effectiveness in the treatment of patients with idiopathic scoliosis [15].

Studies on the effectiveness of the FED method in the treatment of patients with idiopathic scoliosis show a significant improvement in all measured parameters, both in the examination with the scoliometer and with the Zebris system. These changes occurred both in the transverse and frontal planes. It turned out to be important to correct not only individual curves, but also the entire area of the spine in both tested planes. These studies indicated a positive effect on the entire spine, in contrast to the existing therapeutic view on the correction of one curve at the expense of deteriorating the other [16,17].

The use of traditional scoliometer examination and other posture parameters enable the assessment of the effect of the undertaken treatment procedures, mainly focusing not only on the diagnosis, but also on the effectiveness of individual methods and ways of the therapy. However, there are more and more reports indicating that basic examination (e.g., with a scoliometer) is insufficient. The impact of the therapy not only on the rotation of individual curves, but also on the global rotation, should also be evaluated. For this reason, summing parameters were used in the assessment of body posture. These are even less well known, but more and more often they are willingly used to evaluate therapy and its effect on the transverse plane [18–20]. A similar study, assessing the overall effect of therapy on the entire spine, in terms of the frontal plane, involved the scoliotic deformation parameter tested with the Zebris system. The conducted research demonstrated a correlation between these two parameters, despite the fact that they relate to two different transverse and frontal planes.

The project also investigated the impact of FED therapy on scoliotic deformations in terms of its size. The modified SOSORT angular division was used, which divides scoliosis on the basis of size assessed by the Cobb method on the radiograph. The studies showed a significant improvement in all parameters, regardless of the size of the scoliosis.

The examinations showed an improvement in all the tested parameters at various stages of bone maturity (Risser Sign Grade 1–4). Improvement was observed in all patients after the use of the FED method, regardless of the Risser Sign Grade.

The harmfulness of radiological examinations has more and more frequently led to the use of modern computer diagnostics to assess the posture [21–24]. These computer diagnostics allow for a harmless assessment of treatment stages, in terms of posture, especially since they correlate with radiographic images [25]. However, a distinction should be made here regarding when to use these two different examinations: radiological examinations should be used to diagnose and assess the progression of scoliotic deformity, and computer-based monitoring and evaluation should be used to diagnose and assess the treatment course. Computer-based methods are probably an alternative to radiology, but not in all respects. These two examinations differ from each other but should complement each other. Carrying out diagnostic activities on various grounds results in better control of scoliotic deformation progressing to impaired quality of life or to surgery, which often causes complications, and which we would like to avoid in the treatment of patients with idiopathic scoliosis [26].

Due to the nature of the therapy, the patients' follow-up was short-term. However, it would be worth performing repeated examinations at a longer time interval. The FED method is relatively new in Poland, so such studies should be carried out, especially related to the assessment of the impact of the method on the sagittal plane of the posture. It requires further analyses supplemented with long-term follow-up in a larger group of patients. A 3-month and 6-month follow-up examination is planned.

5. Conclusions

All assessed parameters of posture examination, both with the scoliometer and the Zebris system, showed a statistically significant improvement in patients treated with the FED method. Statistical improvement occurred both in boys and girls, as well as in all types of scoliosis. The analysis showed the occurrence of statistically significant correlations between the parameters of the posture examination with a scoliometer and the computer examination. The examinations showed that the FED method had a statistically significant effect on the improvement of all parameters of posture examination, regardless of the size of the scoliotic deformation angle and bone maturity. However, due to the short observation time, this method requires further research with a long follow-up period.

Author Contributions: Conceptualization, S.T.; methodology, S.T.; software, S.T.; validation, S.T., and K.K.; formal analysis, S.T. and K.K.; investigation, S.T.; resources, S.T. and K.K.; data curation, S.T.; writing—original draft preparation, S.T. and K.K.; writing—review and editing, S.T. and K.K.; visualization, S.T. and K.K.; supervision, S.T. and K.K.; project administration, S.T.; funding acquisition, S.T. and K.K. All authors have read and agreed to the published version of the manuscript.

Funding: This research received no external funding.

Institutional Review Board Statement: This study was conducted according to the guidelines of the Declaration of Helsinki, and approved by the Bioethics Committee for Scientific Research at College of Rehabilitation in Warsaw, number 100/2022.

Informed Consent Statement: Informed consent was obtained from all subjects involved in the study.

Data Availability Statement: The datasets analyzed during the current study are available from the corresponding author upon reasonable request.

Conflicts of Interest: The authors declare no conflict of interest.

References

1. Trzcińska, S.; Nowak, Z. FED method in treatment of idiopathic scolioses. *Int. Rev. Med. Pract.* **2020**, *26*, 42–47.
2. Nisser, J.; Smolenski, U.; Sliwniski, G.E.; Schumann, P.; Heinke, A.; Malberg, H.; Werner, M.; Elsner, S.; Drossel, W.G.; Śliwiński, Z.; et al. The FED-Method (Fixation, Elongation, Derotation)—A Machine-supported Treatment Approach to Patients with Idiopathic Scoliosis—Review. *Z. Für Orthopädie Unf.* **2020**, *158*, 318–332. [CrossRef] [PubMed]
3. Cheung, C.W.J.; Zhou, G.Q.; Law, S.Y.; Mak, T.M.; Lai, K.L.; Zheng, Y.P. Ultrasound volume projection imaging for assessment of scoliosis. *IEEE Transact. Med. Imaging* **2015**, *34*, 1760–1768. [CrossRef] [PubMed]
4. Jiang, W.W.; Cheng, C.L.K.; Cheung, J.P.Y.; Samartzis, D.; Lai, K.K.L.; To, M.K.T.; Zheng, Y.P. Patterns of coronal curve changes in forward bending posture: A 3D ultrasound study of adolescent idiopathic scoliosis patients. *Eur. Spine J.* **2018**, *27*, 2139–2147. [CrossRef]

5. Presciutti, S.M.; Karukanda, T.; Lee, M. Management decisions for adolescent idiopathic scoliosis significantly affect patient radiation exposure. *Spine J.* **2014**, *14*, 1984–1990. [CrossRef]
6. Oakley, P.A.; Ehsani, N.N.; Harrison, D.E. The Scoliosis Quandary: Are Radiation Exposures From Repeated X-Rays Harmful? *Dose Response* **2019**, *17*, 1559325819852810. [CrossRef]
7. Trzcińska, S.; Kiebzak, W.; Wiecheć, M.; Śliwiński, Z. Compensation Mechanism in Treatment of idiopathic Scoliosis with the FED Method—Preliminary results. *Pol. J. Physiother.* **2017**, *17*, 6–14.
8. Lapuente, J.; Sastre, S.; Barrios, C. Idiopathic scoliosis under 30 degrees in growing patients. A comparative study of the F.E.D. method and other conservative treatments. *Stud. Health Technol. Inform.* **2002**, *88*, 258–269.
9. Sastre, S. Treatment of scoliosis—F.E.D method. *Pol. J. Physiother.* **2007**, *7*, 223–231.
10. Sastre, S.; Laquente, J.; Salinas, F.; Quiros, S.; Raimondi, P. Conservative Treatment of Scoliosis with F.E.D.: The Results of 867 Cases. Clinical Study. *Biomechanics*. Available online: https://www.researchgate.net/publication/275654301_The_Results_of_867_cases (accessed on 28 August 2022).
11. Sastre, S.; Lapuente, J.P.; Santapau, C.; Bueno, M. Dynamic Treatment of Scoliosis (The Results of 174 Cases). In *Research into Spinal Deformities*; IOS Press: Amsterdam, The Netherlands, 1999; Volume 59, pp. 171–174.
12. Kiebzak, W.; Dwornik, M.; Kiljański, M.; Trzcińska, S. Efficacyof FED therapy in grade 2 idiopathic scoliosis. *Pol. J. Physiother.* **2017**, *17*, 140–147.
13. Śliwiński, Z.; Kufel, W.; Halat, B.; Michalak, B.; Śliwińska, B.; Śliwiński, G. Radiological progress report of curing scoliosis according to the fed method based on own material. *Scoliosis* **2014**, *9* (Suppl. S1), 14. [CrossRef]
14. Trzcińska, S.; Nowak, Z. An analysis of scoliosis deformity in the computer study Zebris as an assessment of FED method effectiveness in treatment of idiopathic scolioses. *Pol. Med. J.* **2020**, *48*, 174–178.
15. Trzcińska, S.; Koszela, K.; Kuszewski, M. Effectiveness of the FED Method in the Treatment of Idiopathic Scoliosis of Girls Aged 11–15 Years. *Int. J. Environ. Res. Public Health* **2021**, *19*, 65. [CrossRef] [PubMed]
16. Trzcińska, S.; Kuszewski, M.; Koszela, K. Analysis of Posture Parameters in Patients with Idiopathic Scoliosis with the Use of 3D Ultrasound Diagnostics—Preliminary Results. *Int. J. Environ. Res. Public Health* **2022**, *19*, 4750. [CrossRef] [PubMed]
17. Białek, M.; Kotwicki, T.; M'hango, A.; Szulc, A. Angle of trunk rotation in primary and compensatory scoliotic curve in children after individual rehabilitation with FITS method. *Ann. Acad. Med. Siles.* **2007**, *61*, 45–48.
18. Kotwicki, T.; Kinel, E.; Chowańska, J.; Bodnar-Nanuś, A. POTSI, Hump Sum and Sum of Rotation—new surface topography parameters for evaluation of scoliotic deformity of the trunk. *Pol. J. Physiother.* **2008**, *8*, 231–240.
19. Chowanska, J.; Kotwicki, T.; Rosadzinski, K.; Śliwiński, Z. School screening for scoliosis: Can surface topography replace examination with scoliometer? *Scoliosis* **2012**, *7*, 9. [CrossRef]
20. Goldberg, C.J.; Kaliszer, M.; Moore, D.P.; Fogarty, E.E.; Dowling, F.E. Surface topograpfy Cobb angles and cosmetic change in scoliosis. *Spine* **2001**, *26*, 55–63. [CrossRef]
21. Oakley, P.A.; Navid Ehsani, N.; Harrison, D.E. 5 Reasons Why Scoliosis X-Rays Are Not Harmful. *Dose Response* **2020**, *18*, 1559325820957797. [CrossRef]
22. Loughenbury, P.R.; Gentles, S.L.; Murphy, E.J.; Tomlinson, J.E.; Borse, V.H.; Dunsmuir, R.A.; Gummerson, N.W.; Millner, P.A.; Rao, A.S.; Rowbotham, E.; et al. Estimated cumulative X-ray exposure and additional cancer risk during the evaluation and treatment of scoliosis in children and young people requiring surgery. *Spine Deform* **2021**, *9*, 949–954. [CrossRef]
23. Ronckers, C.M.; Land, C.E.; Miller, J.S.; Stovall, M.; Lonstein, J.E.; Doody, M.M. Cancer mortality among women frequently exposed to radiographic examinations for spinal disorders. *Radiat. Res.* **2010**, *174*, 83–90. [CrossRef] [PubMed]
24. Schmitz-Feuerhake, I.; Pflugbeil, S. 'Lifestyle' and cancer rates in former East and West Germany: The possible contribution of diagnostic radiation exposures. *Radiat. Prot. Dosim.* **2011**, *147*, 310–313. [CrossRef] [PubMed]
25. Zheng, Y.P.; Lee, T.T.; Lai, K.K.; Yip, B.H.; Zhou, G.Q.; Jiang, W.W.; Cheung, J.C.; Wong, M.S.; Ng, B.K.; Cheng, J.C.; et al. A reliability and validity study for Scolioscan: A radiation-free scoliosis assessment system using 3D ultrasound imaging. *Scoliosis Spinal Disord* **2016**, *11*, 13. [CrossRef] [PubMed]
26. Latalski, M.; Starobrat, G.; Fatyga, M.; Sowa, I.; Wójciak, M.; Wessely-Szponder, J.; Dresler, S.; Danielewicz, A. Wound-Related Complication in Growth-Friendly Spinal Surgeries for Early-Onset Scoliosis-Literature Review. *J. Clin. Med.* **2022**, *11*, 2669. [CrossRef]

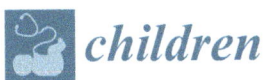

Article

Health-Related Quality of Life after Fractures of the Distal Forearm in Children and Adolescents—Results from a Center in Switzerland in 432 Patients

Thoralf Randolph Liebs *, Alex Lorance, Steffen Michael Berger, Nadine Kaiser and Kai Ziebarth

Inselspital, Department of Paediatric Surgery, University of Bern, 3010 Bern, Switzerland
* Correspondence: liebs@liebs.eu; Tel.: +41-31-632-21-11

Abstract: (1) Background: We aimed to evaluate the health-related quality of life (HRQoL) in children with fractures of the distal forearm and to assess if HRQoL was associated with fracture classification; (2) Methods: We followed up on 432 patients (185 girls, 247 boys) who sustained a fracture of the distal radius or forearm from 1/2007 to 6/2007, 1/2014 to 6/2014, and 11/2016 to 10/2017. Patients filled in the Quick-DASH (primary outcome) and the Peds-QL; (3) Results: The radius was fractured in 429 and the ulna in 175 cases. The most frequent injury of the radius was a buckle fracture (51%, mean age 8.5 years), followed by a complete metaphyseal fracture (22%, 9.5 years), Salter-Harris-2 fracture (14%, 11.4 years), greenstick fracture (10%, 9.3 years), Salter-Harris-1 fracture (1%, 12.6 years), and other rare injuries. The most common treatment was closed reduction and an above-elbow cast in 138 cases (32%), followed by a cast without reduction (30%), splint (28%), and K-wire fixation and cast (9%). Definite treatment was performed initially in 95.8%, a new cast or cast wedging was performed in 1.6%, and revision surgery was performed in 2.5%. There were no open reductions and no plate fixations. After a mean follow-up of 4.2 years, patients with buckle fractures had a mean Quick-DASH of 3.3 (scale of 0–100) (complete fracture: 1.5; greenstick: 1.5; SH-1: 0.9; SH-2: 4.1; others: 0.9). The mean function score of the PedsQL ranged from 93.0 for SH-2 fractures to 97.9 for complete fractures; (4) Conclusions: In this cohort of 432 children with fractures of the distal forearm, there was equally good mean mid- and long-term HRQoL when assessed by the Quick-DASH and the PedsQL. There was a trend for children with complete metaphyseal fractures reporting better HRQoL than patients with buckle fractures or patients with Salter-Harris II fractures, however, these differences were not statistically significant nor clinically relevant.

Keywords: fracture; forearm; radius; ulna; surgery; conservative treatment; health-related quality of life

Citation: Liebs, T.R.; Lorance, A.; Berger, S.M.; Kaiser, N.; Ziebarth, K. Health-Related Quality of Life after Fractures of the Distal Forearm in Children and Adolescents—Results from a Center in Switzerland in 432 Patients. *Children* **2022**, *9*, 1487. https://doi.org/10.3390/children9101487

Academic Editors: Axel A. Horsch, Maher A. Ghandour and Matthias Christoph M. Klotz

Received: 30 August 2022
Accepted: 26 September 2022
Published: 28 September 2022

Publisher's Note: MDPI stays neutral with regard to jurisdictional claims in published maps and institutional affiliations.

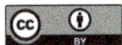

Copyright: © 2022 by the authors. Licensee MDPI, Basel, Switzerland. This article is an open access article distributed under the terms and conditions of the Creative Commons Attribution (CC BY) license (https://creativecommons.org/licenses/by/4.0/).

1. Introduction

In children, fractures of the distal forearm are remarkably common. In most cases, they are the result of a fall on the outstretched hand. These fractures include buckle fractures, greenstick fractures, complete metaphyseal fractures, and fractures involving the growth plate. The latter are commonly classified according to Salter and Harris.

It appears accepted, that non-displaced fractures are treated with a cast, while a long-arm cast is traditionally used for unstable fractures, and a short-arm cast is used for stable fractures [1].

The treatment of displaced distal metaphyseal fractures is less clear. Several aspects have to be taken into account when treating these fractures in children who have open growth plates. These factors include—but are not limited to—the classification of the fracture, the age of the patient, the amount of dislocation in the frontal or lateral plane, the expected remaining growth potential [1], concomitant injuries, and expectations from both the children and the parents. As this list contains factors such as the age of the patient and the remaining growth potential, it is easy to understand that treatment decisions for these fractures are far more complex than in adults, where these parameters are not applicable. Therefore, it is easy to understand, that currently there are no evidence based recommendations regarding the treatment of these injuries depending on patient age, remaining growth, fracture classification and fracture dislocation [2].

Many authors report good results when reducing these fractures with some sort of sedation and/or analgesia and using fixation with a long-arm cast. Some authors recommend an additional K-wire to maintain a reduction in the cast [1]. Even other authors report the use of open reduction and fixation with plates [3,4].

Salter-Harris II fractures are of particular concern as these comprise the majority of physical injuries [5].

In paediatric orthopaedics, traditionally outcome assessment is performed radiographically. For instance, good results are reported when the radiographs demonstrate a good position. However, radiographs might not necessarily capture the subjective outcome assessment of the child. In order to capture the treatment result from the patient's perspective, patient-reported outcome measures (PROMs) have been increasingly used recently. It has been stated that "the ultimate goal of health care is to restore or preserve functioning and well-being related to health, that is health-related quality of life" [6].

There is a lack of studies assessing PROMs in children after they have sustained a fracture of the distal forearm. It is also unknown if the health-related quality of life (HRQoL) differs by fracture classification, fracture severity, or treatment performed.

Therefore, we have initiated this study to evaluate the HRQoL in children who have sustained a fracture of the distal forearm. In addition, we evaluated if HRQoL was associated with fracture classification, fixation method, secondary displacement, or revision surgery.

2. Materials and Methods

This is a retrospective analysis, in which patients who were treated for a distal fracture of the forearm were contacted by postal mail. The regional ethics committees gave their approval to the study protocol (both the ethcis committees of the Paediatric Clinics of Inselspital, University of Bern, and the Ethics Commission of the Canton of Bern).

There are some methodological similarities to sister studies in which the health-related quality of life (HRQoL) after fractures of the femur [7], lateral third of the clavicle [8], fractures of the proximal humerus [9], or supracondylar fractures of the humerus [10] in children and adolescents were assessed.

2.1. Patients

All sequential patients with an age of up to 16 years, who sustained a fracture of the distal radius or forearm from January to June 2007, January to June 2014, and November 2016 to October 2017 and who were treated at our institution were candidates for inclusion in the study. Serving more than a million people, our facility is among the leading pediatric trauma centers in Switzerland.

Patients were identified on the basis of radiological reports within our Picture Archiving and Communication System.

Exclusion criteria were: (1) other significant trauma requiring therapy, (2) initial treatment performed outside our institution, (3) incapacity to complete the questionnaires because of the language barrier or cognitive limitations (Figure 1).

2.2. Radiological Analysis

Initially, all images were assessed by paediatric radiologists. As a second step, all fractures were categorized using the radiological AO classification system [11]. Interobserver bias was prevented by having one of the authors (A.L.), who did not know the patient's clinical outcome, perform this step. Radiographs were also assessed regarding growth arrest. If that author had doubts about his assessment, he contacted the principal author. In all these cases, the doubts could be clarified. Since the author who classified the images gained more and more experience in assessing the images, he reclassified all images a second time, thereby limiting the probability of intraobserver error.

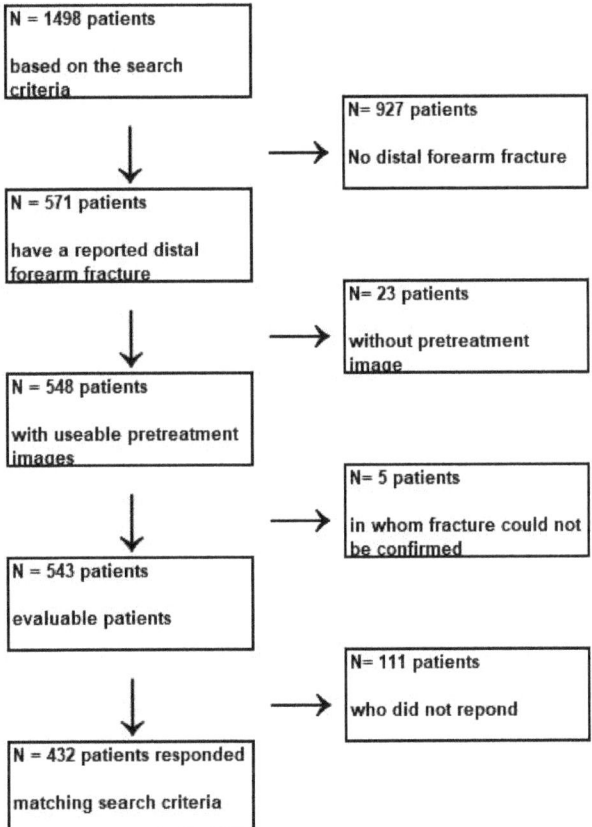

Figure 1. STROBE Participant Flow Chart.

2.3. Data Collection

Starting in February 2018, we mailed study-related information, a consent form, and questionnaires to the participants (or their parents, depending on their age at the time) (Figure 1). Participants who did not reply received three postal-mail-based reminders. To find out why they were not replying, participants who were not yet responding were phoned. At that time, an attempt was made to administer the survey over the phone [10].

As in the sister studies [8–10], we used the disease-specific Quick-DASH (Disabilities of the Arm, Shoulder and Hand) in a validated translation [12,13] as the primary outcome measure. Responses were recorded on a five point Likert scale. Scores were standardised to 0–100, with higher scores indicating more disability. If more than 10% of the items were unanswered, a Quick-DASH score was regarded as missing.

We have chosen the validated translated version of the Paediatric Quality of Life Inventory (PedsQL) as a secondary outcome [14]. Higher scores indicated more physical or social function, and scores ranged from 0–100.

Radiographs and the patient's chart were used to gather information on the patient's demographics, the dates of the injury, the side (right/left), and the chosen treatment. We included questions about handedness and concurrent injuries in the survey [8–10].

We were able to follow up on 432 patients (185 girls, 247 boys) who sustained a fracture of the distal radius or forearm from January to June 2007, January to June 2014, and November 2016 to October 2017, at an average age of 9.3 (SD 3.7) years.

2.4. Treatment Algorithm

2.4.1. Initial Treatment

Non reduction and casting:
If the fracture was not dislocated, we used casting only.

Reduction and casting:
If the fracture was dislocated and the fracture was stable after reduction, we applied an upper-arm cast.

CRPP:
If the fracture was dislocated and the fracture was not stable after reduction, we reduced the fracture and used a percutaneous (unburied) retrograde applied K-wire that was introduced at the tip of the styloid process of the radius and exited the radius proximal of the fracture through the cortex (bicortical fixation). Usually, only one wire was used in order to keep the trauma to the growth-plate to a minimum. A cast was then applied.

If there is adequate pain control and no compromise in perfusion or nerve function, we avoid to perform surgery after midnight and postpone it to the next day [15].

2.4.2. Further Treatment

If the fracture was reduced but no K-wire fixation was used, we perform a radiographic follow-up after 5–7 days in order to exclude a secondary dislocation within the cast.

The cast is usually applied for a period of 4 weeks in patients younger than 10 years and for 5 weeks in patients older than 10 years.

After that time a clinical and radiological follow-up is performed and it is decided if the cast treatment can be discontinued. If a K-wire has been used, typically it can be removed during an outpatient procedure using nitrous oxide and/or nasally applied fentanyl. If the range of motion is restricted, patients are invited back for another appointment after four weeks. Physiotherapy is only taken into consideration at that time. As—in our experience—these cases are rare, they do not justify routine physiotherapy after these common fractures [16].

Neurapraxias are monitored until they resolve spontaneously. Since transient traumatic neurapraxia is frequently noted in this population, these were not considered as complications [10].

2.5. Statistical Analysis

First, we analysed the outcome measures, such as Quick-DASH and PedsQL. Then, we looked for associations between HRQoL and radiological fracture type.

In our dataset, most outcome measures demonstrated a clear ceiling effect—that is, most cases were clustered close to the best conceivable outcome. Such distributions can not be adequately visualized using standard box plots. For this reason, we have selected violin plots instead. In violin plots, the width of the graph represents the probability density of the data (comparable to a mirrored histogram rotated by 90 degrees), allowing a suitable graphical representation [10].

All p-values are two-tailed. We did not perform corrections for multiple comparisons. Statistical analysis was performed using Statistical Package for the Social Sciences (SPSS Inc., Chicago, IL, USA) and R [17].

3. Results

The radius was fractured in 429 cases and the ulna in 175 cases. Both bones were fractured in 173 cases. The most frequent injury of the radius was a buckle fracture (222 children, 51 percent, mean age 8.5 years), followed by a complete metaphyseal fracture (93 children, 22 percent, 9.5 years), Salter-Harris type 2 fracture (62 children, 14 percent, 11.4 years), greenstick fracture (42 children, 10 percent, 9.3 years), Salter-Harris type 1 fracture (5 children, 1%, 12.6 years), and other less frequent injuries (Salter-Harris type 4 (n = 1), Peterson type 1 (n = 2), complex (n = 2)).

The most common treatment was a closed reduction and the application of an above elbow cast in 138 cases (32 percent), followed by a cast without prior reduction (129 children, 30 percent), splint (119 children, 28 percent), and closed reduction with K-wire fixation and above elbow cast (39 cases, 9 percent). Definite treatment was performed initially in 95.8 percent of children, a modification (new cast or cast wedging) was performed in 7 cases (1.6 percent), and revision surgery was performed in 11 cases (2.5 percent). There were no open reductions and there was no plate osteosynthesis (Table 1).

After a mean follow-up of 4.2 years, patients with a buckle fracture had a mean Quick-DASH of 3.3, at a scale of 0–100, with lower values representing better HRQoL (complete fracture: 1.5; greenstick: 1.5; Salter-Harris type 1: 0.9; Salter-Harris type 2: 4.1; others: 0.9). The mean function score of the PedsQL ranged from 93.0 for SH-2 fractures to 97.9 for complete fractures, at a scale of 0–100, with higher values representing better HRQoL (Table 2, Figure 2).

A graphical presentation of the physical and the social function score of the Peds-QL is given in Figures 3 and 4.

There was no statistically significant difference in the association between HRQoL and AO radiological classification or type of surgical treatment. In addition, there were no statistically significant associations between HRQoL and the need for revision surgery in the univariate analysis (Figure 5).

There were no complications requiring interventions, revision surgery, or manipulation. There was no growth arrest.

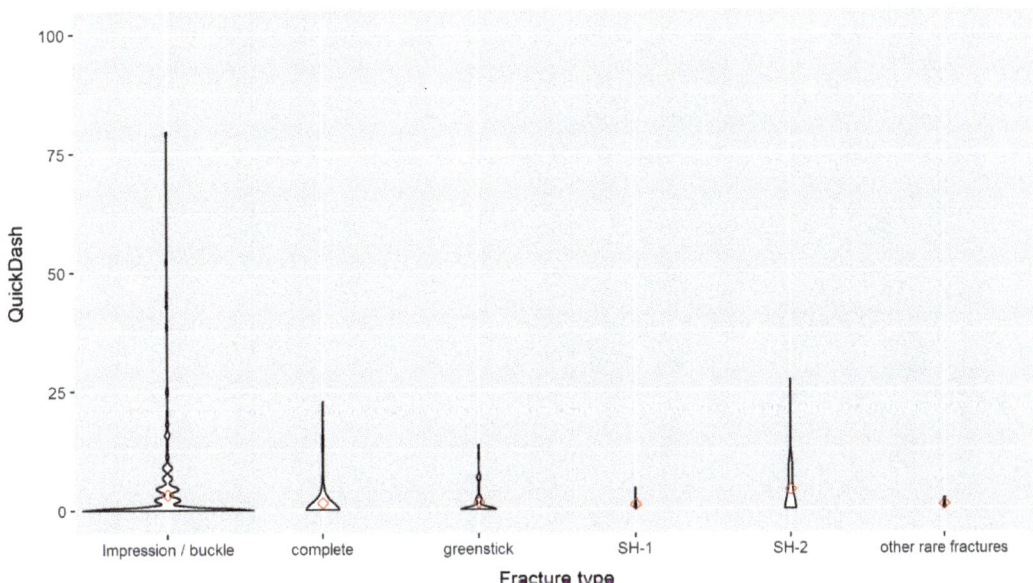

Figure 2. The primary outcome Quick-DASH at follow-up by fracture type of the radius. Since there were considerable ceiling effects, we used violin plots for the graphical presentation. Please see the methods section for a description of the violin plots.

Table 1. Baseline characteristics.

		Type of Radius Fracture																					
		Impression/Buckle				Compete Metaphyseal				Greenstick				SH1				SH2				Other Rare Fractures				Total			
		n	%	Mean	SD	n	%	Mean	SD	n	%	Mean	SD	n	%	Mean	SD	n	%	Mean	SD	n	%	Mean	SD	n	%	Mean	SD
gender	female	112	50%			31	33%			18	43%			1	20%			22	35%			1	20%			185	43%		
	male	110	50%			62	67%			24	57%			4	80%			40	65%			4	80%			244	57%		
Age at the time of injury [years]		222		8.52	3.87	93		9.45	3.36	42		9.29	2.97	5		12.55	1.62	62		11.24	3.07	5		9.95	3.64	429		9.25	3.68
Age at the time of injury	0 to <3 years	23	10%			1	1%			2	5%							4	6%			1	20%			26	6%		
	3 to <6 years	36	16%			18	19%			3	7%							9	15%			1	20%			62	14%		
	6 to <9 years	62	28%			18	19%			14	33%			1	20%			23	37%			1	20%			104	24%		
	9 to <12 years	51	23%			32	34%			15	36%							26	42%			2	40%			123	29%		
	12 years and older	50	23%			24	26%			8	19%			4	80%			26	42%			2	40%			114	27%		
Follow-up duration [years]		222		3.93	4.07	93		4.72	4.63	42		3.79	4.24	5		7.13	6.25	62		4.28	4.44	5		5.47	5.93	429		4.18	4.31
Injured side (right vs. left)	right	82	37%			38	41%			22	52%			4	80%			26	42%			1	20%			173	41%		
	left	134	61%			54	58%			20	48%			1	20%			35	56%			4	80%			248	58%		
	both	4	2%			1	1%											1	2%							6	1%		
Injured side (dominat vs. non-dominant)	non-dominant side	138	63%			48	52%			23	55%			1	20%			42	68%			3	60%			255	60%		
	dominat side	82	37%			45	48%			19	45%			4	80%			20	32%			2	40%			172	40%		
Skin injury	No, the skin was intact	212	96%			87	94%			39	93%			4	80%			56	90%			5	100%			403	94%		
	Yes, there was a graze	9	4%			6	6%			2	5%			1	20%			4	6%							22	5%		
	Yes, a skin suture had to be done									1	2%							2	3%							3	1%		
Vessel injury	No, not that I know of	221	100%			92	99%			42	100%			5	100%			62	100%			5	100%			427	100%		
	Yes, but it was not necessary to suture a vessel or an artery	1	0%			1	1%																			2	0%		
	Yes, it was necessary to perform vascular sutures																												
Numbness in fingers	No	180	81%			68	75%			34	81%			4	80%			37	60%			4	80%			327	77%		
	Yes, less than a week	37	17%			20	22%			8	19%			1	20%			19	31%			1	20%			85	20%		
	Yes, for several weeks	4	2%			1	1%											6	10%							12	3%		
	Yes, for more than 3 months	1	0%			1	1%																			2	0%		
	Yes, still ongoing					1	1%																			1	0%		

Table 2. Results by type of radius fracture.

		Impression/Buckle				Compete Metaphyseal				Greenstick				Type of Radius Fracture SH1				SH2				Other Rare Fractures				Total			
		n	%	Mean	SD	n	%	Mean	SD	n	%	Mean	SD	n	%	Mean	SD	n	%	Mean	SD	n	%	Mean	SD	n	%	Mean	SD
Max. ROM for pronation	90 degrees	213	96%			85	91%			39	93%			5	100%			56	90%			4	80%			402	94%		
	45 degrees	8	4%			8	9%			3	7%							6	10%			1	20%			26	6%		
	0 degrees																												
Max. ROM for supination	90 degrees	218	99%			87	94%			40	95%			5	100%			61	98%			5	100%			416	97%		
	45 degrees	2	1%			6	6%			2	5%							1	2%							11	3%		
	0 degrees	1	0%																							1	0%		
Ability to throw a ball with the injured side	Yes, that is easily possible	209	95%			88	96%			42	100%			5	100%			61	98%			5	100%			410	96%		
	Yes, but just a bit	8	4%			4	4%											1	2%							13	3%		
	No, I am not able to	4	2%																							4	1%		
Impression that the forearm limits the force of the whole arm	not at all	186	84%			78	84%			36	86%			5	100%			39	63%			3	60%			347	81%		
	A little bit	31	14%			15	16%			5	12%							19	31%			1	20%			71	17%		
	moderate	2	1%							1	2%							3	5%			1	20%			7	2%		
	quite	3	1%															1	2%							4	1%		
	very much																												
Satisfaction with cosmetic result	very satisfied	205	94%			73	81%			38	90%			3	60%			45	74%			4	80%			368	87%		
	rather satisfied	11	5%			10	11%			3	7%			2	40%			11	18%			1	20%			38	9%		
	moderately satisfied	1	0%			5	6%			1	2%							3	5%							10	2%		
	A little bit satisfied	1	0%															2	3%							3	1%		
	Not satisfied at all					2	2%																			2	0%		
Current treatment with pain killers	No	190	99%			84	100%			37	97%			3	100%			55	98%			5	100%			374	99%		
	Yes	2	1%							1	3%							1	2%							4	1%		
Point in time when forearm was used regularly	Immediately after treatment	5	2%			1	1%			1	2%															7	2%		
	Immediately after removal of cast	130	59%			43	46%			15	37%			4	80%			26	42%			3	60%			221	52%		
	Other	66	30%			39	42%			17	41%			1	20%			28	45%			2	40%			152	36%		
	Do not know	19	9%			10	11%			8	20%							8	13%							46	11%		
Weeks after forearm was used regularly		222		4.44	2.96	93		8.00	5.72	42		5.59	4.32	5				62		6.38	3.19	5		5.00	4.24	429		5.86	4.26
Revision	definite treatment initially	221	100%			83	89%			42	100%			5	100%			55	89%			5	100%			411	96%		
	modification (cast or cast wedging	1	0%			5	5%											1	2%							7	2%		
	revision surgery					5	5%											6	10%							11	3%		
Quick-DASH (0–100)		222		3.30	8.89	93		1.47	3.87	42		1.46	3.17	5		0.91	2.03	62		4.11	6.13	5		0.91	1.24	429		2.78	7.17
PedsQL, physical function (0–100)		222		9.16	9.01	93		97.88	4.57	42		97.47	4.89	5		95.00	7.19	62		93.04	13.03	5		97.50	3.42	429		96.21	8.70
PedsQL, psychosocial function (0–100)		222		93.04	8.92	93		95.38	8.50	42		95.42	6.35	5		90.00	7.91	62		91.45	11.51	5		87.00	15.29	429		93.44	9.20

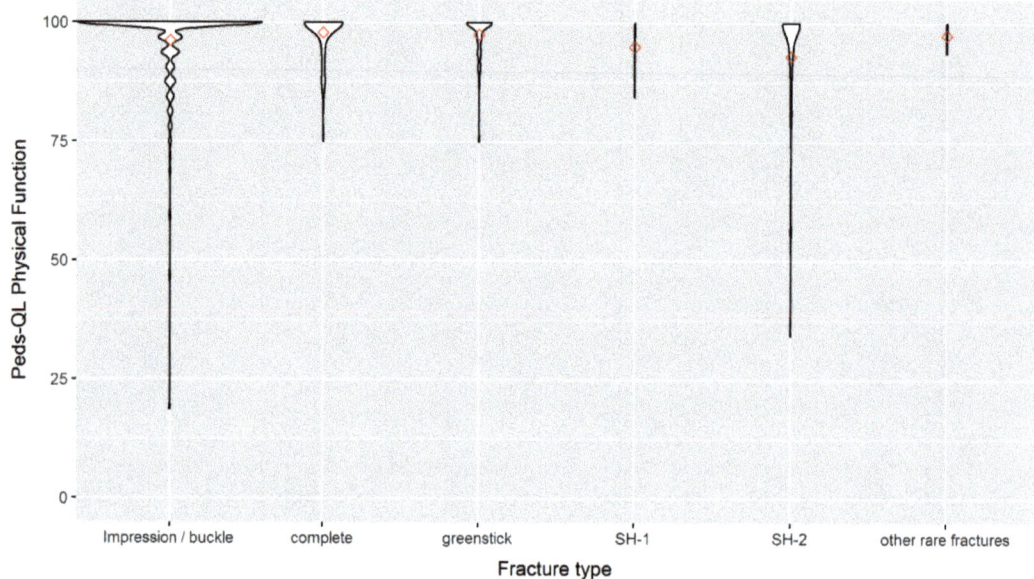

Figure 3. Peds-QL physical function at follow-up by fracture type of the radius.

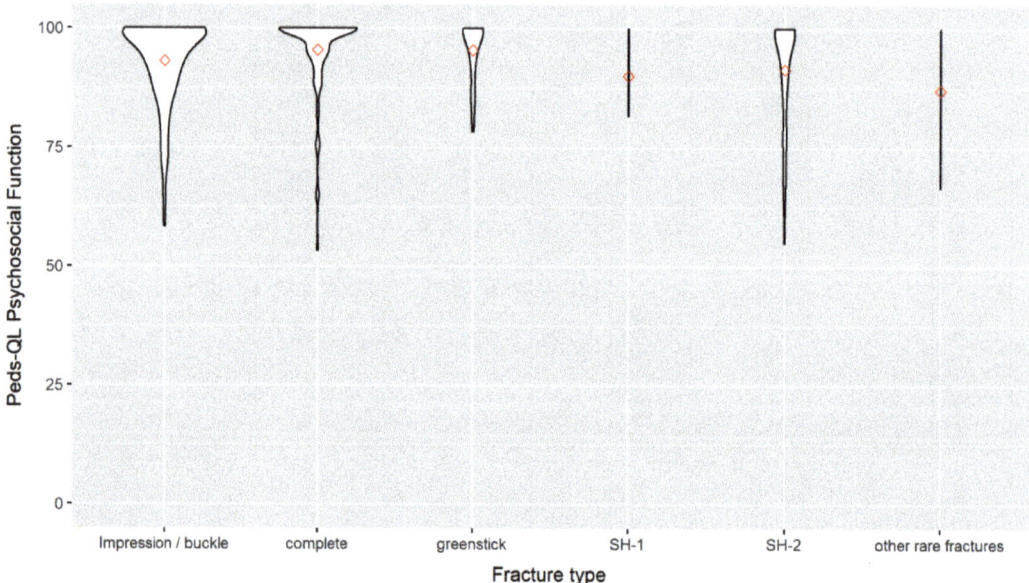

Figure 4. Peds-QL social function at follow-up by fracture type of the radius.

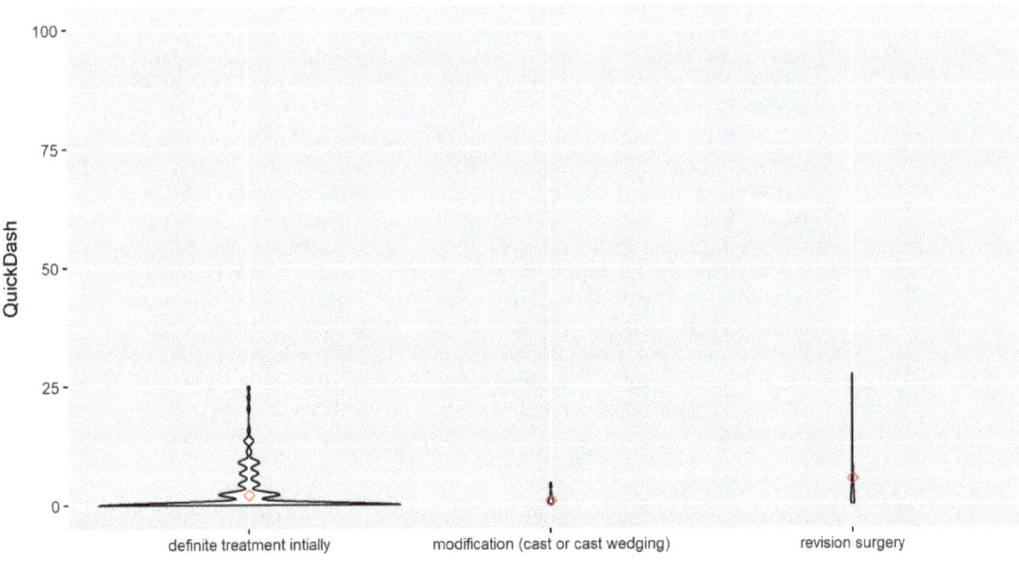

Figure 5. The primary outcome Quick-DASH at follow-up by revision. Please note that patients with impression/buckle fractures are excluded, since a revision is not performed in those fractures.

4. Discussion

This study clearly showed that the treatment protocol described in this study for children with a fracture of the distal forearm is associated with good health-related quality of life (HRQoL) as measured with the Quick-DASH and the Peds-QL at a mean of 4.2 years follow-up. Our analysis of this injury is one of the largest in the literature and one of the few assessing the HRQoL in this population. These excellent results were independent of radiological fracture type, or treatment performed.

4.1. Health-Related Quality of Life and Radiological Fracture Type

The main focus of our study was to report the HRQoL of our population who were treated according to our treatment regime. As could be shown, the results are—on the whole—remarkably good with only minor differences between study groups.

As the most common injury of the radius was a buckle fracture (51%), which is considered to heal without any sequela, we initially considered to exclude this group in our study. However, we reckoned that this group might serve as an appropriate control group since we expected worse HRQoL in the children who sustained other fracture types. To our surprise, patients with buckle fractures had a mean Quick-DASH of 3.3 on a scale of 0–100, which was worse than the HRQoL of the complete metaphyseal fractures (Quick-DASH 1.5), the greenstick fractures (1.5), or the Salter-Harris-1 fractures (0.9). Only the Salter-Harris-2 fracture had a slightly worse HRQoL (4.1) when compared to the buckle fractures. However, it must be noted that the differences are slight and should therefore not be overinterpreted. Further studies are needed to assess if these non-perfect numbers for buckle fractures can be indeed attributed to the fracture, or if it is just random noise that is inherent to the recording of the outcome measure.

If only a cast fixation has been chosen there is a risk of a secondary dislocation. For this reason, we always aim to follow up patients with a risk for a secondary dislocation at 5–7 days after cast application. As could be seen from the results, a modification (new cast or cast wedging) was performed in 7 cases (1.6 percent), and revision surgery was performed in 11 cases (2.5 percent). We, therefore, asked if the HRQoL was inferior in this patient group. As can be seen in Figure 5, there was a good HRQoL in the patients undergoing cast wedging and a slightly inferior HRQoL in the patients who have undergone revision surgery. Further analysis revealed that among that group, patients with a Salter-Harris 2 fracture had slightly worse scores; however, those scores were not statistically significant.

We tried to compare our results to the literature. Unfortunately, we were no able to find many other studies assessing outcome measures such as the Quick-DASH or the Peds-QL in patients who had undergone a fracture of the distal radius or forearm. Musters et al. reported DASH scores for 51 children who underwent either above or below elbow cast for mainly greenstick fractures of the distal forearm and reported DASH scores of 2.1 and 4.4. for these groups [18]. Peterlein et al. [19] reported a remarkably good mean DASH score of 0.4 in 90 patients who had undergone elastic-stable intramedullary nailing (ESIN) of diaphyseal forearm fractures in childhood fractures. In addition, there are two study protocols for fractures of the forearm shaft [20] or metaphyseal [21], but no results yet. Overall, our Quick-DASH is comparable to the few other studies published up to this time, although patient numbers in that studies are much smaller and different fractures were examined.

4.2. Limitations

Our observations must be interpreted in light of several limitations, which apply to the sister studies [7–10] as well: First, as this was a mono-centre study it could be argued that external validity is limited. However, a bias in the run-in phase is unlikely because we are the only hospital in a large geographic area addressing paediatric trauma and we included all consecutive cases, making a high external validity probable [8]. However, given that there is significant diversity in orthopaedic treatments across and within nations, we are aware that no single study is capable of giving full external validity [22]. Second, the radiographs under examination were not specially prepared for this analysis; they were just made routinely. Therefore, the setting of these radiographs is comparable to the situation of the clinician [8]. Since the individual classifying the fractures was unaware of the patient's clinical outcome, the radiological assessment could be viewed as being blinded [8]. Third, due to its retrospective design, this study suffers from methodological weaknesses common in this design. This includes for example no intermediate data points and missing data on the HRQoL prior to the injury. Although the latter is viewed as a methodological flaw in research analyzing adult fractures, this does not always hold true for paediatric fractures because children typically do not have physical limits prior to the injury and we excluded children with prior or concurrent injuries. Therefore, it is reasonable to believe that limitations of the disease-specific outcome measure are in fact attributable to the injury [8]. Fourth, the Quick-DASH has not yet been formally validated in this age group and in some cases the parents filled in the questionnaire based on their assessments of their children's functioning (by proxy). However, the Quick-DASH has been used by numerous authors for the evaluation of paediatric other upper extremity fractures before [23–34]. Consequently it appears, that the DASH/Quick-DASH is most widely utilized outcome measure for paediatric upper extremity fractures. Fifth, our follow-up rate was 80%, which is just the recommended rate for follow-ups. However, most other studies we are aware of have a similar or lower rate of follow-up, e.g., [25,35–37]. To our knowledge, no study that examined distal forearm fractures was able to evaluate the HRQoL in as many children as did our investigation (n = 432). Sixth, although we had a large sample size it is possible that we missed existing associations of HRQoL to fracture patterns or treatment chosen. Given the excellent results of the overall group, which even exhibits a ceiling effect, it is unlikely that any such association would become clinically relevant. Seventh, we analyzed children of different time periods, as we assumed there might be differences over time. However, that topic will be the subject of further analysis in the future.

5. Conclusions

In conclusion, we report that children who sustained a fracture of the distal radius or forearm and who were treated according to this protocol had an excellent health-related quality of life. These findings show that the treatment protocol followed in this study is clear, does not include open reductions or plate fixations, and is associated with excellent treatment outcomes for this frequent injury.

Author Contributions: Conceptualization, T.R.L.; methodology, T.R.L.; validation, A.L., S.M.B., N.K. and K.Z.; formal analysis, T.R.L.; investigation, A.L.; resources, T.R.L., A.L., N.K., K.Z., S.M.B.; data curation, A.L.; writing—original draft preparation, T.R.L.; writing—review and editing, T.R.L., A.L., S.M.B., N.K., K.Z.; visualization, T.R.L.; supervision, T.R.L.; project administration, T.R.L., A.L., S.M.B., K.Z. All authors have read and agreed to the published version of the manuscript.

Funding: This research received no external funding.

Institutional Review Board Statement: The study was conducted in accordance with the Declaration of Helsinki, and approved by both the Institutional Review Board of the Paediatric Clinics of Inselspital, University of Bern, and the Ethics Commission of the Canton of Bern (Basec-Nr: 2016-00011, date of approval: 3 May 2016), both in Switzerland.

Informed Consent Statement: Informed consent was obtained from all subjects or their parents involved in the study.

Conflicts of Interest: The authors declare no conflict of interest.

References

1. Dua, K.; Abzug, J.M.; Sesko, B.A.; Cornwall, R.; Wyrick, T.O. Pediatric Distal Radius Fractures. *Instr. Course Lect.* **2017**, *66*, 447–460.
2. Bašković, M. Acceptable Angulation of Forearm Fractures in Children. *Rev. Esp. Cir. Ortop. Traumatol.* **2022**, S1888-4415. [CrossRef] [PubMed]
3. Di Giacinto, S.; Pica, G.; Stasi, A.; Scialpi, L.; Tomarchio, A.; Galeotti, A.; Podvorica, V.; dell'Unto, A.; Meccariello, L. The challenge of the surgical treatment of paediatric distal radius/forearm fracture: K wire vs plate fixation—Outcomes assessment. *Med. Glas* **2021**, *18*, 208–215.
4. Cha, S.M.; Shin, H.D. Buttress plating for volar Barton fractures in children: Salter–Harris II distal radius fractures in sagittal plane. *J. Pediatr. Orthop. B* **2019**, *28*, 73–78. [CrossRef]
5. Larsen, M.C.; Bohm, K.C.; Rizkala, A.R.; Ward, C.M. Outcomes of Nonoperative Treatment of Salter-Harris II Distal Radius Fractures: A Systematic Review. *Hand* **2016**, *11*, 29–35. [CrossRef]
6. Osoba, D.; King, M. Meaningful differences. In *Assessing Quality of Life in Clinical Trials*; Fayers, P., Hays, R.D., Eds.; Oxford University Press: Oxford, UK, 2005; pp. 243–257.
7. Liebs, T.R.; Meßling, A.; Milosevic, M.; Berger, S.M.; Ziebarth, K. Health-Related Quality of Life after Adolescent Fractures of the Femoral Shaft Stabilized by a Lateral Entry Femoral Nail. *Children* **2022**, *9*, 327. [CrossRef]
8. Liebs, T.; Ryser, B.; Kaiser, N.; Slongo, T.; Berger, S.; Ziebarth, K. Health-related Quality of Life After Fractures of the Lateral Third of the Clavicle in Children and Adolescents. *J. Pediatr. Orthop.* **2019**, *39*, e542–e547. [CrossRef]
9. Liebs, T.R.; Rompen, I.; Berger, S.M.; Ziebarth, K. Health-related quality of life after conservatively and surgically-treated paediatric proximal humeral fractures. *J. Child. Orthop.* **2021**, *15*, 204–214. [CrossRef] [PubMed]
10. Liebs, T.R.; Burgard, M.; Kaiser, N.; Slongo, T.; Berger, S.; Ryser, B.; Ziebarth, K. Health-related quality of life after paediatric supracondylar humeral fractures. *Bone Jt. J.* **2020**, *102-B*, 755–765. [CrossRef]
11. Slongo, T.; Audigé, L.; AO Paediatric Classification Group (Eds.) Distal metaphyseal fractures (13-M). In *AO Pediatric Comprehensive Classification of Long-Bone Fractures (PCCF)*; AO Foundation: Davos, Switzerland, 2007; p. 15.
12. Bot, S.D.; Terwee, C.B.; van der Windt, D.A.; Bouter, L.M.; Dekker, J.; de Vet, H.C. Clinimetric evaluation of shoulder disability ques-tionnaires: A systematic review of the literature. *Ann. Rheum Dis.* **2004**, *63*, 335–341. [CrossRef] [PubMed]
13. Germann, G.; Harth, A.; Wind, G.; Demir, E. Standardisation and validation of the German version 2.0 of the Disability of Arm, Shoulder, Hand (DASH) questionnaire. *Unfallchirurg* **2003**, *106*, 13–19. [CrossRef] [PubMed]
14. Mahan, S.T.; Kalish, L.A.; Connell, P.L.; Harris, M.; Abdul-Rahim, Z.; Waters, P. PedsQL Correlates to PODCI in Pediatric Orthopaedic Outpatient Clinic. *J. Pediatr. Orthop.* **2014**, *34*, e22–e26. [CrossRef] [PubMed]
15. Schmid, T.; Joeris, A.; Slongo, T.; Ahmad, S.S.; Ziebarth, K. Displaced supracondylar humeral fractures: Influence of delay of surgery on the incidence of open reduction, complications and outcome. *Arch. Orthop. Trauma. Surg.* **2015**, *135*, 963–969. [CrossRef] [PubMed]

16. Caruso, G.; Caldari, E.; Sturla, F.D.; Caldaria, A.; Re, D.L.; Pagetti, P.; Palummieri, F.; Massari, L. Management of pediatric forearm fractures: What is the best therapeutic choice? A narrative review of the literature. *Musculoskelet. Surg.* **2020**, *105*, 225–234. [CrossRef] [PubMed]
17. R Development Core Team. *R: A Language and Environment for Statistical Computing*; R Foundation for Statistical Computing: Vienna, Austria, 2008.
18. Musters, L.; Diederix, L.W.; Roth, K.C.; Edomskis, P.P.; Kraan, G.A.; Allema, J.H.; Reijman, M.; Colaris, J.W. Below-elbow cast sufficient for treatment of minimally displaced metaphyseal both-bone fractures of the distal forearm in children: Long-term results of a randomized controlled multicenter trial. *Acta Orthop.* **2021**, *92*, 468–471. [CrossRef]
19. Peterlein, C.-D.; Modzel, T.; Hagen, L.; Ruchholtz, S.; Krüger, A. Long-term results of elastic-stable intramedullary nailing (ESIN) of diaphyseal forearm fractures in children. *Medicine* **2019**, *98*, e14743. [CrossRef]
20. Grahn, P.; Sinikumpu, J.-J.; Nietosvaara, Y.; Syvänen, J.; Salonen, A.; Ahonen, M.; Helenius, I. Casting versus flexible intramedullary nailing in displaced forearm shaft fractures in children aged 7–12 years: A study protocol for a randomised controlled trial. *BMJ Open* **2021**, *11*, e048248. [CrossRef]
21. Laaksonen, T.; Stenroos, A.; Puhakka, J.; Kosola, J.; Kautiainen, H.; Rämö, L.; Nietosvaara, Y. Casting in finger trap traction without reduction versus closed reduction and percutaneous pin fixation of dorsally displaced, over-riding distal metaphyseal radius fractures in children under 11 years old: A study protocol of a randomised controlled trial. *BMJ Open* **2021**, *11*, e045689. [CrossRef]
22. Ackerman, I.N.; Dieppe, P.A.; March, L.M.; Roos, E.M.; Nilsdotter, A.K.; Brown, G.C.; Sloan, K.E.; Osborne, R.H. Variation in age and physical status prior to total knee and hip replacement surgery: A comparison of centers in Australia and Europe. *Arthritis Care Res.* **2009**, *61*, 166–173. [CrossRef]
23. Al Aubaidi, Z.; Pedersen, N.W.; Nielsen, K.D. Radial neck fractures in children treated with the centromedullary Metaizeau technique. *Injury* **2012**, *43*, 301–305. [CrossRef]
24. Lawrence, J.T.; Patel, N.M.; Macknin, J.; Flynn, J.M.; Cameron, D.; Wolfgruber, H.C.; Ganley, T.J. Return to competitive sports after medial epicondyle fractures in adolescent athletes: Results of operative and nonoperative treatment. *Am. J. Sports Med.* **2013**, *41*, 1152–1157. [CrossRef] [PubMed]
25. Isa, A.D.; Furey, A.; Stone, C. Functional outcome of supracondylar elbow fractures in children: A 3- to 5-year follow-up. *Can. J. Surg.* **2014**, *57*, 241–246. [CrossRef] [PubMed]
26. Marengo, L.; Canavese, F.; Cravino, M.; De, R.V.; Rousset, M.; Samba, A.; Mansour, M.; Andreacchio, A. Outcome of Displaced Fractures of the Distal Metaphyseal-Diaphyseal Junction of the Humerus in Children Treated With Elastic Stable Intramedullary Nails. *J. Pediatr. Orthop.* **2014**, *35*, 611–616. [CrossRef]
27. Moraleda, L.; Valencia, M.; Barco, R.; Gonzalez-Moran, G. Natural history of unreduced Gartland type-II supracondylar fractures of the humerus in children: A two to thirteen-year follow-up study. *J. Bone Jt. Surg. Am.* **2013**, *95*, 28–34. [CrossRef]
28. Belthur, M.V.; Iobst, C.A.; Bor, N.; Segev, E.; Eidelman, M.; Standard, S.C.; Herzenberg, J.E. Correction of Cubitus Varus After Pediatric Supracondylar Elbow Fracture: Alternative Method Using the Taylor Spatial Frame. *J. Pediatr. Orthop.* **2016**, *36*, 608–617. [CrossRef]
29. Davids, J.R.; Lamoreaux, D.C.; Brooker, R.C.; Tanner, S.L.; Westberry, D.E. Translation step-cut osteotomy for the treatment of post-traumatic cubitus varus. *J. Pediatr. Orthop.* **2011**, *31*, 353–365. [CrossRef] [PubMed]
30. Smith, J.T.; McFeely, E.D.; Bae, D.S.; Waters, P.M.; Micheli, L.J.; Kocher, M.S. Operative Fixation of Medial Humeral Epicondyle Fracture Nonunion in Children. *J. Pediatr. Orthop.* **2010**, *30*, 644–648. [CrossRef] [PubMed]
31. Schulz, J.; Moor, M.; Roocroft, J.; Bastrom, T.P.; Pennock, A.T. Functional and Radiographic Outcomes of Nonoperative Treatment of Displaced Adolescent Clavicle Fractures. *J. Bone Jt. Surg.* **2013**, *95*, 1159–1165. [CrossRef]
32. Namdari, S.; Ganley, T.J.; Baldwin, K.; Sampson, N.R.; Hosalkar, H.; Nikci, V.; Wells, L. Fixation of Displaced Midshaft Clavicle Fractures in Skeletally Immature Patients. *J. Pediatr. Orthop.* **2011**, *31*, 507–511. [CrossRef]
33. Randsborg, P.-H.; Fuglesang, H.F.S.; Røtterud, J.H.; Hammer, O.-L.; Sivertsen, E.A. Long-term Patient-reported Outcome After Fractures of the Clavicle in Patients Aged 10 to 18 Years. *J. Pediatr. Orthop.* **2014**, *34*, 393–399. [CrossRef]
34. Bogdan, A.; Quintin, J.; Schuind, F. Treatment of displaced supracondylar humeral fractures in children by humero-ulnar external fixation. *Int. Orthop.* **2016**, *40*, 2409–2415. [CrossRef] [PubMed]
35. Ernat, J.; Ho, C.; Wimberly, R.L.; Jo, C.; Riccio, A.I. Fracture Classification Does Not Predict Functional Outcomes in Supracondylar Humerus Fractures: A Prospective Study. *J. Pediatr. Orthop.* **2017**, *37*, e233–e237. [CrossRef] [PubMed]
36. McKee, M.D.; Kim, J.; Kebaish, K.; Stephen, D.J.; Kreder, H.J.; Schemitsch, E.H. Functional outcome after open supracondylar fractures of the humerus. The effect of the surgical approach. *J. Bone Jt. Surg. Br.* **2000**, *82*, 646–651. [CrossRef] [PubMed]
37. Wang, S.I.; Kwon, T.Y.; Hwang, H.P.; Kim, J.R. Functional outcomes of Gartland III supracondylar humerus fractures with early neurovascular complications in children: A retrospective observational study. *Medicine* **2017**, *96*, e7148. [CrossRef]

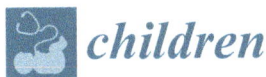

Article

Mid-Term Results of Distal Femoral Extension and Shortening Osteotomy in Treating Flexed Knee Gait in Children with Cerebral Palsy

Andreas Geisbüsch [1,*], Matthias C. M. Klotz [2], Cornelia Putz [1], Tobias Renkawitz [1] and Axel Horsch [1]

1. Department of Orthopedics, Heidelberg University Hospital, 69118 Heidelberg, Germany
2. Marienkrankenhaus Soest, Orthopedics and Trauma Surgery, 59594 Soest, Germany
* Correspondence: andreas.geisbuesch@med.uni-heidelberg.de

Abstract: Background: Distal femoral extension and shortening osteotomy (DFESO) seems to be an effective method for the treatment of flexed knee gait in children with cerebral palsy. Nevertheless, studies investigating the mid- and long-term outcomes after such procedures are lacking in the literature. Therefore, the purpose of this study was to assess the mid-term outcomes regarding sagittal plane kinematics of the knee after DFESO with or without concomitant patella advancement. Furthermore, an evaluation of the postoperative course and possible recurrence of flexed knee gait was planned. **Methods:** In a prospective observational study, 19 patients (28 limbs; mean age 11.8 years (6.7–16.0 years)) were examined using 3-D gait analysis and clinical exam before (E_0) and at a mean of 38 months (E_2: 24–55 months) after surgery. Fifteen patients (22 limbs) had an additional first postoperative gait analysis (E_1) after a mean of 14 (10–20) months after surgery. In these patients, the postoperative changes between the short-term and mid-term gait analyses were evaluated. **Results:** DFESO led to a significant decrease in flexed knee gait with an improvement in sagittal plane kinematics during the stance phase. In addition, a slightly increased anterior pelvic tilt was observed at E_1, and we found a tendency towards stiff knee gait with a decrease in mean knee flexion in swing at E_2. **Conclusions:** DFESO led to a significant improvement in flexed knee gait in children with cerebral palsy. The therapeutic effect seems to be lasting on mid-term follow-up with a slight overall tendency to recurrence.

Keywords: distal femoral extension; shortening osteotomy; DEFSO; cerebral palsy

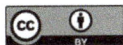

1. Introduction

Flexed knee gait is one of the most common gait patterns in children with cerebral palsy. It impairs gait and leads to increased energy consumption and restriction of ambulation [1]. Apart from the restrictions in gait and self-independence, flexed knee gait may cause anterior knee pain due to increased pressure on the anterior part of the knee and chondromalacia [2]. One of the main pathologic findings in patients showing flexed knee gait is an abnormal tone and/or shortening of the hamstrings [1]. Therefore, lengthening of the hamstrings as a part of single-event multilevel surgery (SEMLS) has been successfully performed for this condition for many years [3–7]. Despite good short- and mid-term results after hamstring lengthening, deterioration in gait and recurrence of flexed knee gait have been reported [8]. A further side effect of hamstring lengthening is an increase in anterior pelvic tilt, which might mediate the recurrence of flexed knee gait [9–11]. Attempts to convert the muscle group into a monoarticular function also showed no improvement in pelvic inclination [8,12]. Over the past years, an increasing number of studies reported the results of treatment of flexed knee gait through distal femoral extension osteotomy with or without shortening of the femur [13–17]. The procedure showed promising short-term results with excellent correction of flexed knee gait [13,18,19]. However, the correction also seems to have an impact on the anterior pelvic inclination [19]. This increase in pelvic tilt might be due to a decreased stabilization of the pelvis due to the relative and functional lengthening of the hamstrings [20]. In addition to that, the tilt of the pelvis also depends on the muscle tone of the rectus femoris, which acts as an antagonist to the hamstrings [8,16]. Nevertheless, in a previous study, Klotz et al. found that simultaneous recession of the rectus femoris could not prevent an increase in anterior pelvic tilt after distal femoral extension and shortening osteotomy [19]. Reports on mid-term and long-term results of DFESO are still scarce [21,22].

Boyer et al. reported the first long-term results of DFESO with patella tendon advancement in crouch gait. They reported a superior effect of DFESO plus patella tendon advancement compared to other methods and significantly less recurrence of flexed knee gait after a period of 13 years [21]. Kuchen et al. reported maintained improvements of sagittal gait kinematics nine years after patellar tendon shortening combined with DFEO [22].

The objective of this study was to assess the mid-term results after distal femoral extension (plus shortening) osteotomy (DFE(S)O) with or without concomitant patella advancement (PA). We sought to evaluate the impact of DFE(S)O on sagittal plane knee joint kinematics, pelvic tilt and general gait quality in patients with cerebral palsy. We hypothesized that DFS(E)O improves sagittal plane gait kinematics, and the changes are maintained until mid-term follow-up (24–60 month). We further hypothesized that DFS(E)O increases pelvic tilt.

2. Methods

2.1. Study Design and Patient Selection

This monocentric prospective observational study evaluates the results of a study population that was treated with DFESO as a part of SEMLS in the Orthopaedic Department of the University Hospital Heidelberg. All included patients had (1) a preoperative three-dimensional (3-D) gait analysis (E_0) prior to the surgical intervention, (2) a GMFCS level I–III (ambulatory walkers), (3) flexed knee gait (defined as a minimum knee flexion during stance of more than one standard deviation compared to an age-matched control group), (4) a bilateral spastic cerebral palsy (BSCP) as the underlying pathology and were (5) between 6 and 16 years old. Patients who underwent surgical treatment or Botulinum toxin injections within the last six months prior to surgery were not considered (exclusion criteria). Patients were considered for mid-term evaluation if postoperative three-dimensional (3-D) gait analysis data were available between 24 and 60 months after surgery (E_2). If an additional 3-D gait analysis was available postoperatively within 18 months, we defined the results as first postoperative control (E_1) to evaluate possible changes between the short-term and mid-term outcomes of these patients. Furthermore, we formed two subgroups of patients that had or had not undergone simultaneous patella tendon advancement in context with the DFESO.

The local ethics committee approved the study.

2.2. Operative Procedure

The indication for DFESO was set in patients with a flexed knee gait and an aberration of more than one standard deviation from the normal collective in the minimum knee flexion during stance in the 3-D gait analysis (less than eight degrees of minimum knee flexion). The amount of correction was defined with the clinical examination of the flexion contracture intraoperatively [19]. The operation was performed as described by Novacheck et al. and Brunner et al. [14,23], with a standard lateral approach to the distal femur. A ventrally based trapezoid-shaped osteotomy of the distal femur was performed, and after correction of the deformity, it was fixed with a plate. The fixation was performed with blade plates (Implantcast, Buxtehude, Germany) in 15 cases, locking plates by Königssee (Königsee Implantate, Allendorf, Germany) in 3 cases, and locking plates of DePuySynthes (DePuySynthes, Westchester, NY, USA) in 1 case. An additional patella advancement was performed in the presence of patella alta. As the surgery was performed within other SELMS procedures, additional surgical interventions were performed if necessary.

2.3. Postoperative Treatment

In accordance with the previously described regime of postoperative treatment after DFESO [19], patients were primarily immobilized in plaster casts with a rigid connection between the casts to ensure an external rotation of the leg of 10–15° degrees. A slight knee flexion of 10° was applied. Early physiotherapeutic treatment was administered in all patients with passive and active mobilization of both the hips and knee joint starting at the first day after surgery. Knee flexion was limited to 40° for two weeks and 60° between the second and fourth postoperative week. All children were treated by a team of orthopedic surgeons in cooperation with physiotherapists and nursing staff with specialized training. All children were referred to rehabilitation institutions specializing in neuromuscular diseases in children after the consolidation of the osteotomy was achieved and weight-bearing was permitted.

2.4. Gait Analysis

Gait analysis and clinical examination were undertaken by physiotherapists and a study nurse specialized in pediatric neuro-developmental therapy. All patients were able to walk freely and asked to walk barefoot on a seven-meter-long walkway at a self-selected speed. Skin-mounted markers were applied to the bony landmarks according to a standard protocol. A Vicon camera system (Vicon®, Oxford Metrics, Oxford, UK) and two piezoelectric force plates (Kistler®, Winterthur, Switzerland) were used, and joint kinematics were calculated with Vicon-Workstation® (Oxford Metrics, Oxford, UK) according to the protocol of Kabada et al. [24]. Kinematic data were acquired for the knee and pelvis. The physical examination recorded the range of motion and popliteal angle.

2.5. Data Acquisition and Evaluation

Nineteen patients (28 limbs) met the inclusion criteria mentioned above and were selected from the motion lab database (Figure 1). All patients had a preoperative analysis (E_0) and received DFESO. Of those, seven children were treated with additional patella tendon advancement (PTA). Table 1 gives an overview of the concomitant procedures performed during the SEMLS procedure. These included bony and soft tissue reconstructions of the hip, or transposition of the rectus femoris, lengthening of the hamstrings, correction of equinus foot through calf muscle lengthening and correction of the hind foot. Fifteen patients (22 limbs) had a three-dimensional gait analysis at short-term follow-up (E_1; up to 18 months after DFESO). All 19 patients were followed for the mid-term evaluation between 24 and 60 months after surgery (E_2). As a first step, we calculated the results of patients between E_0 and E_2 to determine the mid-term results after DFESO. After that, we analyzed the postoperative course by evaluating the results of patients that had an additional short-term examination (E_1). A further subgroup analysis was performed for patients that had undergone DFESO plus PTA. The data were analyzed using SPSS statistics (IBM SPSS Statistics 19, IBM, Ehningen, Germany). To evaluate the normal distribution of the data, the Shapiro–Wilk test was applied. The data were further evaluated using either the Student's t-test in the case of normal distribution of the data or the Wilcoxon signed-rank test if data were not normally distributed. Statistical significance was set at a p-value < 0.05 for Student's t-Test and 0.025 for Wilcoxon signed-rank test. If patients had repeated postoperative gait analysis, an ANOVA for repeated measures with Bonferroni correction or Friedman's test with post hoc analysis were used. To compare the subgroup that received PTA to the non-PTA group Mann–Whitney U-Test was applied.

Table 1. Overview of the retrieved data of patients included in our sample.

Age	FU	GMFCS	Side	DFESO	PTA	Bony Reconstruction Hip	Soft Tissue Surgery of the Hip	Recession or Transposition of Rectus Femoris	Hamstring Lengthening	Additional Derotational Osteotomy	Equinus Correction	Hindfoot Reconstruction
6.7	55.2	I	L	+						+	+	
			R	+						+	+	
11.6	33.6	II	L	+			+	+		+	+	+
			R	+			+	+		+	+	+
11.6	33.5	II	L	+			+	+	+	+	+	
			R	+			+	+	+	+	+	
13.8	31.8	II	L	+								+
			R	+								+
13.4	48	II	L	+						+	+	
			R								+	
12.2	26.4	II	L	+			+	+		+	+	
			R				+	+				
15.4	33.9	II	L	+			+	+			+	
			R	+			+	+			+	
13.5	47.3	II	L	+	+			+	+	+	+	
			R		+			+			+	+
11.1	24.4	II	L	+						+	+	+
			R	+						+	+	+
7.2	26.4	III	L	+			+	+	+		+	+
			R	+				+	+		+	+
8.9	25.1	III	L	+			+			+	+	
			R			+			+		+	
15.8	26.8	III	L	+	+		+			+		
			R				+		+	+		
10	54.8	II	L		+						+	+
			R	+	+					+	+	
9.2	42.3	II	L					+		+	+	
			R	+				+		+	+	
9.3	55	III	L					+		+		
			R	+				+			+	+
16.1	27.8	III	L	+	+					+	+	
			R	+	+						+	
12.3	36.1	III	L		+					+		+
			R	+	+					+		+
12.7	54.6	III	L	+	+					+	+	
			R	+	+					+	+	
14.1	31.3	III	L	+	+	+					+	
			R	+	+						+	+

FU: follow-up; GMFCS: Gross Motor Function Classification System; DEFO: distal femoral extension osteotomy; PTA: patella tendon advancement. Equinus correction = lengthening of the calf muscles. Hindfoot reconstruction included arthrodesis and soft tissue procedures, e.g., muscle transposition.

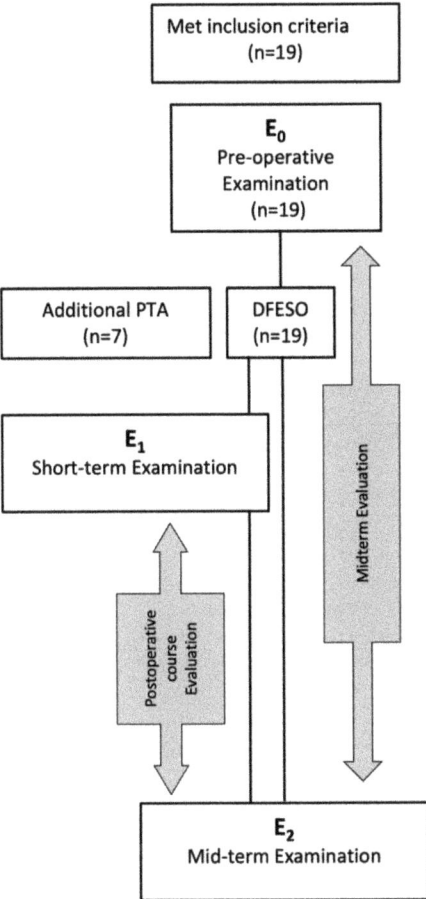

Figure 1. Overview of the different time points of evaluation. E_0: preoperative, E_1: short-term examination 6–18 month postoperative; E_2: mid-term examination 24–60 month postoperative.

3. Results

Overall, 19 patients (28 limbs) could be included in the study and evaluation. The mean age at surgery was 11.8 years (6.7–16.0). All patients had a preoperative gait analysis at a mean of 3.7 (0.5–9) months prior to surgery. The mean mid-term follow-up time (E_2) was 38 (24–55) months. Fifteen patients (22 limbs) had an additional first postoperative gait analysis (E_1) after a mean of 14 (10–20) months after surgery. There was no evidence of non-union or implant failure. All patients were ambulatory walkers, including eight patients with a GMFCS level III, eleven patients with a GMFCS level II and only one patient with a GMFCS level I. Kinematic data of the knee and pelvis, as well as physical examination data, were available in all patients. Apart from the kinematic data of the pelvis, the statistical testing showed normal distribution of the values.

3.1. Kinematic Results

There was a significant change in all sagittal plane kinematic values of the knee at E_2 in comparison to the preoperative values (min. and mean knee flexion in stance, min. knee flexion at initial contact, ROM over 100% GC, mean knee flexion over 100% GC, mean and peak knee flexion in swing) (Table 2 and Figure 2). The mean minimum knee flexion in stance was 38° (SD17°) at E_0 in accordance with the severe flexed knee gait preoperatively. There was a significant improvement in the minimum knee flexion in stance of 16° (SD 17°) from E_0 to E_2 ($p < 0.001$). The mean knee flexion in stance also improved from 46° (SD 19°) preoperatively to 33° (12°) postoperatively (E_2) ($p = 0.001$), while the range of motion showed an overall improvement of almost 10° from E_0 to E_2. We found a significant change in the mean knee flexion over the entire gait cycle from 50° (SD 15°) at E_0 to 37° (SD 9°) at E_2 ($p < 0.001$). In contrast, the mean knee flexion in swing showed a decline from 65° (SD12°) to 58° (8°) ($p = 0.008$). The same effect was seen for peak knee flexion in swing with a significant overall decrease of 7° ($p = 0.008$). The individual case analysis showed an improvement in the min. knee flexion in stance of more than 80% in one case, 60–80% in six cases, 40–60% in five cases, 20–40% in six cases and 10–20% in six cases. Four patients (six limbs) showed a worse minimum knee flexion in stance at E_2 than preoperatively.

Table 2. Overview of the kinematic parameters at the different time points; E_0: preoperative; E_2: 24–60 months postoperative.

Parameter	Context	E_0	E_2	Significance
GDI	Overall	56.3 ± 7.6 (44–76)	70.6 ± 9.8 (49–92)	$p = 0.001$
Walking speed (M/s)	Overall	0.73 ± 0.18	0.84 ± 0.19	$p = 0.04$
Min. knee flexion at initial contact	Overall	46.8° ± 11.6°	31.3° ± 9.5°	$p < 0.001$
	DFESO + PTA	52.1° ± 6.1°	35.2° ± 9.8°	$p = 0.01$
	DFESO	44.4° ± 12.8°	29.5° ± 9.0°	$p = 0.001$
Min. knee flexion in stance	Overall	34.7° ± 18.3°	20.9° ± 10.1°	$p < 0.001$
	DFESO + PTA	41.4° ± 15.5°	25.9° ± 14.2°	$p = 0.021$
	DFESO	35.9° ± 20.1°	22.7° ± 12.2°	$p = 0.003$
Peak knee flexion in swing	Overall	65.2° ± 12.1°	58.5° ± 7.9°	$p = 0.008$
	DFESO + PTA	69.6° ± 9.6°	58.6° ± 8.5°	$p = 0.021$
	DFESO	63.2° ± 12.8°	58.4° ± 7.8°	$p = 0.12$
Mean knee flexion over 100% GC	Overall	49.6° ± 14.2°	37.9° ± 9.4°	$p < 0.001$
	DFESO + PTA	56.3° ± 10.8°	39.2° ± 10.9°	$p = 0.015$
	DFESO	46.5° ± 14.7°	33.2° ± 10.8°	$p = 0.005$
Mean hip flexion in stance	Overall	26.3° ± 10.4°	18.9° ± 8.0°	$p = 0.001$
	DFESO + PTA	30.1° ± 4.6°	23.5° ± 5.5°	$p = 0.86$
	DFESO	24.5° ± 11.9°	16.8° ± 8.2°	$p = 0,007$
Mean pelvic tilt	Overall	13.5° ± 8.4°	12.9° ± 5.6°	$p = 0.72$
	DFESO + PTA	12.6° ± 4.4°	13.7° ± 8.4°	$p = 0.59$
	DFESO	13.9° ± 9.8°	12.6° ± 4.1°	$p = 0.53$

Overall: includes patients with and without PTA (n = 19, 28 limbs); DFESO + PTA (n = 7, 9 limbs); DFESO (n = 12, 19 limbs). Statistical significance was reached when $p < 0.05$.

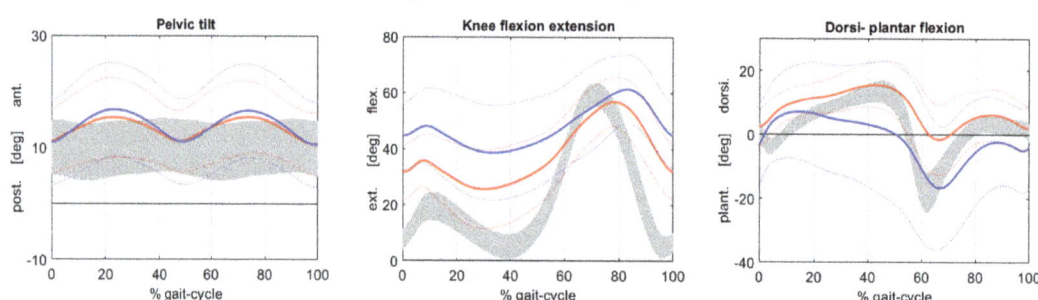

Figure 2. Sagittal plane kinematic graphs illustrating the pelvic tilt, knee flexion and extension and ankle dorsi- and plantar flexion during preoperative (E_0: blue line) and mid-term (E_2: red line) gait analysis. The grey areas represent gait data of an age-matched control group. The x-axis represents gait cycle in percent; y-axis marks the range of motion in degrees. Solid lines represent average values and dashed lines one standard deviation.

The sagittal plane kinematic data of the pelvis revealed a change in the maximum anterior pelvic tilt from 18° (SD 9°) preoperatively to 17° (SD 7°) at E_2. The mean anterior pelvic tilt changed from 14° (SD 8°) to 13° (SD 6°). Both changes were not significant in the analysis ($p = 0.72$ and 0.58).

3.2. Clinical Examination

The preoperative clinical examination revealed a flexion contracture of 15° (SD 7°), which improved by 12° at E_2 ($p < 0.001$). The mean popliteal angle was 42° (SD 23°) at E_0 and showed a significant change towards a full extension of 8° (SD 12°) at E_2 ($p = 0.01$).

3.3. Changes in the Postoperative Course (E_1 to E_2)

Min. knee flexion in stance changed from 21° (SD 13°) to 23° (SD 13°) from E_1 to E_2 ($p > 0.05$). The mean knee flexion in stance and knee flexion at initial contact showed a decline in the postoperative period–mean knee flexion in stance of 5° and knee flexion at initial contact of 3°. The changes were non-significant for both parameters ($p = 0.055$ and $p = 0.06$) (Table 3). Peak knee flexion in swing increased by 5.6° during the postoperative course. The clinical examination revealed an increase in the popliteal angle from 30° (0°–70°) to 34° (15°–60°) from the postoperative to mid-term evaluation. The flexion contracture as measured in the clinical examination changed from 3° (0°–15°) postoperatively to 5° (0–20°) at E_2. This change proved to be non-significant in the post hoc analysis with Bonferroni correction ($p > 0.05$). The mean pelvic tilt showed a non-significant trend toward preoperative values in the mid-term evaluation (E_1: 15° (SD9°) and E_2: 13° (6°)). The same tendency was observed for the maximum pelvic tilt.

Table 3. Overview of the kinematic parameters at the different time points of patients with repeated postoperative gait analysis (n = 15; 22 limbs).

Parameter	Context	E_0	E_1	E_2	Significance
Min. knee flexion in stance	Overall	40.0° ± 17.9°	20.8° ± 13.1°	23.3° ± 12.8°	¶, □
Mean knee flexion in stance	Overall	46.2° ± 21.1°	27.5° ± 11.3°	34.9° ± 11.8°	¶, §, □
Knee flexion at initial contact	Overall	48.2° ± 11.4°	29.6° ± 10.5°	32.8° ± 8.5°	¶, □
Peak knee flexion in swing	Overall	66.4° ± 12.3°	53.0° ± 11.1°	58.6° ± 8.6°	¶, §, □
Mean knee flexion over 100% GC	Overall	51.0° ± 14.9°	32.8° ± 10.5°	38.0° ± 9.8°	¶, □
Mean hip flexion in stance	Overall	27.3° ± 2.4°	21.3° ± 1.9°	21.2° ± 1.5°	¶, □
Mean pelvic tilt	Overall	13.9° ± 9.5°	15.3° ± 9.2°	13.3° ± 6.4°	

E_0: preoperative; E_1: 1–18 month postoperative; E_2: 24–60 month postoperative; ¶: significant change between E_0 and E_2 ($p < 0.05$); □: significant change between E_0 and E_1; §: significant change between E_1 and E_2 ($p < 0.05$).

3.4. Patella Tendon Advancement

There was no significant difference in the severity of flexed knee gait between the PTA and non-PTA groups at E_0 (min. knee flexion in stance: $p = 0.48$, min. knee flexion at initial contact: $p = 0.17$, mean knee flexion: $p = 0.64$). Patients with additional patella tendon advancement (n = 9) showed no significant difference from the non-PTA group (n = 19) in minimum knee flexion in stance, min. knee flexion at initial contact or peak flexion in swing at the mid-term control (E_2) ($p = 0.73, 0.15$ and 0.96). There was also no evidence of a significant difference in maximum pelvic tilt between the groups at E_2.

4. Discussion

Flexed knee gait is one of the most common gait patterns in children and adults with cerebral palsy [1]. It leads to relevant functional restrictions during gait impairing independence and quality of life [25]. Several techniques to improve flexed knee gait have been introduced in the past. Soft tissue procedures, especially lengthening of the hamstrings, have proven to be effective in short-term analysis [3,4,9,26]. However, varying results following hamstring lengthening in long-term evaluation have been published [7,8].

DFESO is an alternative treatment method to address flexed knee gait and fixed flexion deformity. Early reports of the positive effects of the procedure on sagittal plane kinematics of the knee were corroborated by various authors [13–18]. Nonetheless, few studies have investigated the mid- and long-term effects of DFSEO on crouch gait [21,22]. De Morais Filho et al. reported early results with an improvement in sagittal knee joint kinematics after DFEO after 24 months [15] and further evaluated the procedure in combination with patella tendon advancement with a follow-up of 34 months [16]. Sossai et al. found an improvement in minimum knee extension in stance by 22° after 22-month follow-up [17]. The first long-term data were published by Boyer et al. in 2018 comparing the results of DFEO in combination with PTA to non-surgical treatment [21]. Kuchen et al. evaluated the postoperative course in twelve patients that were treated with SELMS due to flexed knee gait. The authors found a maintained improvement of gait kinematics and walking speed after a nine-year follow-up [22].

In this study, we found an improvement in knee kinematics in patients that underwent DFESO with and without PTA, both in short-term and mid-term evaluation. The good results of previous work concerning the short-term outcome [19] could be confirmed with the present data. Furthermore, a lasting improvement in knee kinematics could be measured in the mid-term evaluation after a mean of 38 months. This was also reflected by a substantial improvement in the GDI at mid-term, indicating an overall lasting improvement in gait quality, affirming our first hypothesis. These findings are in keeping with other studies that found lasting improvements after flexed knee gait correction [21,22]. Nonetheless, a tendency towards preoperative flexed knee gait was evident. There was deterioration in all sagittal plane kinematic values of the knee between E_1 (10–24 months postoperative) and E_2 (24–60 months postoperative), but only the changes in mean knee flexion in stance were statistically significant. However, the mean kinematic values of the presented study must be interpreted with caution. While we saw an overall improvement of the kinematic values at E_2, eleven patients showed a minimum knee flexion in stance more than two SD (18°) worse than the control group, suggesting that these patients still walked in crouch gait. Boyer et al. reported a persisting crouch gait in 37% of patients treated with DFEO and PTA in their long-term analysis after eight years [21]. The mid-term results of our study show an even higher percentage of persisting knee flexion gait. In contrast, Kuchen et al. published consistent improvement in gait during follow-up without relevant changes between postoperative, mid- and long-term evaluation [22]. Among other factors, a tightness of the hamstrings during growth leading to recurrence of flexed knee gait must be considered [8]. However, the sample size in this study is too small to allow an evaluation of the influence of age at surgery on the mid-term outcome of DFE(S)O. In addition, the follow-up time of 38 months might not have been long enough for this effect to develop. Numerous concomitant procedures were performed in context with DFESO. Hamstring lengthening was performed in five cases and may have influenced the results of the correction. Healy et al. found that hamstring lengthening is rarely necessary in patients with crouch gait and treatment with DFEOS, as the bony correction itself restored hamstring length and improved hamstring velocity [20]. De Morais Filho et al. reported a larger reduction in knee flexion in stance when additional hamstring lengthening is performed in combination with DFEO and patella tendon shortening, but also noted an increased anterior pelvic tilt in these patients [16]. The patients that received additional hamstring lengthening in our study showed less improvement in knee extension at E_2, but due to the small number of cases the relevance of this finding is questionable. Bony foot corrections to address lever arm dysfunction were also among the most frequent additional procedures. They were often accompanied by equinus correction through calf muscle lengthening in the presence of persisting intraoperative equinus deformity. In these cases, overcorrection, which can lead to calcaneal gait and therefore mediate recurrence of crouch gait, must be carefully avoided [27]. Although we found four patients with increased ankle dorsiflexion postoperatively, only one patient demonstrated calcaneal gait at E2 in combination with a deterioration in sagittal plane knee kinematics.

In a previous study evaluating the short-term outcome of DFESO, a significant increase in the anterior pelvic tilt with possible clinical impact was found [19], corroborating the findings of other authors [13,15] reporting increased anterior pelvic tilt after DFESO [16,28]. In the present study, both mean and maximum pelvic tilt were nearly identical in the preoperative and the mid-term evaluation. A slight increase in the anterior pelvic tilt was observed at E_1, but this tendency was not statistically significant, and the increased tilt vanished in the mid-term control thus dismissing our second hypothesis. However, the increase in pelvic tilt in the immediate postoperative cause might be one of the reasons for the recurrence of flexed knee gait over time, as it can be compensated by increased flexion of the knee [8]. An increased muscle tone in the rectus femoris and psoas muscle may also influence the anterior pelvic tilt, as the balance between hip extension and hip flexion is altered [13,16,29,30]. Böhm et al. identified an increased muscle tone of the rectus femoris as one of the key factors in increased pelvic tilt after correction of crouch gait [29]. The effect was also discussed by de Morais Filho et al., and the authors noted that none of their patients had received an additional rectus femoris transfer [16]. A substantial number of patients in our study received a transposition of the rectus femoris and recession of the psoas. This might explain why anterior pelvic tilt was not as evident in comparison to other studies. In contrast to our data, Stout et al. reported no influence of rectus femoris transfer or psoas lengthening on anterior pelvic tilt in patients that received DFEO and PTA [13]. Furthermore, we observed a slight decrease in the mean and peak knee flexion during swing phase, indicating that DFESO led to a tendency to stiff knee gait, corroborating the results of other authors [17,28]. Sossai et al. reported a decrease in peak knee flexion in swing after patella tendon shortening, although not all patients simultaneously underwent supracondylar extension osteotomy [17]. Park et al. observed a similar effect after a 24-month follow-up when knee flexion deformity is addressed with a femoral shortening osteotomy [28]. During the postoperative course we observed an improvement in the peak knee flexion in swing, although the tendency did not fully compensate for the postoperative loss. An increased walking speed could also have led to a reduced knee flexion in swing. The observed increase in walking speed could therefore have been at least partially responsible for the loss of knee flexion in swing.

In 2018, Broyer et al. published the first long-term data on patients that underwent DFESO + PTA [21]. The authors compared the results of the procedure to patients with crouch gait who did not undergo surgical intervention. They found a significant improvement in static and functional outcome parameters in the DFESO + PTA group after eight years. At the same time, there was a trend towards a slight deterioration in the initial correction. In the present study, a similar effect was found at mid-term evaluation.

DFESO can be performed in combination with PTA in the presence of patella alta. Although differing reports exist [19], previous studies have shown an additional benefit of PTA in patients with flexed knee gait [13,14]. Stout et al. reported an increased correction of 20° when crouch gait is addressed with DFEO and PTA in comparison to DFEO alone [13]. The data of the present study showed no significant difference in the kinematic results between patients that had additional PTA and those who did not. However, it must be critically acknowledged that, due to the sample size in this study, a subgroup analysis is difficult. Only seven patients (nine limbs) received additional PTA, and a positive effect of the procedure on the mid-term outcome might not have been detectable due to the small sample size.

5. Conclusions

The present study indicates that DFESO improves flexed knee gait and has a lasting positive impact on sagittal plane kinematics in children with cerebral palsy and crouch gait. However, further investigations are needed to identify those patients that benefit most from the procedure and explain the detected tendency towards recurrence at mid-term follow-up. The results of the study are limited by the sample size and the retrospective study design. Furthermore, the additional procedures performed might influence the results of the study.

Author Contributions: Conceptualization: A.G.; methodology: A.G.; software: A.G. and M.C.M.K.; validation: A.G. and M.C.M.K.; formal analysis: A.G. and M.C.M.K.; investigation: A.G. and M.C.M.K.; data curation: A.G.; writing—original draft preparation: A.G.; writing—review and editing: A.G., M.C.M.K., A.H., C.P. and T.R.; visualization: A.G., C.P. and A.H. All authors have read and agreed to the published version of the manuscript.

Funding: There was no external funding for the study. Regardless Tobias Renkawitz received research support and personal fees from Arbeitsgemeinschaft Endoprothetik (AE), DGOU, DGOOC, BVOU, DePuy International, Otto Bock Foundation, Deutsche Arthrose Hilfe, Aesculap, Zimmer, Stiftung Oskar Helene Heim Berlin, Vielberth Foundation Regensburg, the German Ministry of Education and Research as well as the German Federal Ministry of Economic Cooperation and Development. Axel Horsch received research support from Arthrose Hilfe and Ipsen.

Institutional Review Board Statement: The study was conducted in accordance with the Declaration of Helsinki, and approved by the ethics committee of the medical faculty, University Heidelberg (date of approval: 10/2009, number: S302/2009 and 02/2016 number: S-017/2016).

Informed Consent Statement: Informed consent was obtained from all subjects involved in the study.

Data availability statement: All of the data analyzed in this manuscript can be provided upon request by contacting the corresponding author.

Conflicts of Interest: The authors declare no conflict of interest.

References

1. Sutherland, D.H.; Davids, J.R. Common gait abnormalities of the knee in cerebral palsy. *Clin. Orthop. Relat. Res.* **1993**, *288*, 139–147.
2. Rodda, J.M.; Graham, H.K.; Nattrass, G.R.; Galea, M.P.; Baker, R.; Wolfe, R. Correction of severe crouch gait in patients with spastic diplegia with use of multilevel orthopaedic surgery. *J. Bone Jt. Surg.* **2006**, *88*, 2653–2664. [CrossRef]
3. Kay, R.M.; Rethlefsen, S.A.; Skaggs, D.; Leet, A. Outcome of medial versus combined medial and lateral hamstring lengthening surgery in cerebral palsy. *J. Pediatric Orthop.* **2002**, *22*, 169–172. [CrossRef]
4. Gordon, A.B.; Baird, G.O.; McMulkin, M.L.; Caskey, P.M.; Ferguson, R.L. Gait analysis outcomes of percutaneous medial hamstring tenotomies in children with cerebral palsy. *J. Pediatric Orthop.* **2008**, *28*, 324–329. [CrossRef]
5. Park, M.S.; Chung, C.Y.; Lee, S.H.; Choi, I.H.; Cho, T.J.; Yoo, W.J.; Park, B.S.; Lee, K.M. Effects of distal hamstring lengthening on sagittal motion in patients with diplegia: Hamstring length and its clinical use. *Gait Posture* **2009**, *30*, 487–491. [CrossRef]
6. Sung, K.H.; Lee, J.; Chung, C.Y.; Lee, K.M.; Cho, B.C.; Moon, S.J.; Kim, J.; Park, M.S. Factors influencing outcomes after medial hamstring lengthening with semitendinosus transfer in patients with cerebral palsy. *J. Neuroeng. Rehabil.* **2017**, *14*, 83. [CrossRef]
7. Õunpuu, S.; Solomito, M.; Bell, K.; DeLuca, P.; Pierz, K. Long-term outcomes after multilevel surgery including rectus femoris, hamstring and gastrocnemius procedures in children with cerebral palsy. *Gait Posture* **2015**, *42*, 365–372. [CrossRef]
8. Dreher, T.; Vegvari, D.; Wolf, S.I.; Geisbusch, A.; Gantz, S.; Wenz, W.; Braatz, F. Development of knee function after hamstring lengthening as a part of multilevel surgery in children with spastic diplegia: A long-term outcome study. *J. Bone Jt. Surg.* **2012**, *94*, 121–130. [CrossRef]
9. DeLuca, P.A.; Õunpuu, S.; Davis, R.B.; Walsh, J.H. Effect of hamstring and psoas lengthening on pelvic tilt in patients with spastic diplegic cerebral palsy. *J. Pediatric Orthop.* **1998**, *18*, 712–718. [CrossRef]
10. Morais Filho, M.C.; Blumetti, F.C.; Kawamura, C.M.; Fujino, M.H.; Matias, M.S.; Lopes, J.A.F. Comparison of the Results of Primary Versus Repeat Hamstring Surgical Lengthening in Cerebral Palsy. *J. Pediatric Orthop.* **2020**, *40*, e380–e384. [CrossRef]
11. de Morais Filho, M.C.; Fujino, M.H.; Kawamura, C.M.; Dos Santos, C.A.; Lopes, J.A.F.; Blumetti, F.C.; Mattar Junior, R. The increase of anterior pelvic tilt after semitendinosus transfer to distal femur in patients with spastic diplegic cerebral palsy. *J. Pediatric Orthop. Part B* **2019**, *28*, 327–331. [CrossRef] [PubMed]
12. Dreher, T.; Vegvari, D.; Wolf, S.L.; Klotz, M.; Muller, S.; Metaxiotis, D.; Wenz, W.; Doderlein, L.; Braatz, F. Long-term effects after conversion of biarticular to monoarticular muscles compared with musculotendinous lengthening in children with spastic diplegia. *Gait Posture* **2013**, *37*, 430–435. [CrossRef] [PubMed]
13. Stout, J.L.; Gage, J.R.; Schwartz, M.H.; Novacheck, T.F. Distal femoral extension osteotomy and patellar tendon advancement to treat persistent crouch gait in cerebral palsy. *J. Bone Jt. Surg.* **2008**, *90*, 2470–2484. [CrossRef] [PubMed]
14. Novacheck, T.F.; Stout, J.L.; Gage, J.R.; Schwartz, M.H. Distal femoral extension osteotomy and patellar tendon advancement to treat persistent crouch gait in cerebral palsy. Surgical technique. *J. Bone Jt. Surg.* **2009**, *91* (Suppl. S2), 271–286. [CrossRef] [PubMed]
15. de Morais Filho, M.C.; Neves, D.L.; Abreu, F.P.; Juliano, Y.; Guimaraes, L. Treatment of fixed knee flexion deformity and crouch gait using distal femur extension osteotomy in cerebral palsy. *J. Child. Orthop.* **2008**, *2*, 37–43. [CrossRef] [PubMed]
16. de Morais Filho, M.C.; Blumetti, F.C.; Kawamura, C.M.; Leite, J.B.R.; Lopes, J.A.F.; Fujino, M.H.; Neves, D.L. The increase of anterior pelvic tilt after crouch gait treatment in patients with cerebral palsy. *Gait Posture* **2018**, *63*, 165–170. [CrossRef]

17. Sossai, R.; Vavken, P.; Brunner, R.; Camathias, C.; Graham, H.K.; Rutz, E. Patellar tendon shortening for flexed knee gait in spastic diplegia. *Gait Posture* **2015**, *41*, 658–665. [CrossRef]
18. Rutz, E.; Gaston, M.S.; Camathias, C.; Brunner, R. Distal femoral osteotomy using the LCP pediatric condylar 90-degree plate in patients with neuromuscular disorders. *J. Pediatric Orthop.* **2012**, *32*, 295–300. [CrossRef]
19. Klotz, M.C.M.; Hirsch, K.; Heitzmann, D.; Maier, M.W.; Hagmann, S.; Dreher, T. Distal femoral extension and shortening osteotomy as a part of multilevel surgery in children with cerebral palsy. *World J. Pediatrics* **2017**, *13*, 353–359. [CrossRef]
20. Healy, M.T.; Schwartz, M.H.; Stout, J.L.; Gage, J.R.; Novacheck, T.F. Is simultaneous hamstring lengthening necessary when performing distal femoral extension osteotomy and patellar tendon advancement? *Gait Posture* **2011**, *33*, 1–5. [CrossRef]
21. Boyer, E.R.; Stout, J.L.; Laine, J.C.; Gutknecht, S.M.; Araujo de Oliveira, L.H.; Munger, M.E.; Schwartz, M.H.; Novacheck, T.F. Long-Term Outcomes of Distal Femoral Extension Osteotomy and Patellar Tendon Advancement in Individuals with Cerebral Palsy. *J. Bone Jt. Surg.* **2018**, *100*, 31–41. [CrossRef] [PubMed]
22. Kuchen, D.B.; Eichelberger, P.; Baur, H.; Rutz, E. Long-term follow-up after patellar tendon shortening for flexed knee gait in bilateral spastic cerebral palsy. *Gait Posture* **2020**, *81*, 85–90. [CrossRef] [PubMed]
23. Brunner, R.; Camathias, C.; Gaston, M.; Rutz, E. Supracondylar osteotomy of the paediatric femur using the locking compression plate: A refined surgical technique. *J. Child. Orthop.* **2013**, *7*, 571–574. [CrossRef] [PubMed]
24. Kadaba, M.P.; Ramakrishnan, H.K.; Wootten, M.E. Measurement of lower extremity kinematics during level walking. *J. Orthop. Res. Off. Publ. Orthop. Res. Soc.* **1990**, *8*, 383–392. [CrossRef]
25. Lundh, S.; Nasic, S.; Riad, J. Fatigue, quality of life and walking ability in adults with cerebral palsy. *Gait Posture* **2018**, *61*, 1–6. [CrossRef]
26. Chang, W.N.; Tsirikos, A.I.; Miller, F.; Lennon, N.; Schuyler, J.; Kerstetter, L.; Glutting, J. Distal hamstring lengthening in ambulatory children with cerebral palsy: Primary versus revision procedures. *Gait Posture* **2004**, *19*, 298–304. [CrossRef]
27. Dreher, T.; Buccoliero, T.; Wolf, S.I.; Heitzmann, D.; Gantz, S.; Braatz, F.; Wenz, W. Long-term results after gastrocnemius-soleus intramuscular aponeurotic recession as a part of multilevel surgery in spastic diplegic cerebral palsy. *J. Bone Jt. Surg.* **2012**, *94*, 627–637. [CrossRef] [PubMed]
28. Park, H.; Park, B.K.; Park, K.B.; Abdel-Baki, S.W.; Rhee, I.; Kim, C.W.; Kim, H.W. Distal Femoral Shortening Osteotomy for Severe Knee Flexion Contracture and Crouch Gait in Cerebral Palsy. *J. Clin. Med.* **2019**, *8*, 1354. [CrossRef]
29. Bohm, H.; Hosl, M.; Doderlein, L. Predictors for anterior pelvic tilt following surgical correction of flexed knee gait including patellar tendon shortening in children with cerebral palsy. *Gait Posture* **2017**, *54*, 8–14. [CrossRef]
30. Wolf, S.I.; Mikut, R.; Kranzl, A.; Dreher, T. Which functional impairments are the main contributors to pelvic anterior tilt during gait in individuals with cerebral palsy? *Gait Posture* **2014**, *39*, 359–364. [CrossRef]

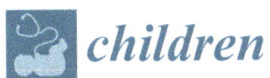

Article

Pediatric Open Long-Bone Fracture and Subsequent Deep Infection Risk: The Importance of Early Hospital Care

Andrew W. Kuhn [1], Stockton C. Troyer [2] and Jeffrey E. Martus [3,*]

1 Department of Orthopedic Surgery, Washington University in St. Louis, St. Louis, MO 63108, USA
2 Washington University School of Medicine in St. Louis, St. Louis, MO 63108, USA
3 Department of Orthopaedic Surgery and Rehabilitation, Vanderbilt University Medical Center, Nashville, TN 37232, USA
* Correspondence: jeff.martus@vumc.org; Tel.: +1-615-343-5875

Abstract: The purpose of the current study was to identify risk factors for deep infection after an open long-bone fracture in pediatric patients. Systematic billing queries were utilized to identify pediatric patients who presented to a level I trauma center from 1998 to 2019 with open long-bone fractures. There were 303 open long-bone fractures, and 24 (7.9%) of these became infected. Fractures of the tibia/fibula ($p = 0.022$), higher revised Gustilo-Anderson type ($p = 0.017$), and a longer duration of time between the injury and hospital presentation ($p = 0.008$) were all associated with the presence of deep infection. Those who went on to have a deep infection also required more operative debridements ($p = 0.022$) and a total number of operative procedures ($p = 0.026$). The only factor that remained significant in multivariable regression was the duration between the injury and hospital presentation (OR 1.01 [95%CI 1.003–1.017]; $p = 0.009$), where the odds of deep infection increased by 1% for every minute of delayed presentation.

Keywords: pediatric; open fracture; infection; trauma; morbidity; orthopedic

1. Introduction

Fractures represent a significant proportion of all pediatric emergency department visits and hospital admissions in the United States, especially for older male adolescents [1,2]. In a study of 3350 children with 3413 limb fractures presenting to one center, distal radius fractures, supra-condylar fractures of the humerus, and forearm shaft fractures were most common, while femur and tibia/fibula fractures also accounted for a large proportion of fractures in other studies [2,3]. Although open fractures are thought to contribute a small percentage (<10%) of all pediatric fractures, they are considered surgical emergencies as they carry a significant risk for infection and associated morbidity [4–6].

Open fractures are typically stratified by the revised Gustilo–Anderson Classification, where the type (I, II, and IIIA-C) is based on wound size and the extent of associated tissue damage [7]. A treatment protocol for open fractures first described and employed by Gustilo and Anderson between 1969 and 1973, portended a significant reduction in infection rates through debridement and copious irrigation, primary closure for type I and II fractures and secondary closure for type III fractures, no primary internal fixation except in the presence of associated vascular injuries, cultures of all wounds, and oxacillin-ampicillin before and for three days postoperatively [7,8]. Some aspects of pediatric open fracture management remain unchanged and are universally accepted across institutions, such as immediate antibiotic administration and tetanus prophylaxis, whereas other facets of care are more controversial and debated, particularly in the setting and management of type I open fractures [9–12].

In an attempt to optimize hospital course and reduce the risk of complications and infection following pediatric open fractures, different aspects of management have been empirically studied including: the initiation and duration of antibiotic treatment [13,14];

Citation: Kuhn, A.W.; Troyer, S.C.; Martus, J.E. Pediatric Open Long-Bone Fracture and Subsequent Deep Infection Risk: The Importance of Early Hospital Care. *Children* **2022**, *9*, 1243. https://doi.org/10.3390/children9081243

Academic Editors: Axel A. Horsch, Maher A. Ghandour and Matthias Christoph M. Klotz

Received: 4 August 2022
Accepted: 16 August 2022
Published: 17 August 2022

Publisher's Note: MDPI stays neutral with regard to jurisdictional claims in published maps and institutional affiliations.

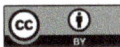

Copyright: © 2022 by the authors. Licensee MDPI, Basel, Switzerland. This article is an open access article distributed under the terms and conditions of the Creative Commons Attribution (CC BY) license (https://creativecommons.org/licenses/by/4.0/).

choice of antibiotics and the utility of preoperative cultures [13–16]; surgical approach for all fractures and nonoperative treatment for type I fractures [12–14,17–26]; time to operative debridement and irrigation [13,14,27–29]; the addition of negative pressure dressings [13,30,31]. Unfortunately, when compared to the management of open fractures in adults, high-level evidence is lacking, and most recommendations are based on case-series and/or historical standards of care [6,13,14]. For instance, the most recent published review and recommendations for antibiotic selection in pediatric open fractures found a paucity of high-level evidence and concluded broadly that Type I open fractures should be treated with a first-generation cephalosporin and for type II and III, additional Gram-negative coverage should be added [32].

The primary aim of this study is to describe trends in management and elucidate pertinent risk factors for developing a deep infection after an open long-bone fracture in pediatric patients. We hypothesized that infection would be more prevalent in higher revised Gustilo–Anderson type open fractures as well as in cases of delayed administration of antibiotic prophylaxis.

2. Materials and Methods

2.1. Patient Identification, Inclusion and Exclusion Criteria

Patients under the age of 18 who presented to Vanderbilt University Medical Center (VUMC) between 1998 and 2019 with an open fracture of a long bone were retrospectively queried with over 1000 ICD9 and ICD10 codes pertaining to open long-bone fractures. Patients were only included if they had a documented open long bone fracture event and adequate data and follow-up. Traumatic amputations were not included in this analysis. If patients did not have documentation of their "date and time of injury", "date and time of admission to an outside facility (OSF)/VUMC", or "date, time, and duration of antibiotics administered", they were excluded. Patients had to have follow-up through deep infection, "healed fracture" (near or complete union), or fracture non-/malunion to be included in this study. If patients were discharged from a surgeon's care and instructed to follow up on an "as needed" basis, they met the necessary endpoint and were considered healed. If a patient had multiple open long bone fractures resulting from the same injury, each was treated as a unique event. Our institutional antibiotic protocol is as follows: Type I or II pediatric open fractures are treated with cefazolin. If allergic to cefazolin, clindamycin is given instead. If allergic to both cefazolin and clindamycin, vancomycin is initiated. For type III or highly contaminated type I or II pediatric open fractures, piperacillin/tazobactam is administered. If allergic to piperacillin/tazobactam, clindamycin or vancomycin is provided, with metronidazole and either ciprofloxacin or gentamicin. Antibiotics are administered within 1 h of arrival. A tetanus vaccine is also offered if not up to date.

2.2. Database Structure and Elements

Demographic and injury characteristics, management decisions, the temporality of various treatments, and outcome variables were collected and based on previously developed data collection instruments (Registry for Orthopaedic Trauma in Children, ROTC). Additional elements that were thought to be possibly associated with infection were included as well. All study data were collected, managed, and built using the REDCap electronic data capture tool hosted at VUMC [33]. REDCap is a secure, web-based application designed to support data capture for research studies, providing: (1) an intuitive interface for validated data entry; (2) audit trails for tracking data manipulation and export procedures; (3) automated export procedures for seamless data downloads to common statistical packages; (4) procedures for importing data from external sources.

For date–time event variables, scanned Emergency Medical Services (EMS), triage notes, other documents and clinical notes, and documentation of different services (e.g., anesthesia care records) and/or procedure notes were utilized to ensure the most accurate date–times possible. For "date and time of discharge", 12:00 p.m. was utilized given the lack of precise timing documented. Deep infections were based on clinical notation and/or direct confirmatory signs (fistula, sinus, wound breakdown, purulent drainage or pus, positive cultures, or histopathological examination). All risk factors were in relation to each patient's endpoint. Each variable was assessed in its relation to developing a deep infection, and how they were defined for the purposes of this study can be found in Table 1. This is a historical cohort in which data from medical records were reviewed and collected. Institutional Review Board (IRB) approval was granted (VUMC; #182036) for this study.

Table 1. Variables Assessed in Relation to Acquiring a Deep Infection After Pediatric Open Long-Bone Fracture.

Characteristic	Coded
Age	(Continuous Measurement)
Sex	Female, Male
Race [a]	White, Non-White
Weight [b]	(Continuous)
Comorbidities [c]	No, Yes
Self-Reported Antibiotic Allergies	No, Yes
Season [d]	Spring, Summer, Fall, Winter
Mechanism of Injury [e]	Low Energy, High Energy
Setting and Contamination Risk [f]	Low Risk, Medium Risk, High Risk
Polytrauma [g]	No, Yes
Multiple Open Fractures	No, Yes
Long-Bone Fractured	Femur, Humerus, Radius/Ulna, Tibia/Fibula
Segment of Long Bone Fractured	Diaphyseal, Metaphyseal/Epiphyseal
Revised Gustilo-Anderson Classification [h]	I, II, IIIA-C
Vascular Compromise/Injury	No, Yes
Nerve Injury	No, Yes
Compartment Syndrome Requiring Fasciotomy	No, Yes
Time to Admission (min)	(Continuous Measurement)
Transferred From Outside Facility	No, Yes
Time to Antibiotics (min)	(Continuous Measurement), < or ≥3 h
Number of Antibiotic Classes Administered	(Count Measurement)
Time to Operative Debridement (h)	(Continuous Measurement), < or ≥6 h
Number of Operative Debridements	(Count Variable)
Time to Definitive Fixation (h)	(Continuous Measurement)
Duration of Antibiotics While Admitted (h)	(Continuous Measurement)
Length of Hospital Stay (days)	(Continuous Measurement)
Discharged with Antibiotics	No, Yes
Discharge Disposition	Home, Rehabilitation/Other
Total Number of Operative Procedures	(Count Measurement)

[a] White or Non-White (Black or African American, Asian, Native Hawaiian or Other Pacific Islander, American Indian or Alaska Native, of Spanish Origin, or Other). [b] Standardized to z-scores based on sex and age-adjusted normative data https://web.emmes.com/study/ped/resources/htwtcalc.htm (accessed on 1 October 2019). [c] Harboring one or more documented systemic, metabolic, skeletal, or psychiatric/neurologic conditions on presentation. [d] Spring (March, April, May), Summer (June, July, August), Fall (September, October, November), Winter (December, January, February). [e] High Energy (MVC, ATV, MCC, other machinery related, crush related, GSW, fall > 10 feet), Low Energy (fall < 10 feet, sport-related, bicycle, monkey bars, trampoline "rough-housing"). [f] High Risk (outside barnyard, fecal, dirty water, dirt/grass, mulch, playground, or a deeply contaminated wound); Medium Risk (outside street, pavement, concrete, hard surface, or surface contamination of the wound); Low Risk (inside with minimal or no wound contamination). [g] Presenting with significant head, chest, abdominal, or other injuries requiring additional work-up and treatment. [h] Designated by the attending orthopaedic surgeon in nearly all cases and based on clinical history, presentation, exam, imaging, and intraoperative findings.

2.3. Statistical Analyses

Pertinent demographics, injury characteristics, management decisions, the temporality of various treatments, and outcomes across cases were described and reported utilizing raw counts, measures of central tendency (mean, median, or mode), and measures of data dispersion (95% confidence intervals, standard errors, inter-quartile ranges) where appropriate. First, univariate logistic regression modeling was conducted to assess the associations between all relevant independent variables and the presence of a deep infection. Associations that reached a threshold of $p < 0.05$ were entered into a multivariable logistic regression model. To account for the rarity of deep infection and the phenomenon of separation, Firth's correction was utilized to adjust for biased estimates by maximizing the penalized likelihood function [34]. Effect sizes were reported as odds ratios (OR) with 95% confidence intervals. All statistics were computed with SPSS v26.0 (IBM; Armonk, NY, USA).

3. Results

3.1. Patient Characteristics

Nine hundred and thirty-six patients were returned from the systematic billing queries, and 291 met the necessary inclusion and exclusion criteria (Figure 1). There were 303 open long-bone fractures, and 24 (7.9%) of these became infected. Patients were, on average, 11.8 (±4.2) years old at the time of presentation. Most were male (65.0%), white (73.3%), and had no documented systemic, metabolic, skeletal, or psychiatric/neurologic comorbidities (73.3%). Around 15% had a self-reported antibiotic allergy. Patients who had a deep infection were typically older (12.4 vs. 11.8 years old), more likely to be male (79.1% vs. 63.8%), and have comorbidities at presentation (37.5% vs. 25.8%). However, none of these or the other collected patient demographic characteristics were significantly associated with deep infection (Table 2).

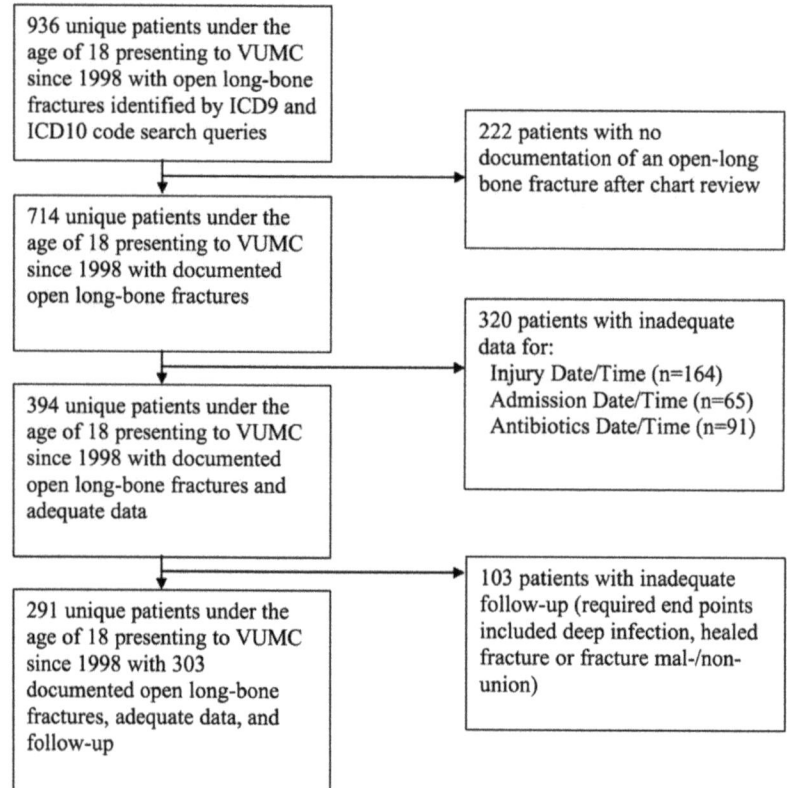

Figure 1. Inclusion and Exclusion Flowchart.

Table 2. Patient Demographic Characteristics.

Characteristic Mean (SD), Median (IQR), or n (%)	No Infection (n = 279)	Deep Infection (n = 24)	TOTAL (n = 303)	OR [95%OR]	p-Value
Age	11.8 (±4.2)	12.4 (±4.7)	11.8 (±4.2)	1.029 [0.934, 1.143]	0.563
Sex					
Female *	101 (36.2)	5 (20.8)	106 (35.0)		
Male	178 (63.8)	19 (79.1)	197 (65.0)	2.015 [0.807, 5.912]	0.139
Race					
White *	205 (73.5)	17 (70.8)	222 (73.3)		
Non-White	74 (26.5)	7 (29.2)	81 (26.7)	1.182 [0.456, 2.801]	0.717
Weight (Standardized Z-Score)	0.4 (±1.2)	0.6 (±1.3)	0.4 (±1.2)	1.182 [0.834, 1.687]	0.349
Comorbidities					
No *	207 (74.2)	15 (62.5)	222 (73.3)		
Yes	72 (25.8)	9 (37.5)	81 (26.7)	1.754 [0.725, 4.051]	0.205
Self-Reported Antibiotic Allergies					
No *	237 (84.9)	19 (79.2)	256 (84.5)		
Yes	42 (15.1)	5 (20.8)	47 (15.5)	1.576 [0.527, 4.051]	0.390

* reference group.

3.2. Open Fracture and Injury Event Characteristics

Most of the fractures occurred in the summer (38.0%) and spring (27.1%), resulting from high-energy mechanisms (56.4%) in high-risk settings (49.1%). A large proportion (40.6%) of patients presented with significant head, chest, abdominal, or other injuries requiring additional work-up and treatment. The most commonly fractured long bone was the radius/ulna (42.9%), followed by the tibia/fibula (32.3%). Most fractures were diaphyseal (71.0%) and type I or II open fractures (70.6%). Vascular compromise/injury (8.6%), nerve injury (12.5%), and compartment syndrome requiring fasciotomy (5.9%) were less frequent. Long-bone fracture was significantly associated with the occurrence of deep infection ($p = 0.022$). The tibia/fibula was significantly more likely to become infected compared to the radius/ulna (OR = 4.00 [1.515–12.05]). Revised Gustilo–Anderson classification was also significantly associated with deep infection ($p = 0.017$), whereas compared to type I, type IIIA-C fractures were at over four times the odds of developing deep infection (OR = 4.411 [1.559, 14.984]) (Table 3).

Table 3. Open Fracture and Injury Event Characteristics.

Characteristic Mean (SD), Median (IQR), or n (%)	No Infection (n = 279)	Deep Infection (n = 24)	TOTAL (n = 303)	OR [95%OR]	p-Value
Season					0.279
Winter *	34 (12.2)	1 (4.2)	35 (11.6)		
Spring	75 (26.9)	7 (29.2)	82 (27.1)	2.284 [0.472, 22.26]	331
Summer	102 (36.6)	13 (54.2)	115 (38.0)	3.028 [0.698, 28.42]	0.154
Fall	68 (24.4)	3 (12.5)	71 (23.4)	1.175 [0.185, 12.47]	0.870

Table 3. Cont.

Characteristic Mean (SD), Median (IQR), or n (%)	No Infection (n = 279)	Deep Infection (n = 24)	TOTAL (n = 303)	OR [95%OR]	p-Value
Mechanism of Injury					
Low Energy *	126 (45.2)	6 (25.0)	132 (43.6)		
High Energy	153 (54.8)	18 (75.0)	171 (56.4)	2.347 [0.974, 6.379]	0.057
Setting and Contamination					0.239
Low Risk *	58 (22.4)	3 (12.5)	61 (21.6)		
Medium Risk	78 (30.1)	5 (20.8)	83 (29.3)	1.171 [0.299, 5.228]	0.822
High Risk	123 (47.5)	16 (66.7)	139 (49.1)	2.232 [0.750, 8.785]	0.158
Polytrauma					
No *	168 (60.2)	12 (50.0)	180 (59.4)		
Yes	111 (39.8)	12 (50.0)	123 (40.6)	1.511 [0.660, 3.463]	0.325
Multiple Open Fractures					
No *	256 (91.8)	23 (95.8)	279 (92.1)		
Yes	23 (8.2)	1 (4.2)	24 (7.9)	0.697 [0.075, 2.900]	0.663
Long-Bone					0.022 **
Tibia/Fibula *	84 (30.1)	14 (58.3)	98 (32.3)		
Femur	35 (12.5)	4 (16.7)	39 (12.9)	0.730 [0.211, 2.117]	0.531
Humerus	35 (12.5)	1 (4.2)	36 (11.9)	0.243 [0.026, 1.048]	0.059
Radius/Ulna	125 (44.8)	5 (20.8)	130 (42.9)	0.250 [0.083, 0.660]	0.005
Segment of Long Bone					
Diaphyseal *	197 (70.6)	18 (75.0)	215 (71.0)		
Metaphyseal/Epiphyseal	82 (29.4)	6 (25.0)	88 (29.0)	0.841 [0.308, 2.038]	0.712
Gustilo-Anderson					0.017 **
I *	112 (40.1)	4 (16.7)	116 (38.3)		
II	91 (32.6)	7 (29.2)	98 (32.3)	2.048 [0.632, 7.434]	0.232
IIIA-C	76 (27.2)	13 (54.2)	89 (29.4)	4.411 [1.559, 14.984]	0.004
Vascular Compromise/Injury					
No *	257 (92.1)	20 (83.3)	277 (91.4)		
Yes	22 (7.9)	4 (16.7)	26 (8.6)	2.512 [0.738, 7.092]	0.130
Nerve Injury					
No *	242 (86.7)	23 (95.8)	265 (87.5)		
Yes	37 (13.3)	1 (4.2)	38 (12.5)	0.413 [0.045, 1.674]	0.246
Compartment Syndrome Requiring Fasciotomy					
No *	264 (94.6)	21 (87.5)	285 (94.1)		
Yes	15 (5.4)	3 (12.5)	18 (5.9)	2.779 [0.684, 8.776]	0.139

* reference group, ** denotes statistical significance.

3.3. Open Fracture Management Characteristics

Most patients presented to an OSF or VUMC a little over an h (64.0 (±44.0) min) from their injury. Close to a third (32.0%) were transferred to VUMC from an OSF for definitive care. Most patients (73.9%) received antibiotics within 3 h of their injury (161.4 (±152.8) min) and received a median of 1 (IQR: 1-2) antibiotic class during their admission. The mean time to operative debridement was a little under 15 h from their injury (14.8 (±11.1) h). Approximately one-fifth (17.9%) of open fractures were operatively debrided within 6 h of injury, and the median number of operative debridements was 1 (IQR 1-1). The time to definitive fixation was a little over a day (24.5 (±36.9) h). The average duration between first and last antibiotic administration while admitted was almost 3 days (69.8 (±102.7) h), and the average length of hospital stays was about 4 days (4.0 (±4.8) days). The majority of patients (94.7%) were discharged home, and around one-fifth (19.9%) were on antibiotics. The total number of operative procedures needed before each patient's endpoint was 1 (IQR 1-1). Those who had longer durations of time between their injury and presentation to either an OSF or VUMC were more likely to become infected (89.9 vs. 61.8 min; OR 1.009 [95%CI 1.003, 1.016]; p = 0.008). The duration of time between injury and presentation to either an OSF or VUMC was significantly correlated with the duration between the injury and first antibiotic administration (r = 0.176, p = 0.002), but not with the duration of time between the injury and first operative irrigation and debridement (r = −0.036, p = 0.538). Those who went on to have deep infections required more operative debridements (p = 0.022) and a greater number of operative procedures (p = 0.026) (Table 4).

Table 4. Open Fracture Management Characteristics.

Characteristic Mean (SD), Median (IQR), or n (%)	No Infection (n = 279)	Deep Infection (n = 24)	TOTAL (n = 303)	OR [95%OR]	p-Value
Time to Hospital (min)	61.8 (±41.2)	89.9 (±64.8)	64.0 (±44.0)	1.009 [1.003, 1.016]	0.008 **
Transferred From OSF					
No *	192 (68.8)	14 (58.3)	206 (68.0)		
Yes	87 (31.2)	10 (41.7)	97 (32.0)	1.594 [0.676, 3.644]	0.280
Time to Antibiotics (min)	161.5 (±157.4)	159.8 (±83.9)	161.4 (±152.8)	1.000 [0.997, 1.002]	0.689
<3 h *	206 (73.8)	18 (75.0)	224 (73.9)		
≥3 h	73 (26.2)	6 (25.0)	79 (26.1)	0.987 [0.361, 2.399]	0.978
Number of Antibiotic Classes Administered	1 (1–2)	2 (1–3)	1 (1–2)	1.271 [0.884, 1.761]	0.185
Time to Operative Debridement (h)	14.5 (±8.5)	18.8 (±27.3)	14.8 (±11.1)	1.021 [0.996, 1.047]	0.093
<6 h *	46 (17.2)	6 (27.3)	52 (17.9)		
≥6 h	222 (82.2)	16 (72.7)	238 (82.1)	0.530 [0.211, 1.486]	0.214
Number of Operative Debridements	1 (1-1)	1 (1-2)	1 (1-1)	1.429 [1.060, 1.893]	0.022 **
Time to Definitive Fixation (h)	23.9 (±36.8)	30.9 (±37.9)	24.5 (±36.9)	1.005 [0.995, 1.012]	0.273
Duration of Antibiotics While Admitted (h)	67.1 (±99.2)	100.3 (±136.1)	69.8 (±102.7)	1.002 [0.999, 1.005]	0.120
Length of Hospital Stay (days)	4.0 (±4.7)	4.8 (±5.7)	4.0 (±4.8)	1.038 [0.954, 1.108]	0.351

Table 4. Cont.

Characteristic Mean (SD), Median (IQR), or n (%)	No Infection (n = 279)	Deep Infection (n = 24)	TOTAL (n = 303)	OR [95%OR]	p-Value
Discharged with Antibiotics					
No *	220 (80.0)	18 (81.8)	238 (80.1)		
Yes	55 (20.0)	4 (18.2)	59 (19.9)	0.967 [0.292, 2.611]	0.950
Discharge Disposition					
Home *	265 (95.3)	21 (87.5)	286 (94.7)		
Rehabilitation/Other	13 (4.7)	3 (12.5)	16 (5.3)	3.203 [0.780, 10.319]	0.099
Number of Operative Procedures	1 (1-1)	1 (1-3)	1 (1-1)	1.278 [1.034, 1.584]	0.026 **

* reference group, ** denotes statistical significance.

3.4. Multivariable Analysis

There were five factors significantly associated with the development of deep infection after an open long bone fracture (Figure 2). When these factors were incorporated into a single multivariable regression model, the only factor that remained significant was the duration of time between the injury event and presentation to an OSF or VUMC, where for every minute that time to hospital presentation was delayed, the odds of deep infection increased by 1% [OR = 1.010 (1.003–1.018); p = 0.006] (Table 5).

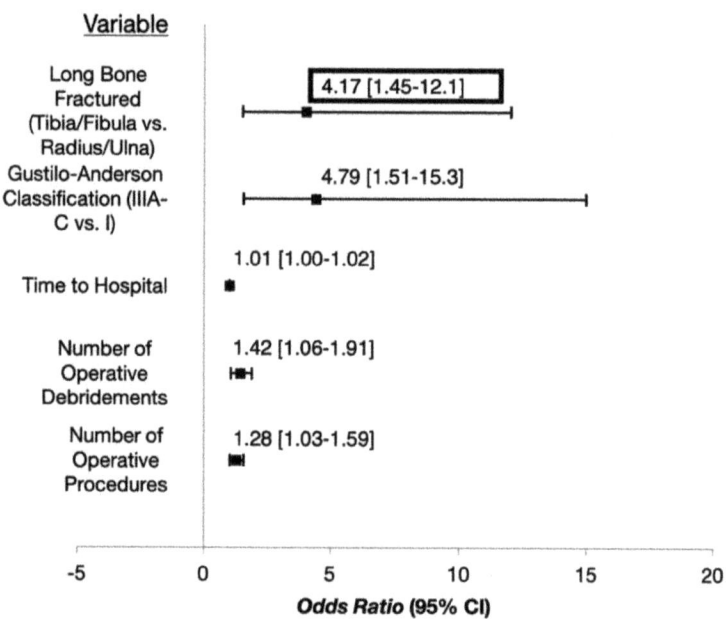

Figure 2. Odds Ratios and 95% Confidence Intervals for Factors Significantly Associated with D-veloping a Deep Infection After Pediatric Open Long-Bone Fractures.

Table 5. Multivariable Analysis for Factors Associated with Developing a Deep Infection After Pediatric Open Long-Bone Fractures.

Characteristic	OR [95% CI]	p-Value
Long-Bone		
Tibia/Fibula *		
Femur	0.508 [0.131, 1.614]	0.262
Humerus	236 [0.025, 1.064]	0.062
Radius/Ulna	0.380 [0.107, 1.178]	0.096
Gustilo-Anderson		
I *		
II	1.169 [0.302, 4.845]	0.822
IIIA-C	2.366 [0.622, 10.074]	0.210
Time to Hospital	1.010 [1.003, 1.017]	0.009 **
Number of Operative Debridements	1.209 [0.621, 2.408]	0.573
Number of Operative Procedures	1.001 [0.581, 1.557]	0.996

* reference group, ** denotes statistical significance.

4. Discussion

The purpose of the current study was to identify factors associated with developing a deep infection in pediatric patients with open long-bone fractures. Five variables were independently associated: (1) Fractures of the tibia/fibula; (2) higher revised Gustilo–Anderson type; (3) a longer duration of time between the injury and presentation to a hospital; (4) a higher number of operative debridements; (5) a higher number of total operative procedures. After incorporating all significant variables into a multivariable regression model, the only variable that remained statistically significant was the duration of time between the injury and presentation to a hospital, where for every additional minute delay in hospital presentation, the odds of infection increased by 1%.

Unfortunately, the literature regarding infection risk after pediatric open fracture is sparse and comprised primarily of small case series or small cohorts addressing a single risk factor [13]. In a recent systematic review of the adult literature, lower extremity open fractures were significantly more likely to develop infectious complications compared to upper extremity fractures [35]. A recent systematic review and meta-analysis of pediatric open fractures found that Gustilo–Anderson type III fractures of the tibia were associated with a lower risk of osteomyelitis than femoral fractures and found the lowest rates of osteomyelitis/infection in upper limb fractures [12]. Our study similarly found that the lower extremity, specifically the tibia/fibula is at greater risk for deep infection after an open fracture in the pediatric population. Additionally, our study demonstrated that the infection risk for type IIIA-C open fractures is four times greater compared to type I open fractures, a trend that was previously demonstrated in a 2009 systematic review by Baldwin et al. [36]. Their pooled analyses revealed that type III open tibia fractures in children were 3.48 times more likely to have an infectious complication compared to type I fractures and 2.28-fold more likely compared to type II. Interestingly, when Luhmann et al. [37] analyzed 65 open forearm fractures in a pediatric sample, fracture type was not associated with infection; however, as the authors note, the study may not have had adequate power to detect statistically significant differences.

Immediate antibiotic administration has been heralded as a mainstay of open fracture management. Patzakis and Wilson [38] demonstrated an infection rate of 4.7% for open fractures when antibiotics were administered within 3 h after injury and a rate of 7.2% when there was a delay of ≥3 h. However, they included both pediatric and adult patients. In the current study of only pediatric patients, the average time to antibiotics was under 3 h [161.5 (±157.4) min] for all patients, and there was no relationship between time to antibiotics and the development of a deep infection when the variable was left as a continuous measure or when patients were binned into two groups, <3 h vs. ≥3 h. However, time to first antibiotic administration was significantly associated (although with a small effect size) with time to hospital presentation in our post hoc correlative analyses, thus supporting the importance of early antibiotic administration. It has also been the classic teaching to debride the wound within 6 h of injury. Time to operative debridement was, on average, 14.5 (±8.5) h. There was no relationship between time to operative debridement and the presence of deep infection when the variable was left as a continuous measure or when patients were binned into two groups, <6 h vs. ≥6 h. These results are similar to two previously published studies by Skaggs et al. [28,29], who looked at 554 and 118 pediatric open fractures, finding that infection rates were not related to time to operative debridement groups of <6 h, 7–24 h, 25+ h and <6, 6–12, 12–24, and 24+ h, respectively. Kelly et al. also found no association between the development of infection and time to surgical debridement in 288 open fractures in pediatric patients [6]. Ibrahim et al. [27], 2014, examined the effect of delayed surgical debridement in pediatric open fractures by conducting a systematic review and meta-analysis. Late surgical debridement was associated with a pooled rate of infection of 2.5%, which was not higher than the infection rate of 4.2% seen for early surgical debridement (<6 h) in children with open fractures. The number of total operative debridements and operative procedures was associated with the presence of a deep infection in our study, which may represent a more correlative than causative relationship.

Even though time to antibiotics and time to operative debridement were not independently associated with the presence of deep infection in this study, the duration of time between the injury event and presentation to a hospital was a risk factor. For every additional minute delay in hospital presentation, the odds of infection increased by 1%. This finding raises more questions than answers and requires further study, given that the data included in this retrospective study were limited in both granularity and power. Factors surrounding immediate open fracture management in the field and in the emergency department should be included in future studies, including the performance and timing of temporary wound coverage with a sterile bandage, bedside irrigation and/or debridement, closed reduction, splinting, etc.

There are other limitations in this study worth declaring. As previously mentioned, a low number of cases required that data be binned and categorized into a smaller number of groups in order to maintain adequate power. Therefore, we could not analyze trends that required greater detail, such as antibiotic type and dosing. This resulted in analyzing antibiotic therapy as a count variable based on the number of different antibiotic classes administered. In a similar manner, we could not analyze factors related to definitive fixation and soft tissue coverage with substantial detail. Our search strategy may also not have identified every patient with an open fracture over the last two decades due to inaccurate billing codes. Lastly, retrospective research relies on reviewing records, which may have contained both factual and temporal inaccuracies. Future prospective and collaborative research should aim to identify additional risk factors for deep infection and clarify the ideal treatment strategy for these injuries. This will advance efforts to minimize complications and optimize outcomes for children who sustain open long-bone fractures.

5. Conclusions

Deep infection was associated with open fractures of the tibia/fibula and higher type open fractures. For every additional minute delay in hospital presentation, the odds of infection increased by 1%, suggesting that early hospital care is a critical factor in the management of these injuries. We recommend that in all cases of potential open fracture, children should present to a hospital as quickly as possible to be evaluated, receive care, and reduce the risk of deep infection.

Author Contributions: Conceptualization, J.E.M.; methodology J.E.M. and A.W.K.; formal analysis, A.W.K.; investigation, J.E.M. and A.W.K.; resources, J.E.M.; data curation, A.W.K.; writing—original draft preparation, A.W.K., S.C.T. and J.E.M.; writing—review and editing, A.W.K., S.C.T. and J.E.M.;

visualization, A.W.K.; supervision, J.E.M.; project administration, J.E.M., A.W.K. and S.C.T. All authors have read and agreed to the published version of the manuscript.

Funding: This research received no external funding.

Institutional Review Board Statement: The study was conducted in accordance with the Declaration of Helsinki and approved by the Institutional Review Board (or Ethics Committee) of VUMC; #182036).

Informed Consent Statement: Not applicable.

Data Availability Statement: The data are available in the results section of the manuscript.

Conflicts of Interest: These data were previously presented at the American Orthopaedic Association Annual Leadership Meeting in 2020.

References

1. Naranje, S.M.; Erali, R.A.; Warner, W.C., Jr.; Sawyer, J.R.; Kelly, D.M. Epidemiology of Pediatric Fractures Presenting to Emergency Departments in the United States. *J. Pediatric Orthop.* **2016**, *36*, e45–e48. [CrossRef] [PubMed]
2. Cheng, J.C.; Shen, W.Y. Limb fracture pattern in different pediatric age groups: A study of 3350 children. *J. Orthop. Trauma* **1993**, *7*, 15–22. [CrossRef] [PubMed]
3. Galano, G.J.; Vitale, M.A.; Kessler, M.W.; Hyman, J.E.; Vitale, M.G. The most frequent traumatic orthopaedic injuries from a national pediatric inpatient population. *J. Pediatric Orthop.* **2005**, *25*, 39–44. [PubMed]
4. Stewart, D.G., Jr.; Kay, R.M.; Skaggs, D.L. Open fractures in children. Principles of evaluation and management. *J. Bone Jt. Surg.* **2005**, *87*, 2784–2798. [CrossRef]
5. Trionfo, A.; Cavanaugh, P.K.; Herman, M.J. Pediatric Open Fractures. *Orthop. Clin.* **2016**, *47*, 565–578. [CrossRef]
6. Kelly, D.; Sheffer, B.; Elrod, R.; Piana, L.; Pattisapu, N.; Nolan, V.; Spence, D.; Sawyer, J. Infections After Open Fractures in Pediatric Patients: A Review of 288 Open Fractures. *J. Surg. Orthop. Adv.* **2022**, *31*, 73–75.
7. Gustilo, R.B.; Anderson, J.T. Prevention of infection in the treatment of one thousand and twenty-five open fractures of long bones. Retrospective and prospective analyses. *J. Bone Jt. Surg.* **2002**, *84*, 682. [CrossRef]
8. Gustilo, R.B.; Anderson, J.T. Prevention of infection in the treatment of one thousand and twenty-five open fractures of long bones: Retrospective and prospective analyses. *J. Bone Jt. Surg.* **1976**, *58*, 453–458. [CrossRef]
9. Lavelle, W.F.; Uhl, R.; Krieves, M.; Drvaric, D.M. Management of open fractures in pediatric patients: Current teaching in Accreditation Council for Graduate Medical Education (ACGME) accredited residency programs. *J. Pediatric Orthop. B* **2008**, *17*, 1–6. [CrossRef]
10. Wetzel, R.J.; Minhas, S.V.; Patrick, B.C.; Janicki, J.A. Current Practice in the Management of Type I Open Fractures in Children: A Survey of POSNA Membership. *J. Pediatric Orthop.* **2015**, *35*, 762–768. [CrossRef]
11. Elia, G.; Blood, T.; Got, C. The Management of Pediatric Open Forearm Fractures. *J. Hand Surg.* **2020**, *45*, 523–527. [CrossRef]
12. Singh, A.; Bierrum, W.; Wormald, J.; Eastwood, D.M. Non-operative versus operative management of open fractures in the paediatric population: A systematic review and meta-analysis of the adverse outcomes. *Injury* **2020**, *51*, 1477–1488. [CrossRef] [PubMed]
13. Pace, J.L.; Kocher, M.S.; Skaggs, D.L. Evidence-based review: Management of open pediatric fractures. *J. Pediatric Orthop.* **2012**, *32* (Suppl. S2), S123–S127. [CrossRef]
14. Godfrey, J.; Pace, J.L. Type I Open Fractures Benefit From Immediate Antibiotic Administration But Not Necessarily Immediate Surgery. *J. Pediatric Orthop.* **2016**, *36* (Suppl. S1), S6–S10. [CrossRef]
15. Kreder, H.J.; Armstrong, P. The significance of perioperative cultures in open pediatric lower-extremity fractures. *Clin. Orthop. Relat. Res.* **1994**, *302*, 206–212. [CrossRef]
16. Tomaszewski, R.; Gap, A. Results of the treatment of the open femoral shaft fractures in children. *J. Orthop.* **2014**, *11*, 78–81. [CrossRef] [PubMed]
17. Allison, P.; Dahan-Oliel, N.; Jando, V.T.; Yang, S.S.; Hamdy, R.C. Open fractures of the femur in children: Analysis of various treatment methods. *J. Child. Orthop.* **2011**, *5*, 101–108. [CrossRef]
18. Aslani, H.; Tabrizi, A.; Sadighi, A.; Mirblok, A.R. Treatment of open pediatric tibial fractures by external fixation versus flexible intramedullary nailing: A comparative study. *Arch. Trauma Res.* **2013**, *2*, 108–112. [CrossRef]
19. Aslani, H.; Tabrizi, A.; Sadighi, A.; Mirbolook, A.R. Treatment of pediatric open femoral fractures with external fixator versus flexible intramedullary nails. *Arch. Bone Jt. Surg.* **2013**, *1*, 64–67.
20. Bazzi, A.A.; Brooks, J.T.; Jain, A.; Ain, M.C.; Tis, J.E.; Sponseller, P.D. Is nonoperative treatment of pediatric type I open fractures safe and effective? *J. Child. Orthop.* **2014**, *8*, 467–471. [CrossRef]
21. Doak, J.; Ferrick, M. Nonoperative management of pediatric grade 1 open fractures with less than a 24-h admission. *J. Pediatric Orthop.* **2009**, *29*, 49–51. [CrossRef]

22. Godfrey, J.; Choi, P.D.; Shabtai, L.; Nossov, S.B.; Williams, A.; Lindberg, A.W.; Silva, S.; Caird, M.S.; Schur, M.D.; Arkader, A. Management of Pediatric Type I Open Fractures in the Emergency Department or Operating Room: A Multicenter Perspective. *J. Pediatric Orthop.* **2017**, *39*, 372–376. [CrossRef]
23. Iobst, C.A.; Spurdle, C.; Baitner, A.C.; King, W.F.; Tidwell, M.; Swirsky, S. A protocol for the management of pediatric type I open fractures. *J. Child. Orthop.* **2014**, *8*, 71–76. [CrossRef] [PubMed]
24. Iobst, C.A.; Tidwell, M.A.; King, W.F. Nonoperative management of pediatric type I open fractures. *J. Pediatric Orthop.* **2005**, *25*, 513–517. [CrossRef] [PubMed]
25. Laine, J.C.; Cherkashin, A.; Samchukov, M.; Birch, J.G.; Rathjen, K.E. The Management of Soft Tissue and Bone Loss in Type IIIB and IIIC Pediatric Open Tibia Fractures. *J. Pediatric Orthop.* **2016**, *36*, 453–458. [CrossRef] [PubMed]
26. Ozkul, E.; Gem, M.; Arslan, H.; Alemdar, C.; Azboy, I.; Arslan, S.G. Minimally Invasive Plate Osteosynthesis in Open Pediatric Tibial Fractures. *J. Pediatric Orthop.* **2016**, *36*, 416–422. [CrossRef]
27. Ibrahim, T.; Riaz, M.; Hegazy, A.; Erwin, P.J.; Tleyjeh, I.M. Delayed surgical debridement in pediatric open fractures: A systematic review and meta-analysis. *J. Child. Orthop.* **2014**, *8*, 135–141. [CrossRef]
28. Skaggs, D.L.; Friend, L.; Alman, B.; Chambers, H.G.; Schmitz, M.; Leake, B.; Kay, R.M.; Flynn, J.M. The effect of surgical delay on acute infection following 554 open fractures in children. *J. Bone Jt. Surg.* **2005**, *87*, 8–12. [CrossRef]
29. Skaggs, D.L.; Kautz, S.M.; Kay, R.M.; Tolo, V.T. Effect of delay of surgical treatment on rate of infection in open fractures in children. *J. Pediatric Orthop.* **2000**, *20*, 19–22. [CrossRef]
30. Dedmond, B.T.; Kortesis, B.; Punger, K.; Simpson, J.; Argenta, J.; Kulp, B.; Morykwas, M.; Webb, L.X. Subatmospheric pressure dressings in the temporary treatment of soft tissue injuries associated with type III open tibial shaft fractures in children. *J. Pediatric Orthop.* **2006**, *26*, 728–732. [CrossRef]
31. Halvorson, J.; Jinnah, R.; Kulp, B.; Frino, J. Use of vacuum-assisted closure in pediatric open fractures with a focus on the rate of infection. *Orthopedics* **2011**, *34*, e256–e260. [CrossRef] [PubMed]
32. Garcia-Lopez, E.; Vutescu, E.S.; Orman, S.; Schiller, J.; Eberson, C.P.; Cruz, A.I. Antibiotic Considerations in the Management of Pediatric Open Fractures: Current Concept Review. *JPOSNA* **2021**, *3*. Available online: https://www.jposna.org/index.php/jposna/article/view/225 (accessed on 3 August 2022).
33. Harris, P.A.; Taylor, R.; Thielke, R.; Payne, J.; Gonzalez, N.; Conde, J.G. Research electronic data capture (REDCap)—A metadata-driven methodology and workflow process for providing translational research informatics support. *J. Biomed. Inform.* **2009**, *42*, 377–381. [CrossRef] [PubMed]
34. Heinze, G.; Ploner, M.; Dunkler, D.; Southworth, H. Firth's Bias-Reduced Logistic Regression, Version 1.23; 2018. Available online: https://search.r-project.org/CRAN/refmans/logistf/html/logistf.html (accessed on 3 August 2022).
35. Kortram, K.; Bezstarosti, H.; Metsemakers, W.J.; Raschke, M.J.; Van Lieshout, E.M.M.; Verhofstad, M.H.J. Risk factors for infectious complications after open fractures; a systematic review and meta-analysis. *Int. Orthop.* **2017**, *41*, 1965–1982. [CrossRef] [PubMed]
36. Baldwin, K.D.; Babatunde, O.M.; Russell Huffman, G.; Hosalkar, H.S. Open fractures of the tibia in the pediatric population: A systematic review. *J. Child. Orthop.* **2009**, *3*, 199–208. [CrossRef] [PubMed]
37. Luhmann, S.J.; Schootman, M.; Schoenecker, P.L.; Dobbs, M.B.; Gordon, J.E. Complications and outcomes of open pediatric forearm fractures. *J. Pediatric Orthop.* **2004**, *24*, 1–6. [CrossRef] [PubMed]
38. Patzakis, M.J.; Wilkins, J. Factors influencing infection rate in open fracture wounds. *Clin. Orthop. Relat. Res.* **1989**, *243*, 36–40. [CrossRef]

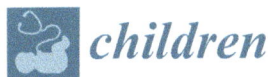

Article

Outcome of Open Reduction Alone or with Concomitant Bony Procedures for Developmental Dysplasia of the Hip (DDH)

Kamal Jamil *[ ], Rostam Saharuddin, Ahmad Fazly Abd Rasid, Abdul Halim Abd Rashid and Sharaf Ibrahim

Department of Orthopaedics & Traumatology, Faculty of Medicine, Universiti Kebangsaan Malaysia, Cheras, Kuala Lumpur 56000, Malaysia
* Correspondence: drkortho@gmail.com

Abstract: Introduction: Developmental dysplasia of the hip (DDH) is commonly managed in a tertiary centre and regularly involves surgical treatment. The aim of this study is to determine the surgical outcome of DDH patient treated with either open reduction alone or combined with bony procedures in our institution. Methods: Medical records of DDH patients treated surgically were reviewed. Patients were divided into two groups: Group A: underwent open reduction (OR) only; and Group B: underwent open reduction with additional bony procedures (ORB), such as pelvic or femoral osteotomy. Modified McKay classification was used to evaluate the clinical outcome, and Severin classification for the radiological outcome. Presence of avascular necrosis and other post-operative complications were recorded. Results: A total of 66 patients (76 hips) were reviewed with the mean age of 11.9 ± 4.8 years. Mean duration of follow up was 8.6 ± 4.7 years (ranged 2 to 23 years). From our sample, 50/66 patients (75.8%) achieved satisfactory clinical outcome, whereas 48/66 patients (72.7%) had satisfactory radiological outcome. A higher proportion of patients achieved satisfactory outcomes in the OR group compared to the ORB group ($p < 0.05$), but no difference was seen in terms of radiological outcome ($p = 0.80$). Overall, 23 hips (34.8%) developed radiographic evidence of avascular necrosis (AVN). Nineteen hips had undergone ORB, although they were mainly (63.2%) Grade I AVN. Incidence of AVN was comparable in both groups ($p = 0.63$), but presence of AVN led to a higher proportion of unsatisfactory clinical and radiological outcome ($p < 0.05$). Other complications included redislocation/subluxation (13.6%) and bleeding (0.1%). Conclusions: Good overall outcome of DDH surgery was achieved in our centre. The OR group may produce a better clinical outcome, but with similar radiological results and AVN rate with the ORB group. The presence of AVN is associated with unsatisfactory clinical and radiological outcomes.

Keywords: developmental dysplasia of the hip; open reduction; pelvic osteotomy; femoral osteotomy; hip dysplasia

Citation: Jamil, K.; Saharuddin, R.; Abd Rasid, A.F.; Abd Rashid, A.H.; Ibrahim, S. Outcome of Open Reduction Alone or with Concomitant Bony Procedures for Developmental Dysplasia of the Hip (DDH). *Children* 2022, 9, 1213. https://doi.org/10.3390/children9081213

Academic Editors: Axel A. Horsch, Maher A. Ghandour and Matthias Christoph M. Klotz

Received: 14 July 2022
Accepted: 30 July 2022
Published: 12 August 2022

Publisher's Note: MDPI stays neutral with regard to jurisdictional claims in published maps and institutional affiliations.

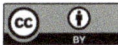

Copyright: © 2022 by the authors. Licensee MDPI, Basel, Switzerland. This article is an open access article distributed under the terms and conditions of the Creative Commons Attribution (CC BY) license (https://creativecommons.org/licenses/by/4.0/).

1. Introduction

The incidence of DDH varies among different regions and population. In Malaysia, the incidence of DDH was reported at 0.7 cases per 1000 births [1]. Other countries which implement universal ultrasonographic screening of DDH reported increasing cases, up to 25 to 50 cases per 1000 birth [2]. Once diagnosed, the aim of the DDH treatment is to provide a concentric and stable hip [2–4]. Early initiation of treatment is essential to allow optimal hip remodelling. If left untreated, the dysplastic hip may lead to dislocation and the child will have an abnormal gait resulting in hip pain. In the long term, early onset of osteoarthritis is expected in these cases [5].

Management of DDH is mainly based on the age of presentation. Pavlik harness can be initiated during the neonatal period. Closed reduction and hip spica are performed between the ages of 6 to 12 months old if the dislocation persisted. Open reduction with or without pelvic and femur osteotomy is reserved for cases of failed closed reduction and for patients with late presentations [3,6]. Successful management of DDH can be reviewed based on the radiographs and clinical assessments.

Treatment by either closed or open reduction has been shown to lead to favourable outcomes in many short- to middle-term studies [7–9]. In a walking-age child with DDH, open reduction with concomitant pelvic osteotomy would provide the best results according to a recent systematic review [10]. Long-term studies suggested that older age at first surgery and complication of avascular necrosis are associated with poor outcomes [5,11]. However, there are not many long-term studies on DDH in Malaysia and to the best of our knowledge there is only one study on the treatment outcome [12]. Therefore, we decided to review the clinical and radiological outcome of the DDH patients that were surgically treated at our centre for the past 20 years. We also want to determine whether an open reduction alone would lead to a similar outcome to a combined surgery with bony procedures.

2. Materials and Methods

Following the approval of the institutional ethics committee board, we retrospectively reviewed the medical records of DDH patients who were surgically treated in our centre since January 1996 to January 2018. All bilateral or unilateral DDH patients operated on during the study period were included in this study. Patients with teratological, paralytic, septic, or traumatic hip dislocations were excluded. All patients included had at least two years of follow-up from the operation date. Figure 1 shows the flowchart of our patient selection and study design.

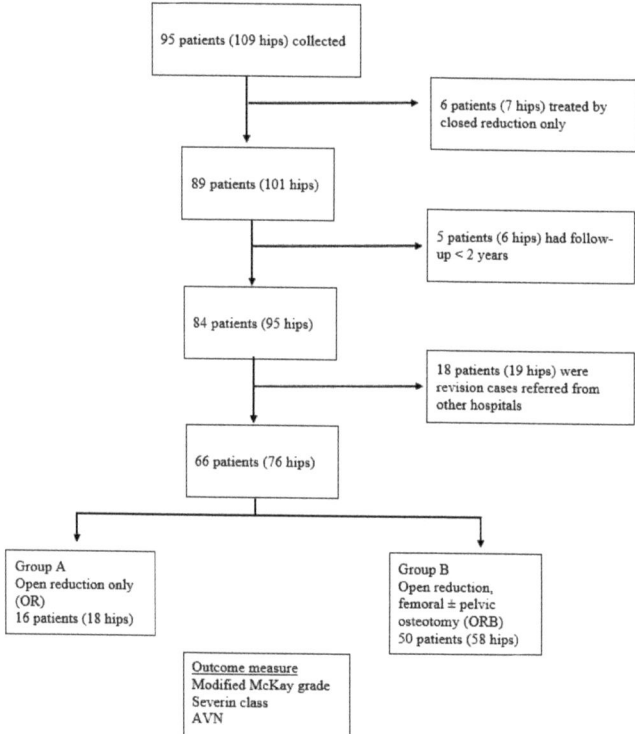

Figure 1. Flowchart of the patient selection and study design.

Patients were divided based on the surgical treatment received. Group A consists of patients who underwent open reduction (OR) only, whilst patients in Group B underwent open reduction with either femoral or pelvic osteotomy (ORB). All patients underwent open reduction with the modified Smith-Petersen approach (anterior approach with bikini skin incision). In cases where there was significant tension of the surrounding soft tissue impeding reduction, femoral shortening was performed following the technique described by Klisic [13]. Pelvic osteotomies (either Salter [14] or Pemberton [15]) were carried out for patients who had poor femoral head coverage following hip reduction. For both groups of patients, the child was immobilized in hip spica for a total duration of 3 months post-operatively. We did not practice pre-operative traction. Surgery was performed by two senior paediatric orthopaedic surgeons (SI and AHR).

The outcome measures were assessed by reviewing the documented clinical data and follow-up radiographs. Modified McKay [16] grading was used to evaluate the clinical outcome of each group. We consider McKay grade I and II ('excellent' and 'good') as 'satisfactory', whereas grade III and IV ('fair and poor') are considered as 'unsatisfactory' outcomes. The Severin [17] classification was used to evaluate the radiological outcome, whereby class I and II were considered 'satisfactory' and class III and IV were 'unsatisfactory'. Intra-operative and post-operative complications were reviewed from the medical records. Any evidence of AVN of the hip was classified using Bucholz and Ogden [18] classification. Data collection was performed by a single researcher. For the purpose of analysis, data on the 'worst' hip were taken for cases with bilateral DDH.

The data collected were analyzed using the SPSS software version 21.0. The chi-square and Fishers' exact test were used for categorical data. The p-value of < 0.05 was considered as statistically significant.

3. Results

A total of 66 patients (76 hips) were selected with the mean age at surgery of 3.8 ± 2.6 years and 11.9 ± 4.8 years at the last follow-up. The mean duration of follow up was 8.6 ± 4.7 years (ranged 2 to 23 years). The majority of patients were females; 57 patients (86.4%) and there were 9 males (13.6%). Table 1 shows the demographic characteristics of the subjects. Group B consisted of children who were significantly older than Group A.

Table 1. Demography of the study subjects. OR = open reduction, ORB = open reduction, femoral procedure ± pelvic osteotomy.

	OR (n = 16)	ORB (n = 50)	p-Value
Age at surgery in years (mean ± SD)	1.5 ± 0.4	4.5 ± 2.5	<0.05
Age at final follow-up (mean ± SD)	8.6 ± 4.6	13.0 ± 4.4	<0.05
Gender: N (%)			0.43 *
Male	1 (1.5%)	15 (22.7%)	
Female	21 (41.2%)	42 (63.6%)	
Laterality: N (%)			0.50 *
Left	7 (10.6%)	28 (10.6%)	
Right	7 (56.9%)	14 (21.2%)	
Bilateral	2 (3.0%)	8 (12.1%)	

* Fisher exact test.

At the latest follow-up visit, the clinical outcome by modified McKay grading revealed that 46 patients (69.7%) were grade I (excellent), four (6.1%) were grade II (good) and 16 (24.2%) were grade III (fair). None of the patients were graded as poor, which is grade IV.

The overall radiological outcome showed that 41 patients (62.1%) had Severin class I, seven patients (10.6%) class II, two (3%) class III and 16 (24.2%) class IV. In total, 23 hips (34.8%) developed radiographic evidence of AVN as classified by Bucholz and Ogden. The majority were grade I (21.2%), followed by grade II (10.6%), and grade III (3%). Figure 2A–C shows a case example of a patient with a satisfactory outcome, while Figure 3 is an example of an unsatisfactory outcome.

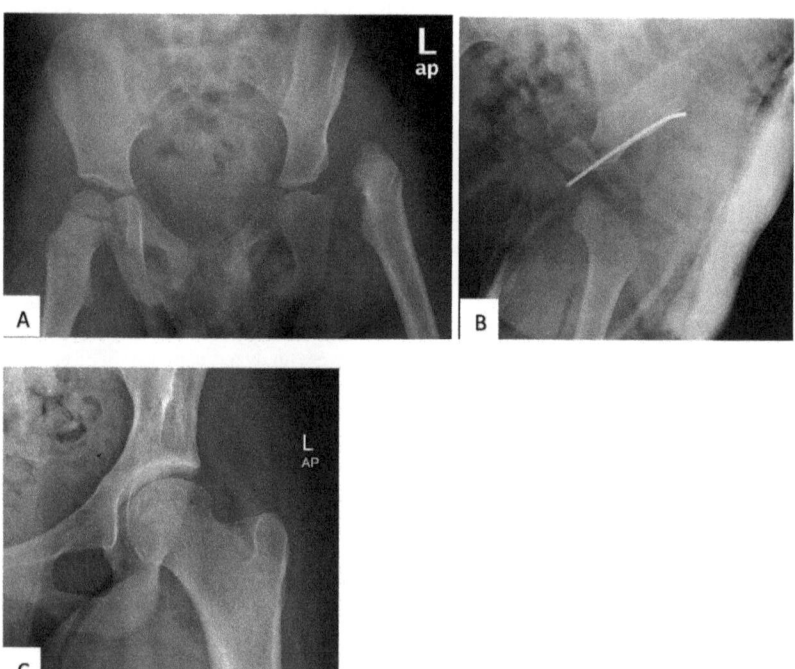

Figure 2. Radiographs of a boy treated with open reduction and Salter osteotomy. He had an excellent clinical outcome (McKay grading). (**A**) Pre-operative anteroposterior pelvic radiograph at age 20 months showing a left hip dislocation and a dysplastic left acetabulum. (**B**) Post-operative hip radiograph shows hip reduction and the Salter osteotomy stabilised with a K-wire. (**C**) Anteroposterior left hip radiograph showing a normal femoral head shape and acetabulum (Severin class I) at age 11 years old.

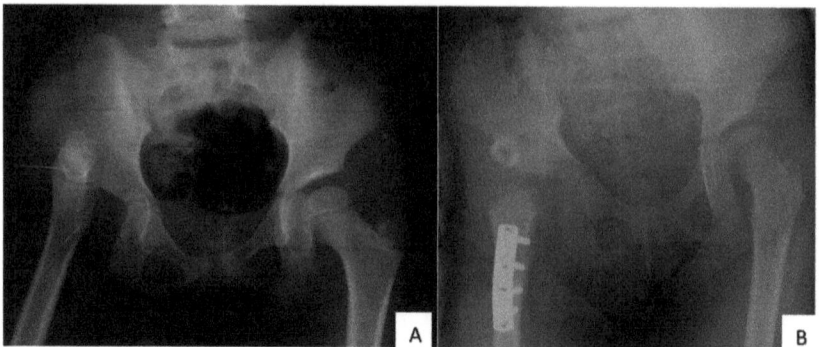

Figure 3. *Cont.*

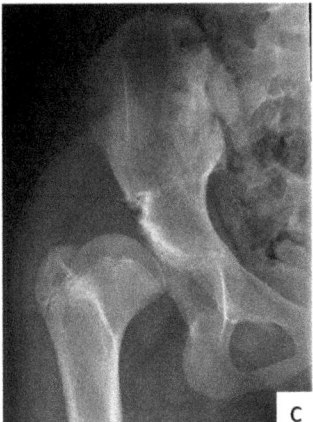

Figure 3. Radiographs of a girl treated with open reduction, femoral shortening, and Salter osteotomy. (**A**) Pre-operative pelvic radiograph at age 6 years old showing a high right hip dislocation and dysplastic acetabulum. (**B**) Post-operative radiograph shows the hip is reduced but retroverted. Salter osteotomy with a bone graft taken from the resected femoral shaft. The K-wire fixing the bone graft has been removed. (**C**) At the age of 13 years, the radiographic outcome is poor (Severin class IV). There are presence of coxa breva, femoral head subluxation, and severe acetabular dysplasia. Her clinical outcome by McKay grading was also poor.

Chi-square test found that the rate of unsatisfactory outcome was significantly lower in the OR group than the ORB ($p < 0.05$) for the clinical outcome (Table 2). However, both groups showed a comparable radiological result by Severin class ($p = 0.80$). There was no difference in the incidence of AVN between both groups ($\chi^2 = 2.66$, $p = 0.63$). Although, presence of AVN led to a higher proportion of unsatisfactory clinical and radiological outcome ($p < 0.05$) (Table 3).

Table 2. Comparison between Group A (OR) and Group B (ORB) according to modified McKay grading and Severin classification. McKay grade I and II (excellent and good) = satisfactory, grade III and IV (fair and poor) = unsatisfactory outcome. The Severin classification class I and II = satisfactory and class III and IV = unsatisfactory. OR = open reduction; ORB = open reduction + femoral procedure with or without pelvic osteotomy.

Group	McKay Grading		Total	χ^2	p-Value
	Satisfactory	Unsatisfactory			
OR	15	1	16		
	(22.7%)	(1.5%)	(24.2%)		
ORB	33	17	50	4.71	<0.05 *
	(50.0%)	(25.8%)	(75.8%)		
Total	48	18	66		
	(72.7%)	(27.3%)			
	Severin Class				
	Satisfactory	Unsatisfactory			
OR	11	5	16		
	(16.7%)	(7.6%)	(24.2%)		
ORB	36	14	50	0.06	0.80
	(54.5%)	(21.2%)	(75.8%)		
Total	47	19	66		
	(71.2%)	(28.8%)			

* Fisher exact test.

Table 3. Correlation between presence of AVN and outcome according to modified McKay grading and Severin classification. McKay grade I and II (excellent and good) = satisfactory, grade III and IV (fair and poor) = unsatisfactory outcome. The Severin classification class I and II = satisfactory and class III and IV = unsatisfactory. AVN = avascular necrosis.

AVN	McKay Grading		Total	χ^2	p-Value
	Satisfactory	Unsatisfactory			
No AVN	36 (53.0%)	8 (12.1%)	43 (65.2%)		
Grade 1	9 (13.6%)	5 (7.6%)	14 (21.2%)	8.32	<0.05 *
Grade 2	4 (6.1%)	3 (4.5%)	7 (10.6%)		
Grade 3	0	2 (3.0%)	2 (3.0%)		
Total	48 (72.7%)	18 (27.3%)	66		
	Severin Class				
	Satisfactory	Unsatisfactory			
No AVN	36 (54.5%)	7 (10.6%)	43 (65.2%)		
Grade 1	6 (9.1%)	8 (12.1%)	14 (21.2%)	13.72	<0.05 *
Grade 2	5 (7.6%)	2 (3.0%)	7 (10.6%)		
Grade 3	0	2 (3.0%)	2 (3.0%)		
Total	47 (71.2%)	19 (28.8%)	66		

* Fisher exact test.

We also investigated whether age at the time of primary surgery would influence the outcome. Comparison between patients operated upon before and after the age of 3 years old revealed that there were no differences in terms of McKay grading ($p = 0.34$), Severin class ($p = 0.23$), and also incidence of AVN ($p = 0.28$).

There were seven patients (eight hips) who had had multiple procedures before the latest follow-up. These patients either had repeat open reduction (one hip) or repeat open reduction with additional femoral/pelvic procedure (seven hips). They also represent the hips which had subluxated (five hips) or redislocated (three hips) in our cohort. Apart from that, nine other patients (11 hips) had history of prior closed reduction (but redislocated) before the index procedure. However, we found that the patients who had multiple procedures showed a comparable outcome with those patients who underwent a single procedure only, in terms of McKay grading ($p = 0.29$), Severin class ($p = 0.38$), and also incidence of AVN ($p = 0.14$). Other complication includes intra-operative blood loss requiring blood transfusion (four hips).

4. Discussion

Our results indicate that the majority of the patients achieved satisfactory clinical (75.8%) and radiological (72.7%) outcome in the medium to long-term, following the surgical treatment with open reduction with or without femoral/pelvic procedure. We construe 'satisfactory' outcome as 'excellent' or 'good' in McKay clinical grading and Severin I and II class for the radiological outcome. Other studies reported their satisfactory outcomes in the range of 70–90%, with various DDH procedures performed and different duration of follow-ups [7,8,19–25]. Many of the authors presented results of a single-stage procedure, combining open reduction with femoral and pelvic osteotomies [7,19–23]. Medium-term studies showed high percentages of satisfactory outcomes (80–90%) for a single-stage procedure, with average duration of follow-up of 3 to 6 years [7,19,24–26]. In long term studies, few researchers have shown comparable results. Varner et al. reviewed 57 patients at skeletal maturity, with a mean duration of 18 years follow-up and found 78% satisfactory radiological outcome [8]. Similarly, Wu et al. achieved about 80% satisfactory clinical and radiological outcome in children treated with open reduction and Pemberton osteotomy at an 11-years-average follow-up [11].

In our study, we found that children who underwent open reduction alone (OR) fared better clinically compared to children who had additional bony procedures (ORB). This is in line with the findings of a recent systematic review which reported that the odds of having a satisfactory clinical and radiological outcome is higher in the OR group [10]. Though, we did not find any difference in the radiological outcome between the groups in our study. The same systematic review also suggested that even though the OR group has a good outcome, they presented with an unacceptably high rates of reoperation, whereby the odds of needing further non-salvage procedures are as high as 10–15 times compared to ORB [10]. We have a relatively small number of patients in the OR group (16 patients), but all of them did not require additional surgeries.

One of the reasons why the OR group might perform better than the ORB is due to the younger age at surgery. It is generally accepted that ORB procedures are indicated for children of at least 18 months old, therefore the age differences compared to the OR group is unavoidable. In a Turkish study, children in the OR group aged below 18 months old had less AVN and reoperation rates in comparison to the ORB group who were older than 18 months [9]. However, there was no differences in their clinical and radiological outcome. Age was also found as an independent risk factor for unsatisfactory hip function in other studies [24,25,27–29]. Older age children have less potential of acetabular remodelling and may require more complex surgery for their treatment. Holman et al. reviewed 57 patients at an average age of 30 years old and found that radiological results at maturity deteriorates in children who were operated after the age of 3 years [5]. We are unable to show this age effect in our study but many of our patients have not reach skeletal maturity at the latest follow-up. Ning et al. further divided their patients into three age groups: 1.5 to 2.5 years, 2.5 to 8 years and above 8 years old during the index surgery [25]. Evaluating a large group of over 800 hips, they found that a single stage procedure at the age between 2.5 to 8 years produced the best radiological outcome with low AVN rates.

AVN is the most serious complication from DDH surgery. Post-operative AVN has been reported to be as low as 0% but up to 67% in various studies [30]. This discrepancy is attributable to the various classifications used to describe this complication. Kalamchi and McEwen [31] and Bucholz and Ogden [18] are the two popular classifications for AVN whereby type I class in both classifications would represent temporary epiphyseal mottling or fragmentation. Type II and above is when the physeal damage is apparent and therefore could possibly lead to growth disturbances and premature arthritis as young adults. Our data show clinically relevant AVN in 13.6% of the cases. We found that the incidence was comparable between the OR and ORB groups, although the presence of AVN was associated with unsatisfactory clinical and radiological outcomes. Our results are in line with the recent systematic review which also failed to find a statistical difference between OR alone and OR with either femoral or pelvic osteotomy in terms of AVN incidence [10]. However, if a single-stage procedure was performed instead (which involved OR with both femoral and pelvic procedures), significantly higher rates of AVN were seen as compared to OR alone. Other studies also associate AVN with unfavourable post-operative outcomes [5,11,24,25,30].

The reason for developing post-operative AVN is still debatable but there are some postulated risk factors. Older age at surgery, higher grade of dislocation, surgical approach (anterior vs medial), performing pelvic osteotomy, and extreme hip position in spica have all been proposed to increase the risk of AVN [26]. Wu et al. investigated the presence of AVN in 167 hips treated with OR and Pemberton osteotomy [11]. They proposed that excessive reduction leading to inferior displacement of the femoral head may compress the lateral epiphyseal artery, thus causing AVN. There is a general belief that performing a femoral shortening can effectively reduce soft tissue tension therefore able to avoid AVN in

DDH surgery, although this has not been proven to be true [10]. Despite that, the procedure may be needed in older children with proximal femoral migration to allow concentric hip reduction. Apart from that, multiple surgeries theoretically would disrupt the blood supply to the hip and lead to AVN. However, we were unable to show that repeated procedures are related to the incidence of AVN in our cohort.

The other challenging complication encountered post operatively is redislocation of the hip. We had 7/66 patients or 10.6% of cases that needed to be re-operated for this reason. Other studies reported their redislocation rates around 0–8% [25,32]. Failure to get the hip reduced deep into the acetabulum is the main reason for redislocation [26]. This may be due to severe joint laxity or increased femoral anteversion. If hip is unstable following reduction and capsulorrhaphy, additional measures such as femoral or pelvic osteotomy might be needed to ensure deep positioning of the femoral head at the primary surgery. Ganger et al. proposed meticulous analysis with CT scan or MRI to assess degree of femoral anteversion, labral abnormality, and acetabular version in redislocated cases [26]. Revision surgery for redislocated hip is technically demanding and should be performed by an experienced surgeon.

The results of this study are based on patients operated upon by two senior orthopaedic surgeons who might have differences in surgical technique but followed a similar treatment algorithm. However, our study is limited by its retrospective design and relatively small number of subjects in the OR group. Measurements on radiographs were performed by a single researcher, but we did not perform reliability study prior to data collection. We also excluded patients who had been operated elsewhere and referred to us, whose results might influence the outcome of this study. We had difficulty in comparing our results with other studies due to the different age groups, duration of follow-up, surgical procedure, and techniques. This issue was also reported by other authors [10,19]. However, our results of 70% satisfactory clinical and radiological outcome with a 13.6% AVN rate is in a broad agreement with other studies [9,22,23,26]. We only included patients with at least 2 years of follow-up, as that is the minimum duration to assess AVN [9]. Although, Domzalski and Synder suggested that vascular changes may not be evident until as late as 11 years after the reduction therefore follow-up less than 10 years may not reflect the true prevalence of AVN [30]. We did not identify the cause of AVN in our study. To reduce the risk of AVN, we believe that the surgical principle in DDH which is 'concentric reduction without tension' should be strictly adhered to, even if additional bony procedures may need to be performed to achieve it. In addition, meticulous surgical technique by highly skilled surgeon is paramount in difficult cases.

5. Conclusions

The outcome of DDH surgery in our centre is comparable to other studies. The OR group may produce a better clinical outcome, but with similar radiological consequence and AVN rate with the ORB group.

Author Contributions: Conceptualization, S.I.; methodology, K.J. and R.S.; software, R.S. and A.F.A.R.; validation, K.J., A.H.A.R. and S.I.; formal analysis, K.J. and R.S.; investigation, R.S. and A.F.A.R.; resources, K.J. and R.S.; data curation, R.S.; writing—original draft preparation, R.S.; writing—review and editing, K.J., A.F.A.R., A.H.A.R. and S.I.; visualization, K.J.; supervision, K.J., A.F.A.R. and A.H.A.R.; project administration, K.J.; funding acquisition, A.H.A.R. All authors have read and agreed to the published version of the manuscript.

Funding: This research received no external funding.

Institutional Review Board Statement: The study was conducted according to the guidelines of the Declaration of Helsinki and approved by the Institutional Review Board (Universiti Kebangsaan Malaysia: JEP-2020-325).

Informed Consent Statement: Patient consent was waived due to the retrospective study design.

Data Availability Statement: The data presented in this study are available on request from the corresponding author. The data are not publicly available because they contain potentially identifying or sensitive patient information.

Conflicts of Interest: The authors declare no conflict of interest.

References

1. Boo, N.; Rajaram, T. Congenital dislocation of hips in Malaysian neonates. *Singapore Med. J.* **1989**, *30*, 71–368. [PubMed]
2. Kotlarsky, P.; Haber, R.; Bialik, V.; Eidelman, M. Developmental dysplasia of the hip: What has changed in the last 20 years? *World J. Orthop.* **2015**, *6*, 886–901. [CrossRef] [PubMed]
3. Murphy, R.F.; Kim, Y.-J. Surgical management of pediatric developmental dysplasia of the hip. *J. Am. Acad. Orthop. Surg.* **2016**, *24*, 615–624. [CrossRef] [PubMed]
4. Vaquero-Picado, A.; González-Morán, G.; Garay, E.G.; Moraleda, L. Developmental dysplasia of the hip: Update of management. *EFORT Open Rev.* **2019**, *4*, 548–556. [CrossRef]
5. Holman, J.; Carroll, K.L.; Murray, K.A.; MacLeod, L.M.; Roach, J.W. Long-term follow-up of open reduction surgery for developmental dislocation of the hip. *J. Pediatr. Orthop.* **2012**, *32*, 121–124. [CrossRef]
6. Weinstein, S.L.; Mubarak, S.J.; Wenger, D.R. Developmental hip dysplasia and dislocation: Part II. *J. Bone Joint Surg.* **2003**, *85*, 2024–2035. [CrossRef]
7. Bhuyan, B.K. Outcome of one-stage treatment of developmental dysplasia of hip in older children. *Indian J. Orthop.* **2012**, *46*, 548–555. [CrossRef]
8. Varner, K.E.; Incavo, S.J.; Haynes, R.J.; Dickson, J.A. Surgical treatment of developmental hip dislocation in children aged 1 to 3 years: A mean 18-year, 9-month follow-up study. *Orthopedics* **2010**, *33*, 1–5. [CrossRef]
9. Yorgancıgil, H.; Aslan, A.; Demirci, D.; Atay, T. Effect of Age and Surgical Procedure on Clinical and Radiological Outcomes in Children with Developmental Dysplasia of the Hip: A Comparative Study. *J. Acad. Res. Med.* **2016**, *6*, 177–182. [CrossRef]
10. Kothari, A.; Grammatopoulos, G.; Hopewell, S.; Theologis, T. How does bony surgery affect results of anterior open reduction in walking-age children with developmental hip dysplasia? *Clin. Orthop. Relat. Res.* **2016**, *474*, 1199–1208. [CrossRef]
11. Wu, K.-W.; Wang, T.-M.; Huang, S.-C.; Kuo, K.N.; Chen, C.-W. Analysis of osteonecrosis following Pemberton acetabuloplasty in developmental dysplasia of the hip: Long-term results. *J. Bone Joint Surg.* **2010**, *92*, 2083–2094. [CrossRef] [PubMed]
12. Asim, A.; Saw, A.; Nawar, M. Treatment of Developmental Dysplasia of the Hip: Shortand Mid-term Outcome. *Malay. Orthop. J.* **2011**, *5*, 17–20.
13. Klisic, P.; Jankovic, L. Combined procedure of open reduction and shortening of the femur in treatment of congenital dislocation of the hips in older children. *Clin. Orthop. Relat. Res.* **1976**, *119*, 60–69. [CrossRef]
14. Salter, R.B. Role of innominate osteotomy in the treatment of congenital dislocation and subluxation of the hip in the older child. *J. Bone Joint Surg.* **1966**, *48*, 1413–1439. [CrossRef] [PubMed]
15. Pemberton, P.A. Pericapsular osteotomy of the ilium for treatment of congenital subluxation and dislocation of the hip. *J. Bone Joint Surg.* **1965**, *47*, 65–86. [CrossRef] [PubMed]
16. Mckay, D.W. A comparison of the innominate and the pericapsular osteotomy in the treatment of congenital dislocation of the hip. *Clin. Orthop. Relat. Res.* **1974**, *98*, 124–132. [CrossRef]
17. Severin, E. Contribution to the knowledge of congenital dislocation of the hip joint. *Acta Chir. Scand.* **1941**, *84*, 163.
18. Bucholz, R. Patterns of ischemic necrosis of the proximal femur in nonoperatively treated congenital hip disease. In *The Hip Proceedings of the Sixth Open Scientific Meeting of the Hip Society*; CV Mosby: Maryland Heights, MI, USA, 1978; pp. 43–63.
19. El-Sayed, M.M. Single-stage open reduction, Salter innominate osteotomy, and proximal femoral osteotomy for the management of developmental dysplasia of the hip in children between the ages of 2 and 4 years. *J. Pediatr. Orthop. B* **2009**, *18*, 188–196. [CrossRef]
20. Forlin, E.; Da Cunha, L.A.M.; Figueiredo, D.C. Treatment of developmental dysplasia of the hip after walking age with open reduction, femoral shortening, and acetabular osteotomy. *Orthop. Clin.* **2006**, *37*, 149–160. [CrossRef]
21. Galpin, R.D.; Roach, J.; Wenger, D.; Herring, J.; Birch, J. One-stage treatment of congenital dislocation of the hip in older children, including femoral shortening. *J. Bone Joint Surg.* **1989**, *71*, 734–741. [CrossRef]
22. Karakaş, E.; Baktir, A.; Argün, M.; Türk, C.Y. One-stage treatment of congenital dislocation of the hip in older children. *J. Pediatr. Orthop.* **1995**, *15*, 330–336. [CrossRef] [PubMed]
23. Umer, M.; Nawaz, H.; Kasi, P.M.; Ahmed, M. Outcome of triple procedure in older children with developmental dysplasia of hip (DDH). *J. Pak. Med. Assoc.* **2007**, *57*, 591. [PubMed]
24. Li, Y.; Hu, W.; Xun, F.; Lin, X.; Li, J.; Yuan, Z.; Liu, Y.; Canavese, F.; Xu, H. Risk factors associated with unsatisfactory hip function in children with late-diagnosed developmental dislocation of the hip treated by open reduction. *Orthop. Traumatol. Surg. Res.* **2020**, *106*, 1373–1381. [CrossRef] [PubMed]
25. Ning, B.; Yuan, Y.; Yao, J.; Zhang, S.; Sun, J. Analyses of outcomes of one-stage operation for treatment of late-diagnosed developmental dislocation of the hip: 864 hips followed for 3.2 to 8.9 years. *BMC Musculoskelet. Disord.* **2014**, *15*, 401. [CrossRef]
26. Ganger, R.; Radler, C.; Petje, G.; Manner, H.M.; Kriegs-Au, G.; Grill, F. Treatment options for developmental dislocation of the hip after walking age. *J. Pediatr Orthop. B.* **2005**, *14*, 139–150. [CrossRef]

27. Chen, Q.; Deng, Y.; Fang, B. Outcome of one-stage surgical treatment of developmental dysplasia of the hip in children from 1.5 to 6 years old. A retrospective study. *Acta Orthop. Belg.* **2015**, *81*, 375–383.
28. Bursalı, A.; Tonbul, M. How are outcomes affected by combining the Pemberton and Salter osteotomies? *Clin. Orthop. Relat. Res.* **2008**, *466*, 837–846. [CrossRef]
29. Eamsobhana, P.; Kamwong, S.; Sisuchinthara, T.; Jittivilai, T.; Keawpornsawan, K. The factor causing poor results in late developmental dysplasia of the hip (DDH). *J. Med. Assoc. Thai.* **2015**, *98*, S32–S37.
30. Domzalski, M.; Synder, M. Avascular necrosis after surgical treatment for developmental dysplasia of the hip. *Int. J. Orthop.* **2004**, *28*, 65–68. [CrossRef]
31. Kalamchi, A.; MacEwen, G.D. Avascular necrosis following treatment of congenital dislocation of the hip. *J. Bone Joint Surg.* **1980**, *62*, 876–888. [CrossRef]
32. Kamath, S.U.; Bennet, G.C. Re-dislocation following open reduction for developmental dysplasia of the hip. *Int. J. Orthop.* **2005**, *29*, 191–194. [CrossRef] [PubMed]

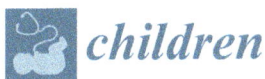

Article

Intraoperative 3D Imaging Reduces Pedicle Screw Related Complications and Reoperations in Adolescents Undergoing Posterior Spinal Fusion for Idiopathic Scoliosis: A Retrospective Study

Antti J. Saarinen [1,2,†], Eetu N. Suominen [1,2,†], Linda Helenius [3], Johanna Syvänen [1], Arimatias Raitio [1] and Ilkka Helenius [2,*]

1 Department of Pediatric Orthopedic Surgery, Turku University Hospital, 20521 Turku, Finland; anjusaa@utu.fi (A.J.S.); ensuom@utu.fi (E.N.S.); johanna.syvanen@tyks.fi (J.S.); arimatias.raitio@fimnet.fi (A.R.)
2 Department of Orthopedics and Traumatology, Helsinki University Hospital, 00260 Helsinki, Finland
3 Department of Anesthesia and Intensive Care, Turku University Hospital, 20521 Turku, Finland; linda.helenius@tyks.fi
* Correspondence: ilkka.helenius@helsinki.fi
† These authors contributed equally to this work.

Abstract: Widely used surgical treatment for adolescent idiopathic scoliosis (AIS) is posterior spinal fusion using pedicle screw instrumentation (PSI). Two-dimensional (2D) or three-dimensional (3D) navigation is used to track the screw positioning during surgery. In this study, we evaluated the screw misplacement, complications, and need for reoperations of intraoperative 3D as compared to 2D imaging in AIS patients. There were 198 adolescents, of which 101 (51%) were evaluated with 2D imaging and 97 (49%) with 3D imaging. Outcome parameters included radiographic correction, health-related quality of life (HRQOL), complications, and reoperations. The mean age was 15.5 (SD 2.1) years at the time of the surgery. Forty-four (45%) patients in the 3D group and 13 (13%) patients in the 2D group had at least one pedicle screw repositioned in the index operation ($p < 0.001$). Six (6%) patients in the 2D group, and none in the 3D group had a neurological complication ($p = 0.015$). Five (5%) patients in the 2D group and none in the 3D group required reoperation ($p = 0.009$). There were no significant differences in HRQOL score at two-year follow-up between the groups. In conclusion, intraoperative 3D imaging reduced pedicle screw-related complications and reoperations in AIS patients undergoing PSI as compared with 2D imaging.

Keywords: scoliosis; O-arm; navigation; pedicle screws; complication; spinal fusion; adolescent idiopathic scoliosis

Citation: Saarinen, A.J.; Suominen, E.N.; Helenius, L.; Syvänen, J.; Raitio, A.; Helenius, I. Intraoperative 3D Imaging Reduces Pedicle Screw Related Complications and Reoperations in Adolescents Undergoing Posterior Spinal Fusion for Idiopathic Scoliosis: A Retrospective Study. *Children* **2022**, *9*, 1129. https://doi.org/10.3390/children9081129

Academic Editors: Axel A. Horsch, Maher A. Ghandour and Matthias Christoph M. Klotz

Received: 12 July 2022
Accepted: 27 July 2022
Published: 28 July 2022

Publisher's Note: MDPI stays neutral with regard to jurisdictional claims in published maps and institutional affiliations.

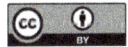

Copyright: © 2022 by the authors. Licensee MDPI, Basel, Switzerland. This article is an open access article distributed under the terms and conditions of the Creative Commons Attribution (CC BY) license (https://creativecommons.org/licenses/by/4.0/).

1. Introduction

Scoliosis is a spinal deformity, which refers to the deviation of the spine greater than 10° in the coronal plane. The most common type of scoliosis is idiopathic scoliosis, which, based on the age of onset, can be classified as infantile, juvenile, and adolescent. Adolescent idiopathic scoliosis (AIS) is the most common form of idiopathic scoliosis, affecting 1–3% of children in the at-risk population of those aged 10–16 years [1,2]. Although most adolescents with AIS will not develop pain or neurologic symptoms, scoliosis can progress to rib deformity and respiratory compromise and can cause significant cosmetic problems and emotional distress. Treatment options for AIS include observation, bracing, and surgery. The goals of treatment for pediatric idiopathic scoliosis are to correct deformity, prevent curve progression, and restore trunk symmetry and balance [1,2].

Posterior corrective surgeries using pedicle screw instrumentation (PSI), which allows curves to be corrected in three dimensions, have become the most popular surgical treatment for scoliosis [3,4]. Pedicle screws provide better deformity correction, improved pulmonary function, reduced blood loss, shorter fusion levels, and reduced operation time compared to prior correction methods [4–8]. Posterior spinal fusion (PSF) is carried out using subperiostal exposure, bilateral facetectomy, and application of bone graft on decorticated posterior spinal bony elements. To address scoliosis the spine is instrumented bilaterally using pedicle screws and these are connected with rods, which allows the straightening of the spine and preventing the curve from progression. PSF with pedicle screws is the gold-standard treatment for AIS. It allows three-dimensional correction of the spinal deformity, and furthermore, with pedicle screw instrumentation provides good correction of the scoliosis with low reoperation rates [3,4]. There is evidence, that patients who underwent posterior spinal fusion with pedicle screws experienced improved back pain and health-related quality of life compared with patients with untreated AIS [5]. In contrast to the comparative efficacy of this technique in correcting scoliosis, screw placement has increased risks of causing complications, such as neurological or vascular injuries [6,7].

High screw density helps restore thoracic kyphosis and correct spinal rotation [8]. Computer tomography (CT)—based navigation methods have improved results on the radiographic outcomes and reduced the number of misplaced screws significantly [9,10]. C-arm fluoroscopic imaging has been used for years and has enabled relatively accurate placement of pedicle screws. However, the C-arm system only provides two-dimensional (2D) fluoroscopic images, for which additional artificial correction during the operation is required in cases with severe deformities due to scoliosis. The flexibility of the growing spine and anatomical deformities caused by AIS reduce navigation accuracy, and even navigated screws are sometimes misplaced [11]. The use of modern three-dimensional (3D) intraoperative imaging and navigation techniques have been introduced for the accurate insertion of pedicle screws (PS) for the growing spine. O-arm (Medtronic Inc, Louisville, KY, USA), which is a cone beam CT that provides 3D imaging is one of the latest intraoperative imaging platforms to allow real-time multidimensional surgical imaging. It has become increasingly popular in the spinal surgery during the last decade [12,13]. Advanced intraoperative CT-based imaging and navigation increase both cost and operation time. Therefore, their use needs to be justified by improved safety and outcome [9].

Our strategy has been to use free-hand pedicle screw insertion and to verify the screw positioning with intraoperative 2D imaging using C-arm, and more recently, 3D imaging using O-arm before the corrective maneuvers. In this study, we aimed to evaluate the complications, need for reoperations, and health-related quality of life (HRQOL) of 3D imaging (O-arm) as compared to 2D imaging (C-arm) in a consecutive series of AIS patients treated with posterior spinal fusion. We hypothesized that intraoperative 3D imaging would reduce pedicle screw-related complications compared to 2D fluoroscopy facilitating the identification of significant pedicle screw malposition.

2. Materials and Methods

This is a retrospective analysis of patients with AIS treated with PSI and evaluated with 2D or 3D intraoperative imaging. Patients were treated in an academic tertiary medical center between 2009–2021. The indication for surgery was a primary curve greater than a Cobb angle of 45°. Patients underwent a posterior spinal fusion with bilateral segmental pedicle screw instrumentation using a combination of vertebral column derotation techniques and selective translation, compression, as well as a distraction [5]. The inclusion criteria of the study were a diagnosed AIS, age between 10–21 years, and posterior spinal fusion with segmental PSI. Exclusion criteria were bleeding disorder, Chiari malformation or syringomyelia in magnetic resonance images, and need for anteroposterior approach or vertebral column resection. All procedures were performed by the same senior orthopedic spine surgeon and patients had a minimum of six months of follow-up (mean 2.0 years, range 0.5–3.2). The study received approval from the Ethics Committee of the Hospital District (ETMK 96/1801/2020).

Intraoperative 3D-imaging scan using the O-arm (Medtronic Inc., Louisville, KY, USA) became available at our institution in 2016. There were 198 consecutive adolescents, of which 101 (51%) were evaluated during 2009–2016 with intraoperative 2D imaging scan (designed as a 2D group) and 97 (49%) were evaluated during 2016–2021 with intraoperative 3D imaging scan (designed as a 3D group). Intraoperative spinal cord (motor evoked and somatosensory potentials) and lumbar nerve root monitoring (electromyography, EMG) were performed in every patient in both study groups. Prospectively collected institutional pediatric spine register was used to acquire data including clinical characteristics, radiographic parameters, health-related quality of life outcomes, and complications.

2.1. Intraoperative Imaging

Pedicle screws in the 2D group were intraoperatively evaluated using traditional methods including posteroanterior and lateral fluoroscopic imaging after all screws were placed. Non-harmonious screws or screws violating bony landmarks were identified. In the 3D group, O-arm spins of every screw were obtained at the end of screw placement. This required typically two different imaging sessions as the height of the one imaging area was limited to five or six levels. Settings included standard thoracic values for the lumbar and lower thoracic area and high-density values in the upper thoracic area.

2.2. Surgical Technique

All patients were treated with bilateral segmental pedicle screw instrumentation for adolescent idiopathic scoliosis. Pedicle screws were inserted using the free-hand technique [5,14] by the senior orthopedic spine surgeon or under his direct supervision. The screw placement was standardized including three pairs of polyaxial screws on top of the construct, uniplanar screws in the midthoracic spine, a single polyaxial screw in the concave apex, and polyaxial screws in the lumbar spine. Screw diameters varied from 4.5 mm to 6.5 mm.

The decision to replace a screw in the 2D group was based on an intraoperative neuromonitoring (IONM) event (decrease of 50% or more in the motor evoked potential) or a pedicle screw violating the bony landmarks on the 2D imaging. Intraoperative neuromonitoring was performed with 15-min interval and at standard procedure time points: before incision, exposure completed, pedicle screws implanted, correction completed, and wound closed. Fluoroscopic 2D imaging was performed after all screws were placed. In the 3D group, intraoperative neuromonitoring events and intraoperative 3D imaging were used for the decision to replace screws. Intraoperative 3D imaging scans were evaluated by the senior surgeon and misplaced screws of 2 mm or more were replaced during the index procedure.

2.3. Scoliosis Research Society-24 (SRS-24) Outcome Questionnaire

The SRS-24 is a disease-specific health-related quality of life (HRQOL) questionnaire used to assess the current state of the patient with AIS and the outcomes of scoliosis surgery. The questionnaire has seven domains: pain, general self-image, function from a back condition, the general level of activity, postoperative self-image, postoperative function, and satisfaction. Each domain score ranges from 1 to 5, with higher scores indicating better patient outcomes. The maximum raw score of SRS-24 is 120 points (corresponding mean maximal score of 5.0 points) [15].

2.4. Statistical Analyses

The normal distribution assumption of the data was verified visually with QQ-plot and with the Shapiro–Wilk test. Descriptive statistics were presented in absolute numbers and percentages or means with standard deviations (SDs) or ranges. Statistical comparisons between the groups were performed with the chi-squared test for categorical parameters and with an independent-samples t-test for continuous variables. All analyses were conducted in JMP® for Macintosh, Version 16.1 (SAS Institute Inc., Cary, NC, USA, 1989–2021). p values < 0.05 were considered statistically significant.

3. Results

The mean age of the patients was 15.5 ± 2.1 years, and the mean Cobb angle of the main curve was 52° ± 8.2° at the time of the surgical procedure, with a remaining curve of 13° ± 4.7° at the final follow-up. There were 1931 pedicle screws in the 3D group and 2048 in the 2D group. There were no significant differences in age, gender, radiographic correction of the deformity, or SRS-24 total score at six months or two-year follow-ups between the two groups (Table 1).

Table 1. Clinical characteristics of the study groups.

Characteristics	3D Group (n = 97)	2D Group (n = 101)	p-Value
Number of pedicle screws	1931	2048	
Age at surgery, years	15.5 (10.5–21.9)	15.5 (10.7–22.5)	0.867
Female gender, n (%)	67 (69%)	75 (74%)	0.418
Follow-up time, years	1.8 (0.50–2.6)	2.1 (0.54–3.2)	<0.001
Major curve, degrees			
Preoperative	52 (45–83)	53 (45–84)	0.138
Postoperative	13 (2–28)	12 (2–24)	
Repositioning of at least one pedicle screw at the index procedure	44 (45%)	13 (13%)	<0.001
SRS-24 total score			
Preoperative	3.7 (2.4–4.6)	3.8 (2.5–4.4)	0.462
6 months follow-up	3.9 (2.4–4.6)	3.8 (2.7–4.7)	0.393
2-year follow-up	4.1 (2.5–4.7)	4.0 (2.9–4.6)	0.271

3.1. Need for Screw Repositioning

In the 3D group, 44 (45%) of the patients had at least one pedicle screw repositioned in the index operation, as compared with 13 (13%) in the 2D group ($p < 0.001$). A total of 70 screws (3.6% of all screws, average 0.73 per patient, range 0–4) were replaced in the index procedure in the 3D group, as compared with 13 (0.63%, average 0.13 per patient, range 0–2, $p < 0.001$) in the 2D group. In the 3D group, 43 of the replaced screws breached the medial wall (61%, mean breach 3.2 mm, range 2–6.5 mm), 17 breached the lateral wall of the pedicle (24%, mean breach 3.6 mm, range 2–6), and 10 the anterior cortex (15%, mean breach 2.7 mm, range 1.1–5 mm) of the vertebrae. Four patients in the 3D group and one in the 2D group had a screw replaced due to a sagittal breach. After screw repositioning, screw placement was verified using 2D imaging in both groups. One patient had transient IONM change (correction maneuver) requiring no replacement of screw in the 3D group. Nine patients in the 2D group had a screw removed intraoperatively due to an IONM signal change.

3.2. Complications

Complications are listed in Table 2. There were no new neurological deficits related to screw misplacement in the 3D group compared to six (5.9%) in the 2D group ($p = 0.015$). The more detailed description of new neurologic deficits and outcomes are represented in Table 3. Five (4.9%) patients in the 2D group required reoperation due to pedicle screw complications compared to no reoperations in the 3D group ($p = 0.009$).

Postoperative CT scans were performed to the six patients with new neurological deficits in the 2D group. Of the five patients requiring screw removal in the 2D group, two were performed during the index procedure and three in a separate procedure. Four patients in the 2D group had a new motor deficit ranging from muscle weakness to paresis. Three of these patients underwent reoperation within 48 h after the index surgery. One patient with fractured L4 pedicle causing chronic pain and atrophy of quadriceps muscles was treated conservatively with frequent monitoring. Two patients in the 2D group developed postural headache due to delayed dural lesions and required reoperation at approximately three months after the initial surgery. None of the patients had deep surgical wound site infection. Three patients in the 2D group, and none of the patients in the 3D group had superficial surgical site infection ($p = 0.043$). None of the patients requiring reoperation had wound-related complications or infections.

Table 2. Complications in the study groups.

Complication	3D Group ($n = 97$)	2D Group ($n = 101$)	p Value
Neurologic complications *	0	6	0.015
Motor deficit	0	4	0.048
Intraoperative monitoring change **	1	9	0.011
Cerebrospinal fluid leak	2	3	0.683
Intraoperative	2	1	0.534
Delayed	0	2	0.100
Surgical site infection			
Superficial	0	3	0.043
Deep	0	0	NA ***

* Includes new postoperative motor deficits as well as postural postoperative headache. ** Decrease of the motor evoked potential of 50% or more intraoperatively. *** Not applicable.

Table 3. New postoperative neurologic deficits and outcome.

Patient	Age at Surgery, Years	Follow-Up Time, Years	Levels	Neurologic Deficit	Actions Taken	Outcome
1	15.2	2.1	T4–L2	Isolated paresis of L5 level	Re-operation. T12 screw compressing cord, screw removed and a local decompression.	Full recovery at follow-up.
2	18.1	2.0	T2–L3	Post-operative muscle weakness in the left lower extremity.	Re-operation. T5 screw compressing cord and screw removed	Full recovery at follow-up.
3	19.2	2.0	T6–L3	Postural headache	Re-operation. Pedicle screw removed, saturation of the dura.	Full recovery at follow-up.
4	16.0	2.1	T5–L4	Motoric denervation in L3 and L4 myotomes according to ENMG	Frequent monitoring	Fracture healed and fragments disappeared in control CT. Mild quadriceps atrophy and pain after exercise at follow-up
5	16.7	2.0	T11–L3	Right sided muscle weakness in lower extremity	Re-operation. T11 pedicle screw removed. Decompression using enlarged posterior column osteotomy presented with no cause. Index operation stopped.	Mild spinal deficit at follow-up. Right side trunk muscle weakness and sensory deficit in lower extremity.
6	15.3	2.0	T6–L3	Postural headache	Re-operation. Pedicle screw removed, saturation of the dura	Full recovery at follow-up.

Four of the patients with neurological complications in the 2D group had a full recovery during the follow-up. Two patients developed a permanent neurological deficit. One patient had persistent mild spinal cord deficit (brisk reflexes) and right-sided motor and sensory impairment on the trunk. Another patient had a fractured pedicle and developed denervation of quadriceps muscle in electromyography, which lead to quadriceps muscle atrophy and chronic pain at follow-up.

4. Discussion

We present findings on the value of advanced intraoperative 3D imaging after free hand pedicle screw placement in adolescent idiopathic scoliosis. Advanced intraoperative 3D imaging reduced pedicle screw-related complications and reoperations in adolescents undergoing pedicle screw instrumentation for idiopathic scoliosis as compared to intraoperative 2D fluoroscopic imaging.

Free-hand pedicle screw instrumentation based on anatomic bony landmarks is fast and effective and carries a relatively low risk for neural deficits. The accuracy of navigation is limited due to movement between the reference and the instrumented level in the mobile growing spine often resulting in lateral deviation of the screw tip [9]. Patients with pedicle screws placed with CT-guided navigation have a lower rate of severely malpositioned screws and unplanned returns to the operating room than patients with pedicle screws placed with freehand/fluoroscopic technique [16–18]. A study on spinal navigation showed a significant shortening of the operation time as more experience was gained, thus demonstrating a positive effect on the learning curve [19].

There exist previous studies reporting the value of navigation-based pedicle screw instrumentation in this spinal condition [11,20]. CT scan is the standard imaging method for evaluating pedicle screw breaches. Plain radiographs have poor reliability in detecting pedicle screw breaches. A cadaveric study on intraoperative 3D-imaging scans reported high accuracy on significant breaches, but lower accuracy on breaches under 2 mm due to artifact signals [10]. However, minor breaches are considered probable safe zone [21]. Kobayashi et al. reported similar radiation exposure in intraoperative and preoperative CT scans suggesting that low dose protocol might help reduce the overall intraoperative dosage when compared to fluoroscopy [22]. Intraoperative 3D imaging reduces the radiation dosage for the surgical team, as it allows more efficient radiation protection.

Insertion of pedicle screws in pediatric patients is challenging due to the small osseous elements of the growing spine. The rotational deformity further complicates the estimation of the screw positioning [23]. However, the elastic nature of immature pedicles allows enlargement of the bony walls, and therefore, screws up to 115% of the pedicle diameter can be implanted [7]. Studies with computer tomography (CT) have reported a wide range of misplaced screws. The largest study of 2020 screws reported a 20.3% perforation rate [24]. Most of the moderate breaches of the pedicle are asymptomatic and overall, PSI has a relatively low complication rate in pediatric scoliosis surgery [6,24]. However, delayed complications caused by previously unrecognized breaches have been reported [25–27]. The surgical operations on the spine have gradual learning curves and there are many intraoperative difficulties and complications which can be encountered. Advanced intraoperative 3D imaging provides a useful aid for less experienced surgeons, as it provides immediate feedback and extra information during the surgery.

A recent study based on prospective adolescent idiopathic scoliosis database found an overall 0.4% incidence of return to the operating room due to screw malposition between years 2003 and 2017. Return to OR for screw malposition changed from 2003 to 2017 (1–0.2%) [28]. Moderate evidence shows CT guidance has lower point estimates of breach rates than free-hand methods at 7.9% compared with 9.7–17.1%. Screw-related complication rates are conflicting at 0% in CT navigation compared with 0–1.7% in 13 low- and moderate-quality studies [29,30].

Long-term outcomes of asymptomatic misplaced pedicle screws have not been extensively reported. In the literature, delayed postural headaches have been reported three months after the index procedure [26,31]. The intraoperative dural lesion is usually noticed during the screw placement due to cerebrospinal fluid leakage. The reports of delayed cerebrospinal fluid leak may indicate perforation of the dura over time by moderately breached screws. We hypothesize that most pedicle screw complications could be prevented by intraoperative evaluation of the screw positioning using 3D imaging after screw placement.

In our study, the screw revision rate was 3.9%. This is in accordance with literature. Larson et al. [11] reported high accuracy of pedicle screws inserted with intraoperative CT based navigation with a screw revision rate of 3.9%, but even after navigated screw insertion, a control CT scan was performed. In their study, the screw revision rate was significantly higher in pediatric than in adult patients. In the study of Sembrano et al. 602 pedicle screws were evaluated with an intraoperative CT scan and 2.8% were intraoperatively revised [32]. The HRQOL was assessed using the SRS-24 questionnaire. Despite the neurological complications in the 2D group, there were no statistically significant differences in 6 months or 2-year follows ups.

Further research is needed on the use and accuracy of navigation in pediatric spine. Evaluation of free-hand pedicle screws using advanced 3D imaging provides an intermediate method to maintain both effectiveness and safety of pedicle screw instrumentation in adolescents undergoing surgery for idiopathic scoliosis.

Limitations

The current study was a retrospective evaluation of the value of advanced intraoperative 3D imaging on the safety of freehand pedicle screw placement in consecutive series of adolescents undergoing posterior spinal fusion for idiopathic scoliosis. Ideally, such evaluation should be performed in a randomized clinical trial. It is possible that the reduced number in the reoperations and complications in the 3D group might reflect the learning curve of the surgical team. However, the use of intraoperative 3D-imaging revealed significant number of pedicle screw breaches which were corrected during the index surgery. As CT scans were not routinely available for the 2D group, no comparison could be made in the accuracy of the screw placement between the groups. The study design was a single center, single surgeon series including 198 consecutive patients from 2009 to 2021 and not all patients had a minimum two-year follow-up. Clinical (complications), radiographic, and health-related quality of life data was based on a prospective spine register. The current study did not include cost-effectiveness analysis which should be investigated in the future.

5. Conclusions

Intraoperative 3D-imaging reduced pedicle screw related complications and reoperations in adolescents undergoing pedicle screw instrumentation for idiopathic scoliosis as compared with traditional intraoperative fluoroscopic 2D imaging. However, the improved clinical outcome was not reflected by better health-related quality of life at the final follow-up. Furthermore, 3D imaging provides immediate educational feedback for less experienced surgeons.

Author Contributions: Conceptualization, I.H. and A.R.; methodology, A.J.S. and E.N.S.; writing—original draft preparation, A.J.S. and E.N.S.; writing—review and editing, J.S., L.H., A.R. and I.H.; supervision, I.H., funding acquisition, I.H. All authors have read and agreed to the published version of the manuscript.

Funding: A.S. has received funding from the Finnish Research Foundation for Orthopaedics and Traumatology, Clinical Research Institute HUCH, Turku University Foundation, and the University of Turku for this study. E.S. has received funding from Clinical Research Institute HUCH. L.H. has obtained research grants from Finska Läkaresällskapet. A.R. has received research grants from Paulo Foundation, Finland. I.H. has received funding from Finnish State Funding, Medtronic (ERP-2020-12238), Stryker (S-I-027), Nuvasive (HUCH grant 70295), and Cerapedics (HUCH grant 70304) to Institution.

Institutional Review Board Statement: The study was conducted in accordance with the Declaration of Helsinki, and approved by the Institutional Review Board of Turku University Hospital District (ETMK 96/1801/2020, date of approval 21 January 2021).

Informed Consent Statement: Informed consent was obtained from all subjects involved in the study.

Data Availability Statement: Study data can be obtained from the corresponding author for a reasonable request.

Acknowledgments: Open access funding provided by University of Helsinki.

Conflicts of Interest: I.H. has following conflict of interest: Consultant for Medtronic; grants and research funding to Institution received from Medtronic International, Stryker, Nuvasive, Cerapedics, and Finnish State Funding via Helsinki and Turku University Hospitals.

References

1. Weinstein, S.L.; Dolan, L.A.; Cheng, J.C.; Danielsson, A.; Morcuende, J.A. Adolescent Idiopathic Scoliosis. *Lancet* **2008**, *371*, 1527–1537. [CrossRef]
2. Altaf, F.; Gibson, A.; Dannawi, Z.; Noordeen, H. Adolescent Idiopathic Scoliosis. *BMJ* **2013**, *346*, f2508. [CrossRef] [PubMed]
3. Ledonio, C.G.T.; Polly, D.W.J.; Vitale, M.G.; Wang, Q.; Richards, B.S. Pediatric Pedicle Screws: Comparative Effectiveness and Safety: A Systematic Literature Review from the Scoliosis Research Society and the Pediatric Orthopaedic Society of North America Task Force. *JBJS* **2011**, *93*, 1227–1234. [CrossRef] [PubMed]
4. Kim, Y.J.; Lenke, L.G.; Cho, S.K.; Bridwell, K.H.; Sides, B.; Blanke, K. Comparative Analysis of Pedicle Screw Versus Hook Instrumentation in Posterior Spinal Fusion of Adolescent Idiopathic Scoliosis. *Spine* **2004**, *29*, 2040–2048. [CrossRef]
5. Helenius, L.; Diarbakerli, E.; Grauers, A.; Lastikka, M.; Oksanen, H.; Pajulo, O.; Löyttyniemi, E.; Manner, T.; Gerdhem, P.; Helenius, I. Back Pain and Quality of Life After Surgical Treatment for Adolescent Idiopathic Scoliosis at 5-Year Follow-up: Comparison with Healthy Controls and Patients with Untreated Idiopathic Scoliosis. *JBJS* **2019**, *101*, 1460–1466. [CrossRef]
6. Hicks, J.M.; Singla, A.; Shen, F.H.; Arlet, V. Complications of Pedicle Screw Fixation in Scoliosis Surgery: A Systematic Review. *Spine* **2010**, *35*, E465. [CrossRef]
7. Suk, S.-I.; Kim, W.-J.; Lee, S.-M.; Kim, J.-H.; Chung, E.-R. Thoracic Pedicle Screw Fixation in Spinal Deformities: Are They Really Safe? *Spine* **2001**, *26*, 2049–2057. [CrossRef]
8. Delikaris, A.; Wang, X.; Boyer, L.; Larson, A.N.; Ledonio, C.G.T.; Aubin, C.-E. Implant Density at the Apex Is More Important Than Overall Implant Density for 3D Correction in Thoracic Adolescent Idiopathic Scoliosis Using Rod Derotation and En Bloc Vertebral Derotation Technique. *Spine* **2018**, *43*, E639–E647. [CrossRef]
9. Cawley, D.; Dhokia, R.; Sales, J.; Darwish, N.; Molloy, S. Ten Techniques for Improving Navigated Spinal Surgery. *Bone Jt. J.* **2020**, *102-B*, 371–375. [CrossRef]
10. Santos, E.R.G.; Ledonio, C.G.; Castro, C.A.; Truong, W.H.; Sembrano, J.N. The Accuracy of Intraoperative O-Arm Images for the Assessment of Pedicle Screw Postion. *Spine* **2012**, *37*, E119. [CrossRef]
11. Larson, A.N.; Santos, E.R.G.; Polly, D.W.J.; Ledonio, C.G.T.; Sembrano, J.N.; Mielke, C.H.; Guidera, K.J. Pediatric Pedicle Screw Placement Using Intraoperative Computed Tomography and 3-Dimensional Image-Guided Navigation. *Spine* **2012**, *37*, E188. [CrossRef]
12. Schouten, R.; Lee, R.; Boyd, M.; Paquette, S.; Dvorak, M.; Kwon, B.K.; Fisher, C.; Street, J. Intra-Operative Cone-Beam CT (O-Arm) and Stereotactic Navigation in Acute Spinal Trauma Surgery. *J. Clin. Neurosci.* **2012**, *19*, 1137–1143. [CrossRef]
13. Jin, M.; Liu, Z.; Liu, X.; Yan, H.; Han, X.; Qiu, Y.; Zhu, Z. Does Intraoperative Navigation Improve the Accuracy of Pedicle Screw Placement in the Apical Region of Dystrophic Scoliosis Secondary to Neurofibromatosis Type I: Comparison between O-Arm Navigation and Free-Hand Technique. *Eur. Spine J.* **2016**, *25*, 1729–1737. [CrossRef]
14. Kuklo, T.R.; Lenke, L.G.; O'Brien, M.F.; Lehman, R.A.J.; Polly, D.W.J.; Schroeder, T.M. Accuracy and Efficacy of Thoracic Pedicle Screws in Curves More Than 90°. *Spine* **2005**, *30*, 222–226. [CrossRef]
15. Haher, T.R.; Gorup, J.M.; Shin, T.M.; Homel, P.; Merola, A.A.; Grogan, D.P.; Pugh, L.; Lowe, T.G.; Murray, M. Results of the Scoliosis Research Society Instrument for Evaluation of Surgical Outcome in Adolescent Idiopathic Scoliosis: A Multicenter Study of 244 Patients. *Spine* **1999**, *24*, 1435. [CrossRef]
16. Baky, F.J.; Milbrandt, T.; Echternacht, S.; Stans, A.A.; Shaughnessy, W.J.; Larson, A.N. Intraoperative Computed Tomography–Guided Navigation for Pediatric Spine Patients Reduced Return to Operating Room for Screw Malposition Compared With Freehand/Fluoroscopic Techniques. *Spine Deform.* **2019**, *7*, 577–581. [CrossRef]
17. Ughwanogho, E.; Patel, N.M.; Baldwin, K.D.; Sampson, N.R.; Flynn, J.M. Computed Tomography–Guided Navigation of Thoracic Pedicle Screws for Adolescent Idiopathic Scoliosis Results in More Accurate Placement and Less Screw Removal. *Spine* **2012**, *37*, E473. [CrossRef]
18. Fichtner, J.; Hofmann, N.; Rienmüller, A.; Buchmann, N.; Gempt, J.; Kirschke, J.S.; Ringel, F.; Meyer, B.; Ryang, Y.-M. Revision Rate of Misplaced Pedicle Screws of the Thoracolumbar Spine–Comparison of Three-Dimensional Fluoroscopy Navigation with Freehand Placement: A Systematic Analysis and Review of the Literature. *World Neurosurg.* **2018**, *109*, e24–e32. [CrossRef]
19. Nakanishi, K.; Tanaka, M.; Misawa, H.; Sugimoto, Y.; Takigawa, T.; Ozaki, T. Usefulness of a Navigation System in Surgery for Scoliosis: Segmental Pedicle Screw Fixation in the Treatment. *Arch. Orthop. Trauma Surg.* **2009**, *129*, 1211–1218. [CrossRef]
20. Feng, W.; Wang, W.; Chen, S.; Wu, K.; Wang, H. O-Arm Navigation versus C-Arm Guidance for Pedicle Screw Placement in Spine Surgery: A Systematic Review and Meta-Analysis. *Int. Orthop.* **2020**, *44*, 919–926. [CrossRef]
21. Kim, Y.J.; Lenke, L.G.; Bridwell, K.H.; Cho, Y.S.; Riew, K.D. Free Hand Pedicle Screw Placement in the Thoracic Spine: Is It Safe? *Spine* **2004**, *29*, 333–342. [CrossRef]

22. Kobayashi, K.; Ando, K.; Ito, K.; Tsushima, M.; Morozumi, M.; Tanaka, S.; Machino, M.; Ota, K.; Ishiguro, N.; Imagama, S. Intraoperative Radiation Exposure in Spinal Scoliosis Surgery for Pediatric Patients Using the O-Arm® Imaging System. *Eur. J. Orthop. Surg. Traumatol.* **2018**, *28*, 579–583. [CrossRef]
23. Şarlak, A.Y.; Buluç, L.; Sarısoy, H.T.; Memişoğlu, K.; Tosun, B. Placement of Pedicle Screws in Thoracic Idiopathic Scoliosis: A Magnetic Resonance Imaging Analysis of Screw Placement Relative to Structures at Risk. *Eur. Spine J.* **2008**, *17*, 657–662. [CrossRef]
24. Kwan, M.K.; Chiu, C.K.; Gani, S.M.A.; Wei, C.C.Y. Accuracy and Safety of Pedicle Screw Placement in Adolescent Idiopathic Scoliosis Patients: A Review of 2020 Screws Using Computed Tomography Assessment. *Spine* **2017**, *42*, 326–335. [CrossRef]
25. Wegener, B.; Birkenmaier, C.; Fottner, A.; Jansson, V.; Dürr, H.R. Delayed Perforation of the Aorta by a Thoracic Pedicle Screw. *Eur. Spine J.* **2008**, *17*, 351–354. [CrossRef]
26. Floccari, L.; Larson, A.N.; Stans, A.A.; Fogelson, J.; Helenius, I. Delayed Dural Leak Following Posterior Spinal Fusion for Idiopathic Scoliosis Using All Posterior Pedicle Screw Technique. *J. Pediatr. Orthop.* **2017**, *37*, e415–e420. [CrossRef]
27. Suh, S.-W.; Kim, G.-U.; Lee, H.-N.; Yang, J.H.; Chang, D.-G. Delayed Presentation of Infected Common Iliac Artery Pseudoaneurysm Caused by Malpositioned Pedicle Screw after Minimally Invasive Scoliosis Surgery. *Eur. Spine J.* **2019**, *28*, 68–72. [CrossRef]
28. Swany, L.; Larson, A.N.; Garg, S.; Hedequist, D.; Newton, P.; Sponseller, P.; Harms Study Group. 0.4% Incidence of Return to OR Due to Screw Malposition in a Large Prospective Adolescent Idiopathic Scoliosis Database. *Spine Deform.* **2022**, *10*, 361–367. [CrossRef]
29. Chan, A.; Parent, E.; Narvacan, K.; San, C.; Lou, E. Intraoperative Image Guidance Compared with Free-Hand Methods in Adolescent Idiopathic Scoliosis Posterior Spinal Surgery: A Systematic Review on Screw-Related Complications and Breach Rates. *Spine J.* **2017**, *17*, 1215–1229. [CrossRef]
30. Dede, O.; Ward, W.T.; Bosch, P.; Bowles, A.J.; Roach, J.W. Using the Freehand Pedicle Screw Placement Technique in Adolescent Idiopathic Scoliosis Surgery: What Is the Incidence of Neurological Symptoms Secondary to Misplaced Screws? *Spine* **2014**, *39*, 286–290. [CrossRef]
31. Albayram, S.; Ulu, M.O.; Hanimoglu, H.; Kaynar, M.Y.; Hanci, M. Intracranial Hypotension Following Scoliosis Surgery: Dural Penetration of a Thoracic Pedicle Screw. *Eur. Spine J.* **2008**, *17*, 347. [CrossRef] [PubMed]
32. Sembrano, J.N.; Polly, D.W.; Ledonio, C.G.T.; Santos, E.R.G. Intraoperative 3-Dimensional Imaging (O-Arm) for Assessment of Pedicle Screw Position: Does It Prevent Unacceptable Screw Placement? *Int. J. Spine Surg.* **2012**, *6*, 49–54. [CrossRef] [PubMed]

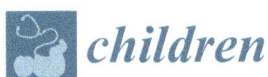

Review

Outcome Prognostic Factors in MRI during Spica Cast Therapy Treating Developmental Hip Dysplasia with Midterm Follow-Up

Katharina Susanne Gather [1,*], Ivan Mavrev [1], Simone Gantz [1], Thomas Dreher [2], Sébastien Hagmann [1] and Nicholas Andreas Beckmann [1]

1. Clinic for Orthopedics and Trauma Surgery, Center for Orthopedics, Trauma Surgery and Spinal Cord Injury, Heidelberg University Hospital, Schlierbacher Landstrasse 200a, 69118 Heidelberg, Germany; ivan.mavrev@gmx.de (I.M.); simone.gantz@med.uni-heidelberg.de (S.G.); sebastien.hagmann@med.uni-heidelberg.de (S.H.); nicholas.beckmann@med.uni-heidelberg.de (N.A.B.)
2. Pediatric Orthopedics and Traumatology, Children's University Hospital Zurich, Steinwiesstrasse 75, 8032 Zurich, Switzerland; thomas.dreher@kispi.uzh.ch
* Correspondence: katharina.gather@med.uni-heidelberg.de; Tel.: +49-6221-56-35491

Abstract: Closed reduction followed by spica casting is a conservative treatment for developmental dysplasia of the hip (DDH). Magnetic resonance imaging (MRI) can verify proper closed reduction of the dysplastic hip. Our aim was to find prognostic factors in the first MRI to predict the possible outcome of the initial treatment success by means of ultrasound monitoring according to Graf and the further development of the hip dysplasia or risk of recurrence in the radiological follow-up examinations. A total of 48 patients (96 hips) with DDH on at least one side, and who were treated with closed reduction and spica cast were included in this retrospective cohort study. Treatment began at a mean age of 9.9 weeks. The children were followed for 47.4 months on average. We performed closed reduction and spica casting under general balanced anaesthesia. This was directly followed by MRI to control the position/reduction of the femoral head without anaesthesia. The following parameters were measured in the MRI: hip abduction angle, coronal, anterior and posterior bony axial acetabular angles and pelvic width. A Graf alpha angle of at least 60° was considered successful. In the radiological follow-up controls, we evaluated for residual dysplasia or recurrence. In our cohort, we only found the abduction angle to be an influencing factor for improvement of the DDH. No other prognostic factors in MRI measurements, such as gender, age at time of the first spica cast, or treatment involving overhead extension were found to be predictive of mid-term outcomes. This may, however, be due to the relatively small number of treatment failures.

Keywords: spica cast; closed reduction; developmental hip dysplasia; hip luxation; MRI

Citation: Gather, K.S.; Mavrev, I.; Gantz, S.; Dreher, T.; Hagmann, S.; Beckmann, N.A. Outcome Prognostic Factors in MRI during Spica Cast Therapy Treating Developmental Hip Dysplasia with Midterm Follow-Up. *Children* **2022**, *9*, 1010. https://doi.org/10.3390/children9071010

Academic Editor: Vito Pavone

Received: 20 May 2022
Accepted: 3 July 2022
Published: 7 July 2022

Publisher's Note: MDPI stays neutral with regard to jurisdictional claims in published maps and institutional affiliations.

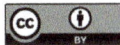

Copyright: © 2022 by the authors. Licensee MDPI, Basel, Switzerland. This article is an open access article distributed under the terms and conditions of the Creative Commons Attribution (CC BY) license (https://creativecommons.org/licenses/by/4.0/).

1. Introduction

The estimated incidence of developmental dysplasia of the hip (DDH) in infants varies geographically from 0.1–30 per 1000 newborns, depending on the population [1–3]. Unrecognized and untreated DDH can lead to premature osteoarthritis and is responsible for up to one-third of hip replacements in adults younger than 60 years [1]. The exact etiology of DDH remains unknown and is likely multifactorial, with its pathophysiology reflecting a combination of primary abnormal acetabular development and secondary abnormal interaction between the femoral head and the acetabulum during perinatal life [4]. Specifically, previous studies have shown that breech intrauterine position, family history of DDH and female gender are the most important risk factors for DDH [1,5]. Other risk factors such as first-born, oligohydramnios, overly restrictive swaddling practices and foot abnormalities have been linked to DDH, but the evidence is weaker [2,5].

Detected at an early age by ultrasound, developmental hip dysplasia (DDH) can be very effectively treated by conservative means, even in severe cases. Success rates of

90.4–99.8% have been shown for the Tübinger splint, the Pavlik harness, or casts, and as such are considered first-line therapy in neonates [6–9]. These splints or casts exploit the huge potential for growth and remodeling of the newborn hip [10]. The goal of treatment in these cases is to achieve and maintain concentric reduction of the hip joint to promote femoral head coverage, and congruent acetabular and femoral head development. Treatment is guided by the age at presentation and the severity of the disease [11]. Later, once the ossification center has formed in the femoral head, the sonographic possibilities become limited and AP X-ray of the pelvis provides superior diagnostic information [12]. Here, the acetabular index is the relevant parameter up to the age of 4. Beginning at the age of 4, the centre-edge angle (CE angle), according to Wiberg, becomes increasingly relevant [13].

In German-speaking countries, conservative therapy is usually guided by ultrasound of the hip. In these regions, the Graf technique has prevailed (see also Section 2.3 Measurements).

The algorithm varies in the case of spica casting. Some prefer leaving window in the cast to perform a transinguinal ultrasound [14–16]. This additional window reduces the stability of the cast, which is why others prefer magnetic resonance imaging (MRI) to evaluate the position of the femoral head after closed reduction and cast application [17–21]. Further available imaging methods are X-ray or computer tomography (CT) scans [22–24]. Reported rates of recurrent dislocation identified on cross-sectional imaging after closed reduction range from 6% to 15% [12]. Although the sensitivity and specificity of CT and MRI for detecting dislocation have been found to be equivalent [25], MRI has the advantage of not exposing the sensitive developing tissues to ionizing radiation and providing superior soft-tissue resolution and enhancement profiles. Specifically, in cases of abnormal post-reduction hips, MRI can identify obstacles to reduce and detect unexpected complications [12]. Due to the unnecessary radiation exposure and no proper display of the cartilaginous hip, we prefer MRI after closed reduction and spica cast application. Even though the correct centre of the femoral head is the main concern, several indices can be measured in MRI. Jaremko et al. evaluated several of these for dysplasia on infant hip MRI (see Section 2.3 Measurements) [26]. Indices of hip dysplasia and adequacy of reduction differ between modalities, including ultrasound, radiography, CT, MRI and arthrography with limited cross-correlation. Jaremko comprehensively adapted all available DDH indices from CT and other modalities to MRI, and tested which could be feasibly measured on MRI, assessed interobserver variability, and correlated indices to each other [26].

Using these indices, our aim was to find parameters on the first MRI after closed reduction and spica cast application correlating with the outcome. In this regard, we looked for prognostic factors predicting the expected success of treatment. To our knowledge, there are no comparable studies to this topic so far.

By means of the parameters measurable in MRI, we wanted to find out whether they can predict conservative therapy success or failure in terms of residual dysplasia or recurrence rate.

2. Patients and Methods

2.1. Patients Population

In this retrospective cohort study, we included all 48 patients (96 hips) with DDH on at least on one side, who were consecutively treated with closed reduction and spica cast between 2005 and 2016 at our institution. The diagnosis was confirmed by an ultrasound in our department. Moreover, 84/96 (87.5%) were female and 12 (12.5%) were male; 54.2% (26/48) were bilateral and 45.8% (22/48) had DDH on one side. Since a spica cast always retains both hips, the healthy opposite sides were also retained in the patients affected on only one side—no reduction was necessary, nor occurred on the healthy side. This ultimately resulted in 69 hips with DDH and 27 healthy hips being treated with a spica cast.

Initial Graf types were type 1a or 1b 27/96 (27.2%), type 2a 9/96 (9.1%), type 2b 3/96 (3.0%), type 2c 12/96 (12.1%), type D 12/96 (12.1%), type 3a 21/96 (21.2%), type 3b 3/96 (3.0%) and type 4 7/96 (7.1%) [27–29]. One patient had no initial ultrasound in our data.

Six patients (12.5%) had received overhead extension prior to spica casting. Furthermore, 3/6 had at least on one site Graf type 4, 1 type 3b and 1 patient had a type 2c hip at initial presentation to our outpatient department after having been treated with overhead extension and spica cast in different hospitals before (the hip was initially Graf type 4). The remaining patient had already started ossification of the unstable decentred femoral head upon initial presentation to our outpatient department at the age of 5 months. We initiated an overhead extension because of the age of the child and the instability of the hip.

Patients with neurogenic or syndromic hip dysplasia were excluded. The exact age at diagnosis could not be determined adequately because the records are incomplete. We were not able to retrospectively verify the time of initial diagnosis for each patient, which was generally made prior to presentation to our department. The treatment began at our department at a mean child age of 9.9 weeks (s = 6.0) (range 4 to 33 weeks). Treatment of male patients started at a mean of 7.3 weeks (s = 2.2) and female patients at 10.3 weeks (s = 6.3) of age. This difference was highly significant ($p = 0.003$). A follow-up was 47.4 months on average (s = 34.5). 9/48 (18.8%) children had a known risk factors for DDH with a breech presentation and/or positive family history.

2.2. Treatment Technique

All patients received a Graf hip ultrasound at our institution to confirm the diagnosis. In cases of an unstable hip (type IIc unstable or more according to Graf's classification) on at least one side, we performed closed reduction and spica casting (see Figures 1 and 2). The patients were deemed too old to try a Tübingen splint when they presented to our outpatient clinic. Cooper et al. and Seidl et al. described the Tübingen splint as a successful option for very young infants. The standard therapy for unstable hips at this age is the spica cast [30,31]. The duration of the cast therapy was determined according to the patient's age and the severity of the disease. The standard therapy was two serial casts of 3 weeks duration. Afterwards, an ultrasound reevaluation was performed. If the DDH was still severe, a further spica cast was applied again for an additional 3 weeks if necessary. If DDH was deemed mild, or the alpha angle was less than the target of 64° or more, a Tübingen splint was applied; if an alpha angle of 64° or more was measured, the treatment was stopped. If a severe DDH was initially present in a very young infant, a 3-week cast therapy was sometimes carried out and then an ultrasound reevaluation performed to decide if the standard two rounds of 3-week treatment spica cast should be continued, or if another option, such as a Tübingen splint was sufficient.

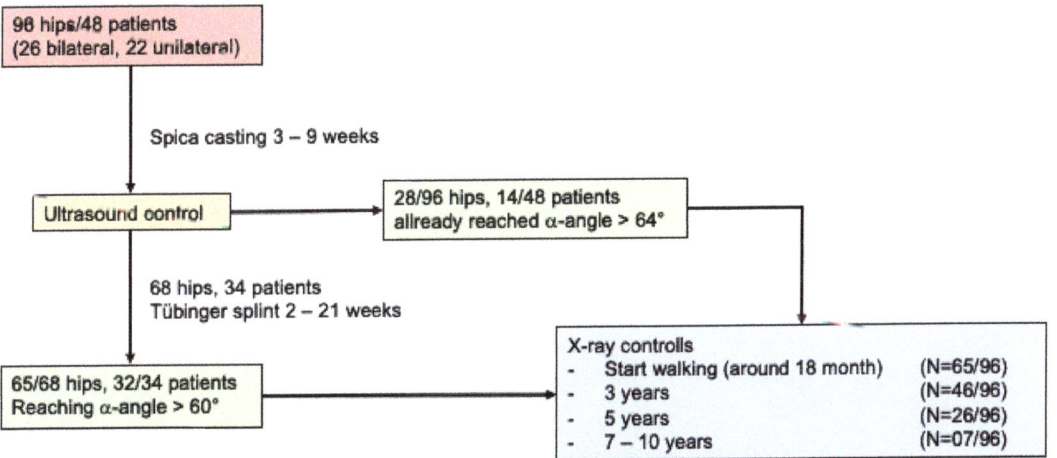

Figure 1. Shows the therapy algorithm of our treatment.

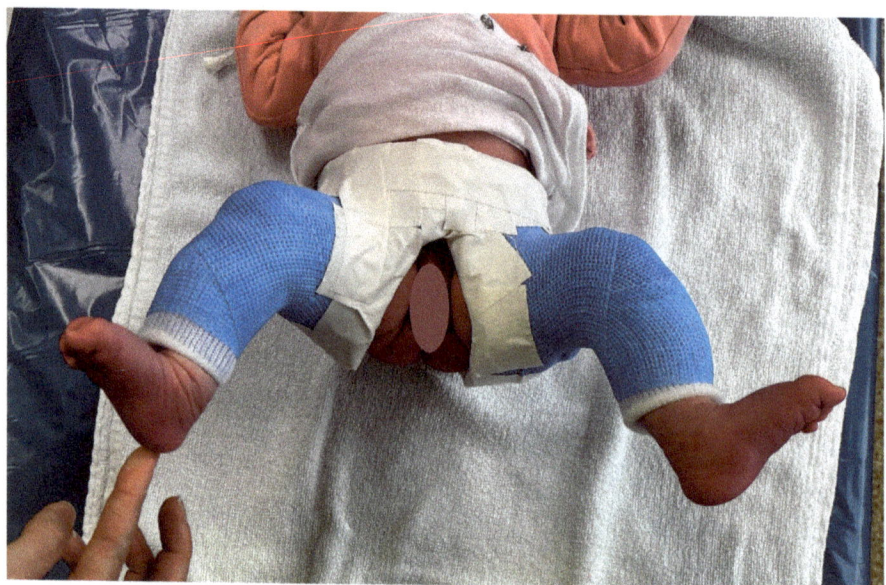

Figure 2. Shows a patient in a spica cast with hip abduction and flexion.

To reach a good result, the reduction was performed under general balanced anaesthesia with laryngeal masks. In all cases, MRI was performed directly after closed reduction to control the position/reduction of the femoral head without additional anaesthesia by taking advantage of residual anaesthesia. In unsteady infants, positioning aids were used, such as a light sandbag to support the spica cast, to additionally minimize movement artefacts in MRI. For MRI sequences see Table 1. The spica cast was renewed after 3 weeks once or twice depending on the initial severity of DDH.

Table 1. Post spica cast pelvic MRI protocol parameters, FOV field of view, fs fat saturation, PD proton density, TE echo time, TR repetition time.

Sequence	FOV (mm)	Voxel Size (mm)	Slice Thickness (mm)	Gap (%)	Foldover Direction	TR (ms)	TE (ms)	Acquisition Matrix
Cor PD tse 320	160	0.5 × 0.5 × 2.0	2.0	10	RL	1500	24	160
Cor T2 tseRB 320	200	0.6 × 0.6 × 2.0	2.0	10	FH	3180	97	200
Axial T2 tseRB fs 320	200	0.6 × 0.6 × 2.0	2.0	20	RL	2900	73	200
Axial T2 tseRB 320	200	0.6 × 0.6 × 2.0	2.0	20	RL	3400	97	200
Axial PD tseR 320	200	0.6 × 0.6 × 2.0	2.0	20	RL	1800	22	200
Sag PD tse 384 re/li	160	0.5 × 0.4 × 2.0	2.0	10	AP	1500	35	160

After the scheduled spica cast therapy, an ultrasound was carried out to reevaluate the hip. If the alpha angle was still below 64°, the therapy was continued with a Tübingen splint until the desired maturation of the hip occurred. The Tübingen hip flexion splint is a removable orthosis that fixes the squat position of the hip and was invented by Prof. Bernau for the treatment of stable hip joints [32]. In this study, treatment control was performed using ultrasound with the technique described by Graf. An alpha angle of at least 60° (Graf Typ I) was required to end therapy (treatment goal was defined as an alpha angle over 64°, but in cases where a type 1 hip had been achieved some parents opted to end further treatment). Afterwards, the children were followed-up according to our in-house standards by means of X-ray until the end of growth. The patients presented 2–3 months after the start of walking, around the age of 3, shortly before starting school, before the pubertal growth spurt and at the end of growth (see Figure 1). This way, recurrences could be detected accordingly and the development of the hip could be observed. Mild dysplasia was further observed and partly treated with a nighttime abduction wedge. If the CE angle was less than 15°, surgical reconstruction was indicated.

2.3. Measurements

Ultrasound was performed with the Graf technique [33,34]. The child is placed in a lateral position in a positioning tray and examined with a linear ultrasound transducer. This is applied to the greater trochanter in the longitudinal axis of the child and produces a frontal section through the acetabulum. After anatomical identification and usability testing, the α- and β-angles are determined (see Figure 3). The tangent to the os ilium is the baseline for both angle determinations. Two guide lines are added to this baseline to measure the bony acetabular roof angle α (bone angle) and the cartilaginous acetabular roof angle β (cartilage angle). For the latter, a connecting line (display line) is drawn between the bony acetabular notch (turnover point) and the centre of the acetabular labrum. The bony notch is located at the point where the acetabulum changes its profile from concave to convex. For the α-angle, a tangent is drawn to the bony acetabulum starting from the lower edge of the os ilium.

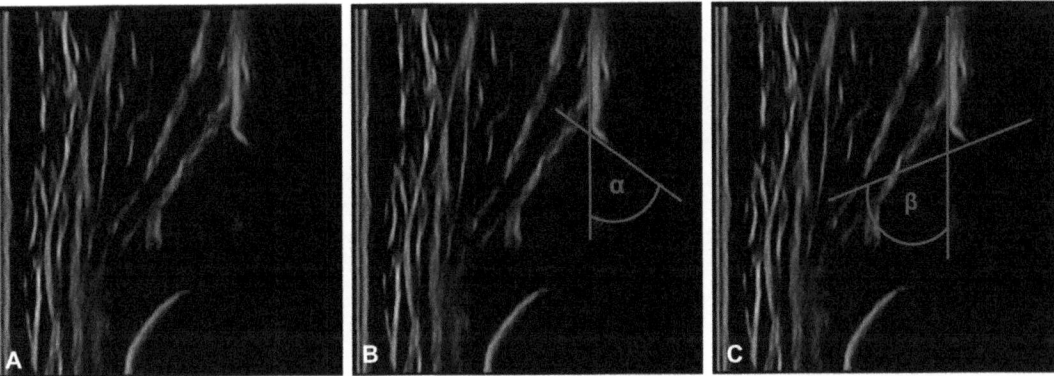

Figure 3. Shows the measurement of the α- and β-angle. (**A**) plain ultrasound image for anatomical identification and usability testing. (**B**) The tangent to the os ilium is the baseline for both angle determinations. For the α-angle, a tangent is drawn to the bony acetabulum starting from the lower edge of the os ilium (**C**) For the latter, a connecting line (display line) is drawn between the bony acetabular notch (turnover point) and the center of the acetabular labrum. The bony notch is located at the point where the acetabulum changes its profile from concave to convex. The angle between the two lines is called β-angle.

Alpha and beta angle were measured initially and after ending spica cast therapy, and until ending treatment or ossification of the femoral head. If the femoral head already ossified during follow-up we performed X-rays instead of ultrasound to follow-up. This usually happens around 8 months of age. 6 children were lost to follow-up at the first planned X-ray after they had begun walking. All other children showed femoral head ossification by the follow-up time. An angle of 64° or more was rated as excellent, 60–63.9 as good, and below this as poor. The aim was to achieve a type I hip according to Graf, which accordingly has an alpha angle of at least 60° and thus to achieve a normal hip.

For MRI indices, we used those described by Jaremko et al. (see Figure 4) [26]. First the hip abduction angle (Abd.) is measured in the axial T1 phase on the image with the largest diameter of the femoral heads. This is defined as the angle between a perpendicular line to Hilgenreiner's line and the line along the mid femoral shaft. The coronal acetabular angle (CorAcet) is measured on the coronal image on which the acetabular roof is steepest. This image must also contain a substantial portion of the femoral head. CorAcet is defined as the angle between Hilgenreiner's line and a line to the superior bony edge of the acetabulum. For the Pelvic width (PelvWid), we used the image showing the widest distance between medial ischial walls at the pelvic inlet. The width is a measure of the inner distance between the inner edge of left and right cortex. Similarly Jaremko et al., we used the axial image on which the acetabulum appears deepest to measure the anterior and posterior bony axial acetabular angles (AxAcet and AxPAcet). This image also contained a substantial part of the femoral head. The AxAcet is the angle between Hilgenreiner's line and a line joining the anterior edge of the bony acetabulum to the lateral edge of the triradiate cartilage. The AxPAcet is measured similarly at the posterior joint line [26].

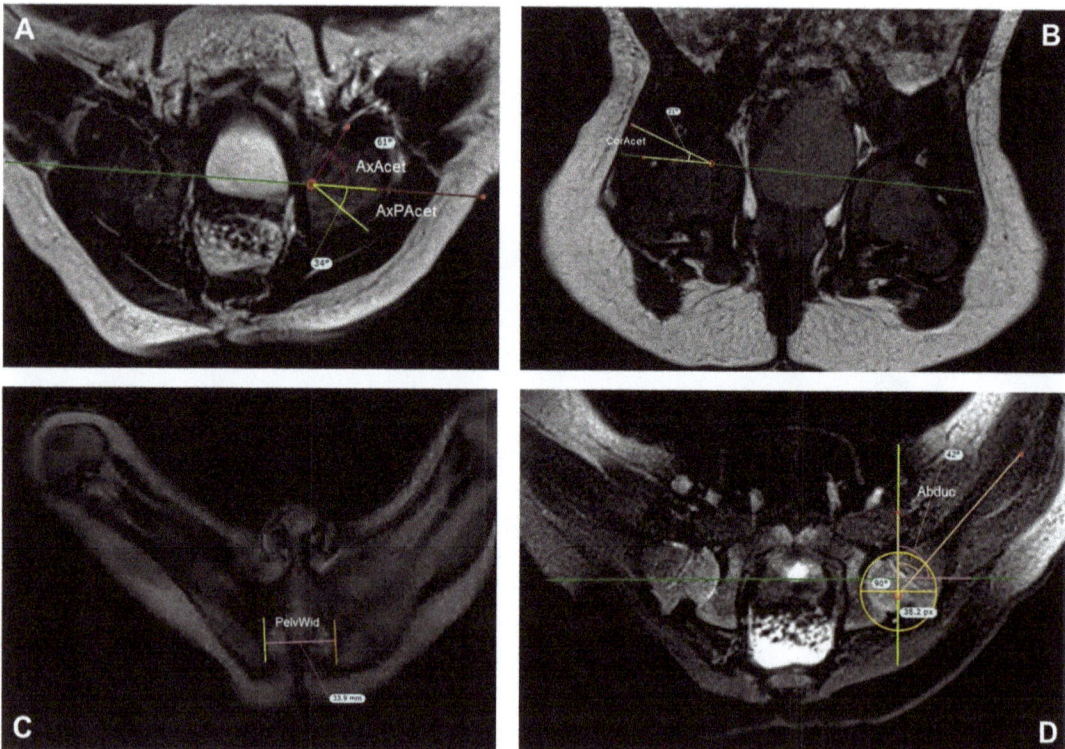

Figure 4. Overview of the measurement technic in the MRI described by Jaremko and performed in TraumaCad. (**A**) AxAcet/AxPAcet: Select the axial image for which the acetabular cup appears deepest. The bony anterior acetabulum index (red) is the angle is made between Hilgenreiner's line (green) and a line joining the anterior edge of the bony acetabulum to the lateral edge of the triradiate cartilage. The bony posterior acetabular index (yellow) is measured similarly at the posterior joint line. (**B**) CorAcet: Select Slice were the acetabular roof is steepest. Angle (yellow) between Hilgenreiner's line (green) and a line joining the superior edge of the bony acetabulum to the lateral edge of the triradiate cartilage. (**C**) PelvWid: widest distance between medial ischial walls at the pelvic inlet, below the hip joints (**D**) Abduc: On the slice showing the largest diameter of the most normally positioned femoral bead, draw Hilgrainer's line (green) between anterior lateral edges of triradiate cartilage in the same fashion as on the coronal images. Abduc angle (orange) is the angle between the line along the mid femoral shaft and a perpendicular to Hilgenreiner's line. (AxAcet AxPAcet = anterior/posterior bony axial acetabular angles, CorAcet = coronal acetabular angle, PelvWid = Pelvic width, Abduc = hip abduction angle) [26].

After ending spica casting, further follow-up was performed using X-ray. Children with DDH should be followed-up radiologically until growth completion, due to late recurrence. If no signs of DDH are present during follow-up, further follow-up at walking age, after 8–10 years and after the end of growth is recommended [35]. In our cases, severe DDH was present, so spica cast therapy was necessary and therefore the control intervals were reduced to walking age, again after 3 and 5 years, and after 10 years. Due to the study period and follow-up time frame, no patient has reached skeletal maturity at this point.

The centre edge angle as described by Wiberg (CE-angle) and the Acetabular Index (AI) were measured and we evaluated for further pathology, such as signs of beginning avascular femoral head necrosis. Although the CE-angle is not validated for children under 4 years age, it was used for comparison with other authors. Of particular interest was the further development of the hips and the femoral head coverage after successful post-maturation: Do the children develop a recurrence of hip dysplasia or do they remain mature without signs of bony DDH? This was evaluated and staged using the AC and CE angle relative to the patient age according to Tönnis [33].

All MRI and radiographic measurements were performed with TraumaCad Version 2.5 (Brainlab Ltd., Petah Tikva, Israel).

2.4. Statistical Analysis

All of the statistical analyses were conducted using SPSS (version 28; SPSS; Chicago, IL, USA). Descriptive statistics, including arithmetic mean value and standard deviation, were calculated. Data is given as mean ± standard deviation (SD) and ranges, if not indicated otherwise.

T-Tests and Pearson's chi-squared-tests were used for group statistics. Prognostic factors were calculated with linear regression tests. Differences were considered significant if the p-value was <0.05.

3. Results

The mean duration of treatment was 11.3 weeks (S = 4.9). The treatment involved a mean of 6.0 weeks (3–9 weeks) cast and 5.3 weeks with Tübinger splint. There was no significant difference between male and female patients. After removing the cast, 70.8% (68/96) needed additional therapy with Tübinger splint depending on sonographic measurements. The others already reached an alpha angle of >64° after cast therapy and did not need any additional splint. These patients were primarily unilaterally affected infants. For initial Graf type see Table 2.

Table 2. In the ultrasound evaluation after spica cast therapy, 28 hips already showed an alpha angle of at least 64° and therefore did not require any further therapy. The following table shows the distribution of the initial Graf types of these patients.

Initial Graf Type	28 Hips Reached Alpha Angle of 64° or More after Spica Casting
1	10/28
2a	3/28
2c	4/28
3a	5/28
D	4/28
Unknown (no initial ultrasound)	2/28

There was a positive correlation between having had an overhead extension and the need of a Tübinger splint after spica cast ($p = 0.014$).

One patient (both hips) needed surgical treatment during the follow-up period. A total of 3 patients (3 hips) still have a residual dysplasia and may require additional surgery at a later date, such as acetabuloplasty and derotation-varisation-osteotomy (DVO). The following measured parameters were not associated with surgery (either performed or recommended): gender, age at time of starting therapy, Graf Type, alpha-angle at the end of therapy or MRI measurements.

3.1. Sonographic Evaluation

The sonographic alpha- and beta-angle measured at the beginning and end of therapy separated by sex are summarized in Table 3. The difference of both angles (alpha and beta) was highly significant with $p < 0.001$. No significant correlation was noted between the first alpha-angle and the first radiologic measurements (CE-angle, AI, ACM, HAS). The initial Graf Type had no influence on the duration of the therapy in total, nor on further surgical treatment. However, the duration of spica cast therapy positively influences the alpha angle at the end of therapy ($p = 0.003$, beta = 0.869). No other measured parameter was shown to have a significant positive correlation. An alpha angle of 64° or more was rated as excellent, 60–63.9 as good, and below as poor.

Table 3. Shows ultrasound parameters at the beginning and end of therapy in total and separated by sex and age in weeks at time of beginning therapy. Alpha = alpha angle defined by Graf. Beta = beta angle defined by Graf.

		Mean Start Cast	Standard Deviation	Mean End Therapy	Standard Deviation
	In total	52.2	9.8	65.6	3.3
alpha	female	52.2	9.6	65.7	3.4
	male	51.8	11.4	64.5	1.8
	In total	74.2	9.3	63.9	6.8
beta	female	74.0	9.9	64.0	7.0
	male	75.1	7.9	63.7	5.8

No significant difference in alpha-angle or Graf Type was noted between the male and female patients. There was a difference in age at time of starting the therapy between both sexes ($p = 0.003$). Girls were treated on average 3 weeks later than boys. No significant differences were found in duration of the therapy ($p = 0.646$) or the alpha angle at the end of therapy.

A total of 3 hips in 2 patients (2/48, 4.1%) did not reach an alpha angle of 60° at the end of therapy. One was getting too old to continue immobilisation with regard to the motor development. The parents of the other patient declined further treatment with a spica cast or Tübinger splint to finish treatment.

3.2. Magnetic Resonance Imaging Measurements

Table 4 gives a summary of the measurements shown in the MRI. 31/48 (64.6%) patients had a second MRI, which was carried out after receiving the second spica cast. All of the MRI scans showed a concentric reduction of the femoral head within the acetabulum.

Table 4. Summary of the magnetic resonance imaging (MRI) measurements in the first and last MRI. Abd = hip abduction angle. AxAcet = axial anterior acetabular angle. AxPAcet = axial posterior acetabular angle. CorAcet = coronal acetabular angle. PelvWid = pelvic width.

	Mean First MRI	Standard Deviation	Mean Second MRI	Standard Deviation
Abd	53.5 (39.3–66.2)	5.2	53.4 (29.0–62.1)	6.7
AxAcet	49.6 (32.8–68.2)	7.1	50.0 (32.8–62.4)	6.6
AxPAcet	46.8 (36.1–63.5)	6.0	46.8 (4.6–69.1)	9.3
CorAcet	25.6 (11.8–44.9)	6.6	24.2 (11.7–47.6)	7.8
PelvWid	35.8 (28.7–51.0)	5.0	38.2 (32.0–52.0)	5.1

There was no significant difference of the measured angles depending on sex. There was a positive correlation between pelvic width and age at time of first spica cast ($p < 0.001$).

All of the measured parameters had no significant influence on the alpha angle at the end of therapy (outcome). Two parameters influenced duration of therapy, first AxPAcet ($p = 0.028$, beta $= -0.218$) and the Abduction ($p = 0.003$, beta $= -0.304$) in the first MRI.

3.3. Radiographic Evaluation

Two patients had no initial ultrasound examination because of age at time of presentation and an already ossified femoral head (25 and 33 weeks). During further follow-up after Spica cast and subsequent additional Tübinger splint we performed anterior-posterior X-rays of the total pelvis after 1.5, 3, 5 and 10 years. Means are shown in Table 5. Moreover, 42/48 patients had at least one follow-up X-ray. Table 5 shows radiographic parameters of AI and CE angle during follow-up separated by the result of the last sonography. Figure 5 shows development of AI and CE-angle over time of follow-up. Factors influencing the outcome of congenital hip dysplasia were found at 3-year follow-up, but not at the others, perhaps due to loss to follow-up after 5 and 10 years. Abduction had a positive effect of the development of AI measured at 3 years age in our cohort ($p = 0.044$, beta $= -0.609$). No other positive effects were found to be statistically significant.

Table 5. Shows radiographic measurements with mean and standard deviation of X-ray measurements of AI and CE angle after 1.5, 3, 5 and 10 years of follow-up separated by the result of the last sonography. CE-angle = centre edge angle by Wiberg. AI-angle = acetabular index. n = number.

Years		Excellent ($\alpha \geq 64°$) n		Good ($\alpha < 64°$) n		Poor ($\alpha < 60°$) n	
1.5–2	AI	65	28.6 (s = 4.0)	10	29.5 (s = 4.2)	1	26.0
	CE		11.3 (s = 8.3)		8.8 (s = 8.8)		18.0
3	AI	46	25.1 (s = 4.8)	9	24.11 (s = 5.6)	1	22.0
	CE		16.4 (s = 5.6)		17.8 (s = 5.6)		21.0
5	AI	26	19.2 (s = 4.3)	8	21.5 (s = 5.2)	1	17.0
	CE		18.4 (s = 4.0)		18.38 (s = 3.8)		20.0
10	AI	7	16.3 (s = 3.9)	3	15.33 (s = 5.9)	0	
	CE		22.6 (s = 5.4)		24.33 (s = 4.7)		

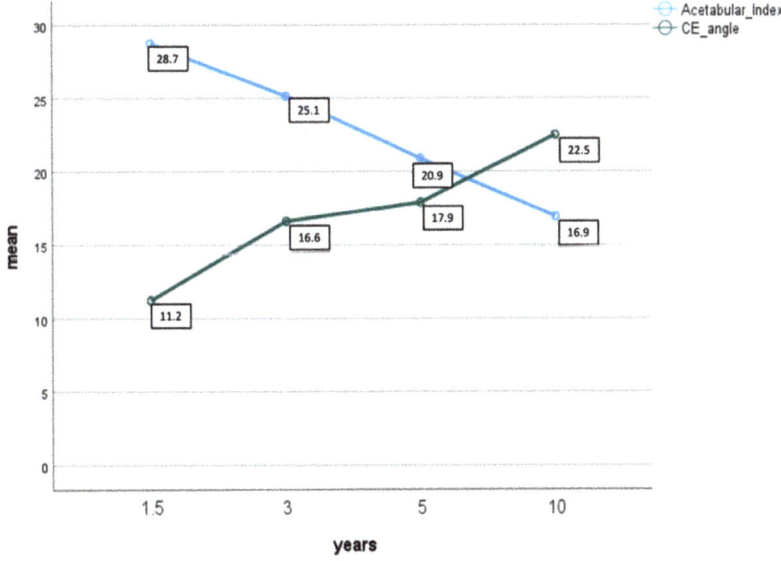

Figure 5. Shows mean development of acetabular index (light blue) and CE angle (green) during follow-up after 1.5, 3, 5 and 10 years.

3.4. Complications

There were no complications such as avascular necrosis of the hip. 11.4% (11/96) hips had delayed remodelling of the femoral head. All showed a spherical femoral head at the end of individual follow-up.

4. Discussion

The aim of this study was to explore possible prognostic factors in spica cast MRI to predict the expected outcome. We included both hips, including ones without signs of DDH, in order to compare all evaluated hips irrespective of DDH severity in order to detect possible prognostic factors. Furthermore, spica cast and Tübinger splint treatment always involves both hips.

Published cohorts have ranged in size from 21–110 patients, allowing for a comparison with the results in this cohort of 49 patients [15,36–40]. The mean age at time of starting treatment in this study was 9.9 weeks and therefore far below most reported ages, which generally started treatment around 6 to 24 months of age or even older [20,36–38]. The poorer outcome and higher rates of AVN in some studies might be associated with older age at time of immobilization [39,41–43]. The absence of AVN in our population may also be due to short cast immobilization period compared to the literature and younger age of our patients [21,36,44,45].

During the follow-up, there was a reduction in the number of patients after the first radiological control up to the 10-year control. This was due to several reasons. Firstly, not all patients were able to complete the possible follow-up period. On the other hand, some parents refused further radiographs of their children after an unremarkable radiographic control or forget/neglected to attend the further appointments. Some may also have moved and/or are performing the checks somewhere else.

We achieved a good outcome compared to the literature, which may be a result of the younger patient age when initializing treatment. Furthermore, 1 of 49 patients underwent surgery and 3 of 49 had residual dysplasia requiring treatment during our follow-up (8.1% in total, 4/49), which is comparable to the literature, reporting unsuccessful closed reduction in 9–31.16% of cases [11,37,40,46]. The girl who underwent surgery had a normal history with treatment beginning at 6 weeks of age for an unstable 2c hip on the left side. After treatment with a spica cast and a Tübingen splint, a Graf type 1 hip was found on both sides. However, X-ray examinations showed an increasing recurrence on both sides during the follow-up, so that surgical hip reconstruction with derotation varisation shortening osteotomy and Dega acetabuloplasty was carried out. Further checks showed no further recurrence of DDH. The three others with residual dysplasia showed the following characteristics: One was pretreated externally with an abduction treatment and presented to our clinic at 22 weeks of age. After initial therapy, the subsequently prescribed abduction wedge was not tolerated at night. After 3 years, there was a persistent DDH on the left side, but no further presentation to our outpatient clinic. The second patient showed a right-sided recurrence of the DDH in the first X-ray control after successful initial treatment from the 8th week of life. After an abduction wedge was prescribed, she was lost to follow-up. In case of the last girl, after successful initial conservative therapy, a mild dysplasia was observed in the 5-year follow-up, which is still being observed.

To our knowledge, we are the first investigate possible prognostic factors on MRI after spica cast placement to predict the expected outcome. We measured several parameters which had been shown by Jaremko et al. to be reliable and evaluated several additional parameters which were considered to be of interest. CorAcet and Abduction had moderate reliability. AxAcet and AxPAcet were rated as unreliable, but were still considered of interest for this study. Pelvwidth was the only very reliable parameter Jaremko et al. had noted. This is more a parameter of age than of DDH, and in this study acted as an additional indirect test of a correlation between age at therapy initiation and outcome. Jaremko described other parameters studied as time-consuming or not clinically relevant [26], so we decided not to measure them. After casting, all hips were centered. Jaremko et al.

described a large number of subluxated hips on MRI in their study, and half of the patients received open reduction or pelvic osteotomies before spica casting. In addition, the average age in their collective was 10 months (0–2 years), well above ours. These are only the main differences between the two groups of patients and illustrate the limitations of comparability between Jaremko et al. and our results.

In our patients, none of the MRI parameters showed a prognostic correlation with the sonographic outcome at the end of therapy. Despite MRI measurements, we also compared sonographic measurements and staging as well as age, sex, and radiographic parameters during follow-up. Here, we found that abduction had a positive effect of the development of AI at 3 years follow-up in our cohort ($p = 0.044$, beta = -0.609). This underlines the relevance of deep centering of the femoral head in the acetabulum for improved development of the hip. Care must be taken to retain the femoral head circulation by avoiding severe abduction.

An additional outcome influencing factor was the duration of cast therapy. The longer the cast was applied, the larger the alpha angle ($p = 0.003$, beta = 0.869).

None of the other measured values were shown to have an influence or predictive value on the expected outcome. This may be due to the relatively small cohort size and the small number of treatment failures. A larger cohort size may reveal that some of these other parameters do have prognostic value.

Limitations: this is a retrospective study without a control group. The relatively short follow-up of 47.4 months on average may have been too short to recognize further prognostic parameters.

5. Conclusions

In our cohort, we found the abduction angle to be the only influencing factor for improved development of the DDH. No other prognostic factors in MRI measurements, such as gender, age at time of the first spica cast, or treatment involving overhead extension were found to be predictive of mid-term outcome. Mild residual dysplasia in the first follow-up X-ray warrants further observation.

Author Contributions: Conceptualization, K.S.G. and T.D.; methodology, K.S.G., I.M. and T.D.; software, K.S.G.; validation, K.S.G. and I.M.; formal analysis, K.S.G., I.M., S.G. and N.A.B.; data curation, K.S.G. and I.M.; writing—original draft preparation, K.S.G.; writing—review and editing, K.S.G. and N.A.B.; visualization, K.S.G.; supervision, S.H. and N.A.B.; project administration, S.H. and N.A.B. All authors have read and agreed to the published version of the manuscript.

Funding: For the publication fee we acknowledge financial support by Deutsche Forschungsgemeinschaft within the funding program "Open Access Publikationskosten" as well as by Heidelberg University.

Institutional Review Board Statement: The study was conducted in accordance with the Declaration of Helsinki, and approved by the Institutional Ethics Committee of University of Heidelberg (protocol code S-538/2015; 3 December 2015).

Informed Consent Statement: Informed consent was obtained from all subjects involved in the study for the clinical treatment. Due to the retrospective evaluation of data collected in everyday clinical practice, no study-related consent had to be obtained from patients and guardians. No study-related additional examinations requiring informed consent were necessary.

Data Availability Statement: The data are not publicly available due to data privacy of the patients.

Conflicts of Interest: The authors declare no conflict of interest.

References

1. Vaquero-Picado, A.; González-Morán, G.; Gil Garay, E.; Moraleda, L. Developmental dysplasia of the hip: Update of management. *EFORT Open Rev.* **2019**, *4*, 548–556. [CrossRef]
2. Harsanyi, S.; Zamborsky, R.; Krajciova, L.; Kokavec, M.; Danisovic, L. Developmental Dysplasia of the Hip: A Review of Etiopathogenesis, Risk Factors, and Genetic Aspects. *Medicina* **2020**, *56*, 153. [CrossRef]
3. Zhang, S.; Doudoulakis, K.J.; Khurwal, A.; Sarraf, K.M. Developmental dysplasia of the hip. *Br. J. Hosp. Med.* **2020**, *81*, 1–8. [CrossRef]
4. Lee, M.C.; Eberson, C.P. Growth and development of the child's hip. *Orthop. Clin.* **2006**, *37*, 119–132. [CrossRef]
5. Yang, S.; Zusman, N.; Lieberman, E.; Goldstein, R.Y. Developmental Dysplasia of the Hip. *Pediatrics* **2019**, *143*, e20181147. [CrossRef]
6. Ziegler, J.; Thielemann, F.; Mayer-Athenstaedt, C.; Günther, K.P. The natural history of developmental dysplasia of the hip. A meta-analysis of the published literature. *Orthopade* **2008**, *37*, 515–516, 518–524. [CrossRef]
7. Weinstein, S.L. Natural history and treatment outcomes of childhood hip disorders. *Clin. Orthop. Relat. Res.* **1997**, *344*, 227–242. [CrossRef]
8. Wedge, J.H.; Wasylenko, M.J. The natural history of congenital disease of the hip. *J. Bone Jt. Surg. Br. Vol.* **1979**, *61*, 334–338. [CrossRef]
9. Pavone, V.; Testa, G.; Riccioli, M.; Evola, F.R.; Avondo, S.; Sessa, G. Treatment of Developmental Dysplasia of Hip with Tubingen Hip Flexion Splint. *J. Pediatr. Orthop.* **2015**, *35*, 485–489. [CrossRef]
10. Tschauner, C.; Klapsch, W.; Baumgartner, A.; Graf, R. Maturation curve of the ultrasonographic alpha angle according to Graf's untreated hip joint in the first year of life. *Z. Orthop. Ihre Grenzgeb.* **1994**, *132*, 502–504. [CrossRef]
11. Jadhav, S.P.; More, S.R.; Shenava, V.; Zhang, W.; Kan, J.H. Utility of immediate postoperative hip MRI in developmental hip dysplasia: Closed vs. open reduction. *Pediatr. Radiol.* **2018**, *48*, 1096–1100. [CrossRef]
12. Barrera, C.A.; Cohen, S.A.; Sankar, W.N.; Ho-Fung, V.M.; Sze, R.W.; Nguyen, J.C. Imaging of developmental dysplasia of the hip: Ultrasound, radiography and magnetic resonance imaging. *Pediatr. Radiol.* **2019**, *49*, 1652–1668. [CrossRef] [PubMed]
13. Nelitz, M.; Guenther, K.P.; Gunkel, S.; Puhl, W. Reliability of radiological measurements in the assessment of hip dysplasia in adults. *Br. J. Radiol.* **1999**, *72*, 331–334. [CrossRef] [PubMed]
14. Eberhardt, O.; Zieger, M.; Wirth, T.; Fernandez, F.F. Determination of femoral head position with transinguinal ultrasound in DDH treatment. *Z. Orthop. Unf.* **2009**, *147*, 727–733. [CrossRef]
15. Eberhardt, O.; Zieger, M.; Langendoerfer, M.; Wirth, T.; Fernandez, F.F. Determination of hip reduction in spica cast treatment for DDH: A comparison of radiography and ultrasound. *J. Child. Orthop.* **2009**, *3*, 313–318. [CrossRef]
16. Mehdizadeh, M.; Dehnavi, M.; Tahmasebi, A.; Shishvan, S.A.M.K.; Kondori, N.B.; Shahnazari, R. Transgluteal ultrasonography in spica cast in postreduction assessment of developmental dysplasia of the hip. *J. Ultrasound* **2019**, *23*, 509–514. [CrossRef] [PubMed]
17. Bos, C.F.; Bloem, J.L.; Obermann, W.R.; Rozing, P.M. Magnetic resonance imaging in congenital dislocation of the hip. *J. Bone Jt. Surg. Br. Vol.* **1988**, *70*, 174–178. [CrossRef] [PubMed]
18. Westhoff, B.; Wild, A.; Seller, K.; Krauspe, R. Magnetic resonance imaging after reduction for congenital dislocation of the hip. *Arch. Orthop. Trauma. Surg.* **2003**, *123*, 289–292. [CrossRef] [PubMed]
19. Wirth, T.; Haake, M.; Hahn-Rinn, R.; Walthers, E. Magnetic resonance tomography in diagnosis and therapy follow-up of patients with congenital hip dysplasia and hip dislocation. *Z. Orthop. Ihre Grenzgeb.* **1998**, *136*, 210–214. [CrossRef]
20. Yu, J.; Duan, F.; Guo, W.; Wang, D.; Qin, X.; Fu, G.; Chen, T. Consistency of Indices Obtained via Hip Medial Ultrasound and Magnetic Resonance Imaging in Reduction and Spica Cast Treatment for Developmental Dysplasia of the Hip. *Ultrasound Med. Biol.* **2021**, *47*, 58–67. [CrossRef]
21. Dibello, D.; Odoni, L.; Pederiva, F.; Di Carlo, V. MRI in Postreduction Evaluation of Developmental Dysplasia of the Hip: Our Experience. *J. Pediatr. Orthop.* **2019**, *39*, 449–452. [CrossRef]
22. Mandel, D.M.; Loder, R.T.; Hensinger, R.N. The predictive value of computed tomography in the treatment of developmental dysplasia of the hip. *J. Pediatric Orthop.* **1998**, *18*, 794–798. [CrossRef]
23. Stanton, R.P.; Capecci, R. Computed tomography for early evaluation of developmental dysplasia of the hip. *J. Pediatr. Orthop.* **1992**, *12*, 727–730. [CrossRef]
24. Li, Y.; Zhou, Q.; Liu, Y.; Chen, W.; Li, J.; Canavese, F.; Xu, H. Closed reduction and dynamic cast immobilization in patients with developmental dysplasia of the hip between 6 and 24 months of age. *Eur. J. Orthop. Surg. Traumatol.* **2019**, *29*, 51–57. [CrossRef]
25. Chin, M.S.; Betz, B.W.; Halanski, M.A. Comparison of hip reduction using magnetic resonance imaging or computed tomography in hip dysplasia. *J. Pediatr. Orthop.* **2011**, *31*, 525–529. [CrossRef]
26. Jaremko, J.L.; Wang, C.C.; Dulai, S. Reliability of indices measured on infant hip MRI at time of spica cast application for dysplasia. *HIP Int.* **2014**, *24*, 405–416. [CrossRef]
27. Graf, R. Classification of hip joint dysplasia by means of sonography. *Arch. Orthop. Trauma. Surg.* **1984**, *102*, 248–255. [CrossRef]
28. Graf, R. Fundamentals of sonographic diagnosis of infant hip dysplasia. *J. Pediatr. Orthop.* **1984**, *4*, 735–740. [CrossRef]
29. Graf, R. Hip sonography: 20 years experience and results. *Hip Int.* **2007**, *17* (Suppl. S5), S8–S14. [CrossRef]
30. Cooper, A.P.; Doddabasappa, S.N.; Mulpuri, K. Evidence-based management of developmental dysplasia of the hip. *Orthop. Clin. N. Am.* **2014**, *45*, 341–354. [CrossRef]

31. Seidl, T.; Lohmaier, J.; Hölker, T.; Funk, J.; Placzek, R.; Trouillier, H.H. Reduction of unstable and dislocated hips applying the Tubingen hip flexion splint? *Orthopade* **2012**, *41*, 195–199. [CrossRef]
32. Bernau, A. The Tubingen hip flexion splint in the treatment of hip dysplasia. *Z. Orthop. Ihre Grenzgeb.* **1990**, *128*, 432–435. [CrossRef] [PubMed]
33. Tönnis, D. *Congenital Dysplasia and Dislocation of the Hip in Children and Adults*; Springer: New York, NY, USA, 1987.
34. Graf, R. Hip sonography in infancy. Procedure and clinical significance. *Fortschr. Med.* **1985**, *103*, 62–66.
35. Hefti, F. *Kinderorthopädie in der Praxis*; Springer: Berlin/Heidelberg, Germany, 2015; Volume 3, p. 929.
36. Sankar, W.N.; Gornitzky, A.L.; Clarke, N.M.; Herrera-Soto, J.A.; Kelley, S.P.; Matheney, T.; Mulpuri, K.; Schaeffer, E.K.; Upasani, V.V.; Williams, N.; et al. Closed Reduction for Developmental Dysplasia of the Hip: Early-term Results From a Prospective, Multicenter Cohort. *J. Pediatr. Orthop.* **2019**, *39*, 111–118. [CrossRef]
37. Li, Y.; Guo, Y.; Shen, X.; Liu, H.; Mei, H.; Xu, H.; Canavese, F.; Chinese Multi-Center Pediatric Orthopedic Study Group (CMPOS). Radiographic outcome of children older than twenty-four months with developmental dysplasia of the hip treated by closed reduction and spica cast immobilization in human position: A review of fifty-one hips. *Int. Orthop.* **2019**, *43*, 1405–1411. [CrossRef]
38. Yong, B.; Li, Y.; Li, J.; Andreacchio, A.; Pavone, V.; Pereria, B.; Xu, H.; Canavese, F. Post-operative radiograph assessment of children undergoing closed reduction and spica cast immobilization for developmental dysplasia of the hip: Does experience matter? *Int. Orthop.* **2018**, *42*, 2725–2731. [CrossRef]
39. Haruno, L.S.; Kan, J.H.; Rivlin, M.J.; Rosenfeld, S.B.; Schallert, E.K.; Zhu, H.; Shenava, V.R. Spica MRI predictors for epiphyseal osteonecrosis after closed reduction treatment of dysplasia of the hip. *J. Pediatr. Orthop. B* **2019**, *28*, 424–429. [CrossRef]
40. Zhang, G.; Li, M.; Qu, X.; Cao, Y.; Liu, X.; Luo, C.; Zhang, Y. Efficacy of closed reduction for developmental dysplasia of the hip: Midterm outcomes and risk factors associated with treatment failure and avascular necrosis. *J. Orthop. Surg. Res.* **2020**, *15*, 579. [CrossRef]
41. Xu, M.; Gao, S.; Sun, J.; Yang, Y.; Song, Y.; Han, R.; Lei, G. Predictive values for the severity of avascular necrosis from the initial evaluation in closed reduction of developmental dysplasia of the hip. *J. Pediatr. Orthop. B* **2013**, *22*, 179–183. [CrossRef]
42. Vandergugten, S.; Traore, S.Y.; Docquier, P.-L. Risk factors for additional surgery after closed reduction of hip developmental dislocation. *Acta Orthop. Belg.* **2016**, *82*, 787–796.
43. Terjesen, T.; Horn, J.; Gunderson, R.B. Fifty-year follow-up of late-detected hip dislocation: Clinical and radiographic outcomes for seventy-one patients treated with traction to obtain gradual closed reduction. *J. Bone Jt. Surg.* **2014**, *96*, e28. [CrossRef] [PubMed]
44. Ge, Y.; Cai, H.; Wang, Z. Quality of reduction and prognosis of developmental dysplasia of the hip: A retrospective study. *HIP Int.* **2016**, *26*, 355–359. [CrossRef] [PubMed]
45. Kotlarsky, P.; Haber, R.; Bialik, V.; Eidelman, M. Developmental dysplasia of the hip: What has changed in the last 20 years? *World J. Orthop.* **2015**, *6*, 886–901. [CrossRef]
46. Murray, T.; Cooperman, D.R.; Thompson, G.H.; Ballock, R.T. Closed reduction for treatment of development dysplasia of the hip in children. *Am. J. Orthop.* **2007**, *36*, 82–84. [PubMed]

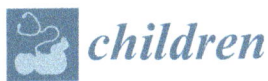

Article

Short Term Radiological Outcome of Combined Femoral and Ilium Osteotomy in Pelvic Reconstruction of the Child

Lorenz Pisecky [1,*], Gerhard Großbötzl [1], Stella Stevoska [1], Matthias Christoph Michael Klotz [2], Christina Haas [1], Tobias Gotterbarm [1], Matthias Luger [1] and Manuel Gahleitner [1]

[1] Department for Orthopedics and Traumatology, Kepler University Hospital GmbH, Johannes Kepler University Linz, Krankenhausstraße 9, 4020 Linz and Altenberger Strasse 96, 4040 Linz, Austria; gerhard.grossboetzl@kepleruniklinikum.at (G.G.); stella.stevoska@kepleruniklinikum.at (S.S.); christina.haas@kepleruniklinikum.at (C.H.); tobias.gotterbarm@kepleruniklinikum.at (T.G.); matthias.luger@kepleruniklinikum.at (M.L.); manuel.gahleitner@kepleruniklinikum.at (M.G.)
[2] Department for Orthopaedics and Traumatology, Marienkrankenhaus Soest GmbH, Widumgasse 5, 59494 Soest, Germany; mcmklotz@gmx.net
* Correspondence: lorenz.pisecky@kepleruniklinikum.at; Tel.: +43-(0)5-7680-83-78478

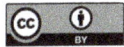

Citation: Pisecky, L.; Großbötzl, G.; Stevoska, S.; Klotz, M.C.M.; Haas, C.; Gotterbarm, T.; Luger, M.; Gahleitner, M. Short Term Radiological Outcome of Combined Femoral and Ilium Osteotomy in Pelvic Reconstruction of the Child. *Children* 2022, *9*, 441. https://doi.org/10.3390/children9030441

Academic Editor: Vito Pavone

Received: 18 February 2022
Accepted: 17 March 2022
Published: 21 March 2022

Publisher's Note: MDPI stays neutral with regard to jurisdictional claims in published maps and institutional affiliations.

Copyright: © 2022 by the authors. Licensee MDPI, Basel, Switzerland. This article is an open access article distributed under the terms and conditions of the Creative Commons Attribution (CC BY) license (https://creativecommons.org/licenses/by/4.0/).

Abstract: Background and Objectives: Reconstruction of the pelvic joint is a common way to address developmental dysplasia of the hip (DDH), as well as neurogenic dislocation of the hip (NDH) and Legg–Calvé–Perthes disease (LCPD) in children. The purpose of this study was to analyze the short-term radiologic outcome after hip reconstructive surgery either treated with sole osteotomy of the femur or in combination with iliac osteotomy in patients with DDH, NDH and LCPD. Materials and Methods: X-rays of 73 children, aged 2–18 years, with DDH, NDH and LCPD after hip reconstructive surgery were measured retrospectively and compared to the preoperative x-rays concerning various parameters to define hip geometry. The surgical procedures were femoral osteotomy (74), Salter innominate osteotomy (27), Pemberton osteotomy (27), open reduction (37), Chiari osteotomy (4). The pre-/postoperative acetabular index (AI), center-edge angle (CE) and Reimers migration index (RMI) were evaluated before and 3 months after surgery. Results: Hip geometry parameters improved significantly (RMI: preop/postop: 62.23% ± 31.63%/6.30% ± 11.51%, $p < 0.001$; CE: 11.53° ± 20.16°/30.58 ± 8.81°, $p < 0.001$; AI: 28.67° ± 9.2°/19.17 ± 7.65°, $p < 0.001$). Sub-group analysis showed a superior RMI in DDH compared with NDH 3 months after surgery (DDH/NDH: 2.77% ± 6.9%/12.94% ± 13.5%; $p = 0.011$). Osteotomy of the iliac bone (Salter innominate, Pemberton, Chiari) resulted in a significant improvement of the postoperative RMI compared to cases without osteotomy of the ilium (7.02 ± 11.1% vs. 16.85 ± 4.71%; $p = 0.035$). Conclusions: Femoral and pelvic osteotomies are effective to improve the radiological pelvic parameters in infants and adolescents with DDH, NDH and LCPD. In addition, the study found that the combination of femoral and pelvic osteotomies led to a better RMI than femoral osteotomy alone. Using the combined ilium and femoral osteotomy, it was possible to show the highest effect on correction of the hip geometry with respect to residual RMI.

Keywords: developmental dysplasia of the hip; neurogenic dislocation of the hip; Legg–Calvé–Perthes disease; combined osteotomy; femur; ilium; varisation derotation osteotomy; Salter; Pemberton; Chiari; open reduction

1. Introduction

In infants and adolescents suffering from developmental dysplasia of the hip (DDH) and neurogenic dislocation of the hip (NDH), surgical treatment is often needed to avoid persistent problems in walking, standing and sitting [1]. Surgical hip joint reconstruction may be needed in children and adolescents with developmental dysplasia of the hip as soon as conservative treatment has failed and residual dysplasia is diagnosed to avoid persistent dysplastic morphology increase the risk of degenerative change [2].

In addition to DDH and NDH, in children with Perthes disease (LCPD) surgical reconstruction of the hip may be necessary to improve the containment. Especially if so-called 'head at risk' signs are present, literature postulates the concept of "super containment" [3–5].

Severe forms of DDH are often related to neuromuscular disorders [6]. In cerebral palsy (CP), different authors could show an incidence of NDH in up to 60% of their patients [7]. Therefore, hip reconstruction is even indicated in cases showing a progressive migration to avoid further dislocation and secondary complications of the hip [8–10].

Especially in adolescents and patients able to walk, therapy is often much more difficult than in smaller children because of shortening of extraarticular soft tissue [11]. Spasticity in neuromuscular disorders correlates with deformation and subluxation of the femur and shortening of the adductor muscle [12]. In most cases, a combination of procedures involving the bone and the soft tissue is needed to achieve complete reduction of the joint [13,14]. Common techniques are open reduction, lengthening of tendons or muscles as well as femoral and pelvic osteotomies [15].

Some surgeons prefer a two-stage approach to the reconstruction of the pelvic geometry and suggest performing surgical reduction and VDRO (varisation derotation osteotomy) first, in combination with an additional osteotomy of the ilium in a subsequent surgical procedure [16]. As long as there are not enough data to show superiority of the combined osseous procedure in patients with misalignment of the pelvic joint, the way of decision-making may still be unclear.

Available literature should have made clear, that a combination of femoral and iliac osteotomy is the proper choice in cases with femoral and iliac deformities. As the discussion is ongoing, whether to perform single or combined osteotomies as well as to perform those osteotomies stepwise and not within a single surgical procedure, the study group wanted to evaluate whether cases treated with combined one step osteotomy show different short term postoperative radiological outcome compared to cases treated with femoral osteotomy alone. The purpose of this study was to highlight the radiologic outcome after pelvic reconstruction either treated with osteotomy of the femur alone or in combination with iliac osteotomy in patients with DDH, NDH and LCPD.

2. Materials and Methods

In a retrospective study, patient files of children (aged 2–18 years) with DDH, NDH and LCPD were searched for hip or pelvic surgeries (open reduction, femoral/pelvic osteotomy ± soft tissue techniques) from 2008 to 2018 at a Central European University Hospital. Ethical approval was obtained from the IRB.

Patients without postoperative spica cast immobilization (3) were ruled out from analysis to reach homogeneity in aftertreatment. 10 patients were lost to follow-up. Finally, 73 patients (male/female: 38/35; 84 hips), aged 7.95 ± 5.18 years, were included. The group was treated by a single experienced pediatric orthopedic surgeon.

Indication for surgery can be seen in Table 1, demographic details and surgical procedures can be seen in Table 2. Included indications for surgery were RMI [17,18] 40 percent or higher or 25–40 percent with progression, classification of Tönnis [19] II or above or AI above the standard of Tönnis (greater than 25 degrees at the age of 2, >23° at 3, >20° at 7) [20]. Tönnis classification II or above for the AI-angle was an indication for surgery in respect of the lateralization of the ossific nucleus and a disruption of the Ménard–Shenton line. Surgery was not performed before the third year of age due to not having enough bone stock for extensive pelvic reconstruction.

The surgeries were carried out under general anesthesia on a radiolucent table using fluoroscopy. The patient was bedded in supine position with slight elevation of surgical site on by placing a foam padding beneath the iliac bone. The entire lower limb and the affected half of the pelvis were washed and draped. Surgical techniques used were open reduction, Chiari iliac osteotomy (4 hips) [21], Salter innominate osteotomy (21 hips) [22] and Pemberton acetabuloplasty (30 hips) [23], VDRO (84 hips) (Table 1) [24]. The surgical approach for open reduction and osteotomy of the ilium was direct anterior as described by Smith-Petersen [25]. A direct lateral approach was used to address the proximal femur for varisation-osteotomy. Beginning with open reduction and VDRO, additional osteotomy of the iliac bone was performed in cases with AI above the Tönnis-standard (Tönnis classification II or higher) and insufficient roofing of the femoral head after VDRO.

Table 1. Joints and surgical procedures [26].

	DDH	NDH	Perthes
N (hips)	31	25	28
age at surgery	5.8 years; 2.9–17; SD 5.7	12.5 years; 5.6–17.8; SD 6.2	7.6 years; 5.2–10.7; SD 1.7
m:f	5:21	11:11	22:3
right:left	10:11	12:7	9:13
bilateral	5	3	3
Surgical procedure in detail			
Femoral osteotomy	31	25	28
Osteotomy of ilium	27	17	12
Salter osteotomy	7	2	12
Chiari osteotomy	2	2	
Pemberton osteotomy	18	12	
Psoas tenotomy		9	1
Adductor tenotomy		8	
Open reduction	16	12	
Hamstring lengthening		7	
Lengthening of extension mechanism		1	

Table 2. Patient groups and surgical procedures in detail [27].

	Sole Osteotomy (Femur)	Combined Osteotomy (Ilium and Femur)
N (patients)	29	44
N (hips)	29	55
Bilateral	0	11
Gender m:f	9:20	28:16
Age at surgery	10.7 years; 5.0–17.8 y; SD 6.4	7.8 years; 2.9–15.1 years; SD 5.3
Location	10 right, 19 left	21 right, 12 left, 11 bilateral
Procedures (n = hips)		
Femoral osteotomy	29	55
Osteotomy of ilium	0	55
Salter osteotomy	0	21
Chiari osteotomy	0	4
Pemberton osteotomy	0	30
Psoas tenotomy	6	4
Adductor tenotomy	5	3
Open reduction	1	27

Table 2. *Cont.*

	Sole Osteotomy (Femur)	Combined Osteotomy (Ilium and Femur)
Hamstring lengthening	0	7
Lengthening of extension mechanism	0	1

The Salter innominate osteotomy was performed until the age of 8, as long as a good flexibility of the symphysis can be assumed. The procedure was not performed bilaterally in one surgical session.

The Pemberton acetabuloplasty was performed in cases with improper rounding of the acetabulum. Furthermore, the triradiate cartilage had to be clearly visible, which limited the procedure up to the age of 8. The procedure was performed bilaterally, if needed.

The Chiari osteotomy was considered to be a salvage procedure in cases with a lack of congruency of the pelvic joint (aspheric, big femoral head and small acetabulum) and progresses skeletal maturity. The procedure was not performed bilateral in one surgical session.

In a total of 55 cases, a combination of the techniques above was performed. Salter and Chiari osteotomies were fixed with three K-wires, Pemberton osteotomies were operated without osteosynthesis.

Osteosynthesis material used to hold the femoral osteotomy was a standard 90° AO blade plate (58 hips) or a 90° locking cannulated blade plate (15 hips).

Casting was performed directly postoperative under general anesthesia. Ten degrees of flexion, 10 degrees of inwards rotation and 20 to 30 degrees of abduction of the hip were tried to maintain within the cast. According to the routine protocol, immobilization was maintained for six consecutive weeks, followed by physiotherapy until full mobilization.

Complications occurring within the first three months after surgery were analyzed under usage of the full medical documentation and classified according to Clavien-Dindo [28]. Necessary unplanned procedures and admissions were collected and sub-group analysis concerning adverse events was carried out.

2.1. Radiological Analysis

The pre- and 3-months postoperative pelvic geometry data were analyzed twice each by author LP and compared statistically. An interval of at least 24 h between the two measurements was chosen. Intra-observer variation for the measurements was calculated using the mean difference, with the 95%-confidence intervals given. Intra-observer reliability rates were calculated using the statistical software Jamovi 1.0. Radiographic investigation consisted of a pelvis AP view in standing position and a lateral view pre- and 3 months postoperatively. AI [29], CE [29] and RMI [29,30] were measured.

2.2. Statistical Analysis

Statistical methods included detailed analysis of the epidemiological data with parameters for arithmetic mean, standard-deviation, median at continuous data and relative frequency for explained variables. The variables of interest for pre- and postoperative pelvic geometry were calculated using Student's t-tests. Sub-group analysis was conducted for AI, CE and RMI pre- and 3 months after surgery. The statistical software Jamovi 1.0 was used.

3. Results

Following surgery, data for pelvic geometry improved in all analyzed groups (DDH, NDH, LCPD), and it was statistically significant (Table 3). The intra-observer reliability rates reached a mean of 0.953 (95%-CI 0.942–0.964).

Table 3. Pelvic geometry [27].

		DDH	NDH	LCPD	Overall
AI	pre	33.90 ± 7.30	29.61 ± 6.10	19.00 ± 5.30	28.67 ± 9.20
	post	19.43 ± 7.20	18.56 ± 8.60	16.71 ± 5.92	19.17 ± 7.65
	diff	14.47 (95%-CI 11.82–17.86)	11.05 (95%-CI 7.00–15.16)	2.29 (95%-CI 0.39–4.00)	9.5 (95%-CI 7.60–11.65)
	p-value	$p < 0.001$	$p < 0.001$	$p = 0.019$	$p < 0.001$
CE	pre	11.73 ± 10.40	14.30 ± 16.60	25.70 ± 6.10	11.53 ± 20.16
	post	31.70 ± 7.20	27.50 ± 12.0	32.90 ± 6.60	30.58 ± 8.81
	diff	19.97 (95%-CI 16.33–36.01)	13.2 (95%-CI 23.72–46.53)	7.2 (95%-CI 4.33–10.07)	19.05 (95%-CI 14.43–24.43)
	p-value	$p < 0.001$	$p < 0.001$	$p < 0.001$	$p < 0.001$
RMI	pre	80.28 ± 27.94	78.00 ± 21.4	27.38 ± 8.38	62.23 ± 31.63
	post	2.77 ± 6.90	12.94 ± 13.5	1.75 ± 4.14	6.30 ± 11.51
	diff	77.51 (95%-CI 65.8–89.43)	65.06 (95%-CI 48.68–73.08)	25.63 (95%-CI 22.36–29.24)	55.93 (95%-CI 48.01–62.85)
	p-value	$p < 0.001$	$p < 0.001$	$p < 0.001$	$p < 0.001$

AI—acetabular index, CE—center edge angle, RMI—Reimers migration index, DDH—developmental dysplasia of the hip, NDH—neurogenic dislocation of the hip, LCPD—Legg-Calvé-Perthes disease, pre—mean preoperative value, post—mean postoperative value, diff—mean difference.

In total, 28 hips showed a dislocation (RMI > 100%) before surgery. After open reduction and acetabular osteotomy, those cases presented a significant decrease of AI from 33.71° ± 7.76° to 19.71° ± 8.16° ($p < 0.001$).

Three months after surgery, children with DDH showed significant decreased RMI compared with children with NDH in a two-sample Student's t-test (2.77 ± 6.90% vs. 12.94 ± 13.50%; $p = 0.011$). More often an osteotomy of the iliac bone (Salter innominate, Pemberton, Chiari) was carried out in patients with DDH than with NDH (27 vs. 17; $p < 0.001$). In cases with combined one step iliac and femoral osteotomy, the residual RMI was significantly lower than in cases with osteotomy of the femur alone (7.02 ± 11.1% vs. 16.85 ± 4.71%; $p < 0.001$) (Table 4, Figures 1 and 2).

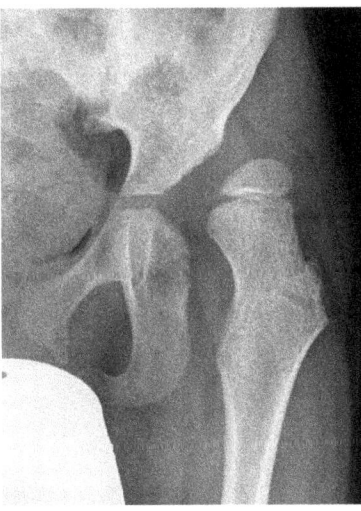 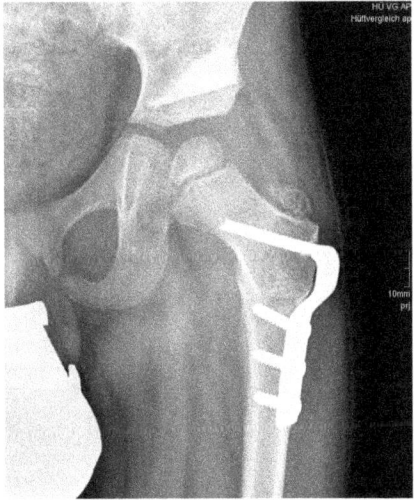

Figure 1. (**left**) Anteroposterior radiograph of a six-year-old male with NDH; (**right**) result 3 months postoperatively.

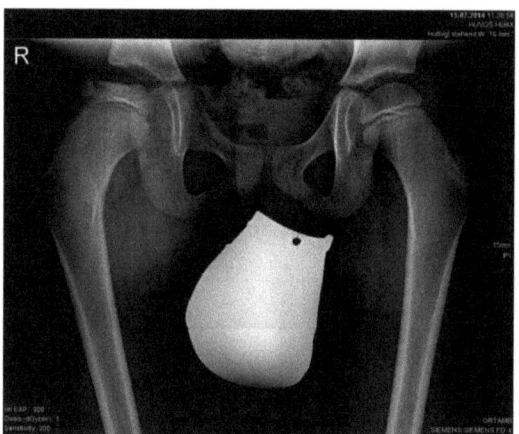 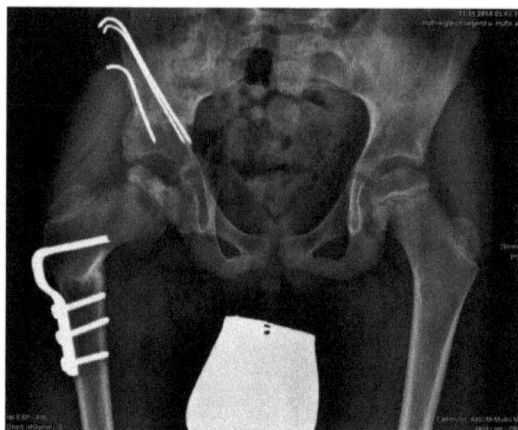

Figure 2. (**left**) Anteroposterior radiograph of a nine-year-old male with LCPD; (**right**): result three months postoperatively.

Table 4. Improvement of RMI with and without osteotomy of the ilium.

		Sole Femoral Osteotomy (N = 29)	Combined Iliac and Femoral Osteotomy (N = 55)
RMI	pre	35.40 ± 14.60	72.00 ± 30.6
	post	16.85 ± 4.71	7.02 ± 11.10
	diff	18.55 (95%-CI 14.05–23.93)	64.98 (95%-CI 57.95–77.3)
	p-value	$p < 0.001$	$p < 0.001$
	diff		9.83 (95%-CI 6.59–15.32)
	p-value		$p < 0.001$

In 30.01% of the patients (22), adverse events were found. Seven superficial skin lesions were counted, three extensive skin lesions, three spasticity of adductors, two subluxations, two dislocations of the cast, one deep infection of the osteosynthesis material, one compliance problem, one reluxation, one delayed bone healing and one spasticity of knee flexors. Classifying the adverse evenly according to Clavien-Dindo, 10 type I, 4 type II, 8 type III, 0 type IV and 0 type V events were seen. Short-term complications were observed nearly equally in the group of NDH (8/23; 34.7%) and in DDH (8/22; 36.4%). Further treatment of the complications included five procedures with three open re-repositions and re-casting as a result of re-dislocation within 12 weeks postoperatively observed on the follow-up x-rays after initial mobilization, one exchange of the osteosynthesis material due to a fracture of the blade plate, one removal of the plate due to deep wound infection involving the osteosynthesis material; three inpatient treatments for pain management and wound care and one admission for high energy shockwave treatment to address the prolonged healing of the bone were necessary. Four children needed intense wound treatment in the outpatient clinic on a regular basis. In no cases did very severe complications with persistent physical damage or even death occurred.

4. Discussion

Techniques in joint-preserving surgery in children and adolescents are demanding for the pediatric orthopedic surgeon. After walking age, treatment of DDH and NDH is difficult due to adaptive shortening of the extra-articular soft tissues, acetabular dysplasia, capsular constriction and increased femoral anteversion. In the literature several methods for reconstruction of the hip are available. In most of the children femoral and pelvic osteotomies are necessary to achieve concentric reduction. In cases of LCPD, the idea of 'super-containment' is well accepted to provide proper roofing for the rebuilding femoral head [3–5]. Realignment of the pelvic joint under usage of pericapsular osseous techniques in combination with or without femoral osteotomy and soft tissue procedures is a common way to treat DDH, NDH and LCPD in children.

The purpose of this study was to evaluate the short-term results of hip reconstructive surgery in young patients with DDH, NDH and LCPD either with ilium osteotomy alone or in combination with femoral osteotomy.

In this study-group the surgical results for reconstruction of the pelvic joint, using the Pemberton-acetabuloplasty, pericapsular osteotomy as described by Salter, Chiari osteotomy and varisation derotation osteotomy of the proximal femur are similar to the prior published data. In total, 84 hips were included in this trial; indications for surgical procedures were DDH, NDH and LCPD. For all three groups, it was possible to present a statistically significant enhancement in pelvic geometry following hip surgery. Therefore, our data suggest that these procedures are suitable to reestablish congruency of the hip in children and adolescents, despite the authors being aware of a progressive deterioration of RMI in cases of pelvic reconstruction at midterm follow-up [27].

The authors noticed that in this cohort, patients with NDH have a lower benefit from surgery in contrast to patients with DDH for the endpoint RMI (12.94% vs. 2.77%; $p = 0.011$). The results for RMI are congruent to previously reported data in children with NDH [14]. Further analysis revealed, that in cases with iliac osteotomy (Salter innominate, Pemberton, Chiari), the residual RMI was notable lower than in cases without (7.02% vs. 16.85%; $p < 0.001$). Iliac osteotomy was performed in 27 out of 31 patients with DDH, which is a notable contrast to the patients with NDH (17 out of 25). In the authors' opinion, the osteotomy of the ilium leads to a significant improvement of RMI and should be performed to achieve congruency of the hip. As to our knowledge this is the first report to present advantages of the combined osteotomy for the endpoint RMI 3 months postoperatively. Clearly, a longer follow-up period is urgently needed to show the sustainability of this effect and will be published by the investigators.

Park et al. performed a similar retrospective trial, in order to find criteria for the one-stage femoral and ilium osteotomy [31]. As major risk factors for surgical failure, the authors revealed a preoperative RMI of 61.8% and above or 5.1% postoperatively. As the discussion is ongoing, in terms of what criterion to choose for concomitant osteotomy of the ilium, the RMI may be one possible option as well as the intraoperative stability of the reduced hip. In the authors' opinion, the criteria of Park et al. involves a well thought-out approach to the discussion whether to perform a sole femoral osteotomy or a combined procedure.

Most notably, and supporting the ongoing dispute of surgical algorithm, Huh et al. pleaded for a stepwise approach to surgical management of decentration of the pelvic joint. At first, a combination of a proximal femoral osteotomy with open reduction and soft tissue techniques should be performed, followed by an osteotomy of the iliac bone in a second surgery, if needed [16]. In the authors' opinion, one reason for thoughts such as this may be the good results of pelvic reconstruction under usage of sole osteotomies, whether femoral or iliac, as published by Czubak et al. 2018 [11], El-Sayed et al. 2015 [32] and Al-Ghamdi et al. did in 2012 [33]. It must be kept in mind, that especially in NDH, a deterioration of RMI is known and therefore the direct postoperative result in those cases should be as stable as possible and a combination of surgical techniques may be needed [14].

In this study, a rate of 30% for adverse events was calculated. Most of those events were easy to handle, which is on one hand comparable to previously published data, but way too high in the authors' opinion [34]. It was expected to see more complications related to the postoperative immobilization such as contractures and superficial skin problems in the NDH group because of the higher muscle tone and the inability to express discomfort underneath the casting. Adverse events were more common in patients with NDH, despite the results not reaching statistical significance.

The heterogeneity of the investigated group as well as the small number of patients are the major limitations of the present study. The surgical techniques are not high-volume procedures, but necessary in a small patient group with demanding diseases.

The major drawback for statistical analysis, the heterogeneity, was accepted because the main result of the study, the improvement of RMI in combined femoral/iliac and sole femoral osteotomy, is not considered to be highly influenced by the underlying illness of the child at the 3-months postoperative follow-up. Clearly, the entity of the disease will make a difference in mid- to long-term follow-up trials. This must be considered when results for longer follow-up periods are given. Additionally, the authors are aware that the mid- to long-term complications may vary in those groups. Therefore, the authors cannot give recommendations for certain surgical procedures concerning long-term postoperative results. To minimize the chance for misinterpretation, all three sub-groups were analyzed separately concerning epidemiological data as well as the postoperative results to give the reader insights in preoperative clinical presentation and group-specific postoperative results. As prospective randomized clinical trials dealing with the described group of patients cannot be easily performed in the daily clinical practice, the authors must accept certain drawbacks in study design.

Furthermore, a limiting factor is the short postoperative follow-up period. The authors decided to evaluate the 3-month follow-up X-rays to achieve comparable short-term results for all evaluated patient groups (DDH, NDH, LCPD). Annual checks for deterioration of pelvic geometry are needed in NDH, as available reports show re-operation rates of 40% [35].

It is necessary to provide mid- and long-term results after hip reconstructive surgery to show long-lasting positive effects on hip geometry and patient outcome. The next step of the study group is to present mid- to long-term results on this topic and we hope to achieve sustainable results with our approach on hip deformities in children.

5. Conclusions

This study summarizes that all described reconstructive methods are feasible to enhance pelvic geometry in children with DDH, NDH and LCPD. In cases with iliac osteotomy, the residual RMI was significantly lower than in cases without.

The combined osteotomy of the ilium and femur led to a significant improvement of RMI compared to femoral osteotomy alone and should be undoubtedly performed in demanding cases. Common complications such as re-dislocation, wound-problems and delayed osseous healing were seen and led to demanding revision-surgery in five cases.

Author Contributions: All authors contributed to the development of the manuscript; L.P., S.S., G.G., M.G., T.G. and M.L. developed the first draft of the manuscript; T.G., C.H. and G.G. performed corrections; L.P., S.S., M.G., M.C.M.K., C.H. and M.L. were responsible for the final manuscript. All authors have read and agreed to the published version of the manuscript.

Funding: This research is part of a long term prospective randomized clinical trial comparing spica cast versus foam split. This clinical trial is funded by the Medical Society of Upperaustria, Dinghoferstraße 4, 4020 Linz, Austria, with a grant of EUR 10,000 attracted by the corresponding author Dr. Lorenz Pisecky.

Institutional Review Board Statement: The study was conducted according to the guidelines of the Declaration of Helsinki, and approved by the Institutional Review Board (Ethikkommission des Landes Oberösterreich; EK1183/2018; 10 February 2019).

Informed Consent Statement: Patient consent was waived due to the retrospective study design.

Data Availability Statement: The used datasets for this study contain potentially identifying or sensitive patient information. The vote of the local review board (Ethikkommission des Landes Oberösterreich, Wagner-Jauregg-Weg 15, 4020 Linz, Austria; Vote number EK Nr: 1183/2018) does not allow general data sharing.

Acknowledgments: Open Access Funding by the University of Linz.

Conflicts of Interest: The authors declare no conflict of interest.

References

1. Huser, A.; Mo, M.; Hosseinzadeh, P. Hip Surveillance in Children with Cerebral Palsy. *Orthop. Clin. N. Am.* **2018**, *49*, 181–190. [CrossRef]
2. Wyles, C.C.; Heidenreich, M.J.; Jeng, J.; Larson, D.R.; Trousdale, R.T.; Sierra, R.J. The John Charnley Award: Redefining the Natural History of Osteoarthritis in Patients With Hip Dysplasia and Impingement. *Clin. Orthop. Relat. Res.* **2017**, *475*, 336–350. [CrossRef]
3. Lloyd-Roberts, G.C.; Catterall, A.; Salamon, P.B. A controlled study of the indications for and the results of femoral osteotomy in Perthes' disease. *J. Bone Jt. Surg. Br.* **1976**, *58*, 31–36. [CrossRef]
4. Poussa, M.; Hoikka, V.; Yrjonen, T.; Osterman, K. Early signs of poor prognosis in Legg-Perthes-Calve disease treated by femoral varus osteotomy. *Rev. Chir. Orthop. Reparatrice Appar. Mot.* **1991**, *77*, 478–482.
5. Thompson, G.H. Salter osteotomy in Legg-Calve-Perthes disease. *J. Pediatr. Orthop.* **2011**, *31*, S192–S197. [CrossRef]
6. Chan, G.; Miller, F. Assessment and treatment of children with cerebral palsy. *Orthop. Clin. N. Am.* **2014**, *45*, 313–325. [CrossRef]
7. Root, L. Surgical treatment for hip pain in the adult cerebral palsy patient. *Dev. Med. Child Neurol.* **2009**, *51* (Suppl. 4), 84–91. [CrossRef] [PubMed]
8. Hagglund, G.; Andersson, S.; Duppe, H.; Lauge-Pedersen, H.; Nordmark, E.; Westbom, L. Prevention of dislocation of the hip in children with cerebral palsy. The first ten years of a population-based prevention programme. *J. Bone Jt. Surg. Br.* **2005**, *87*, 95–101. [CrossRef]
9. Hagglund, G.; Alriksson-Schmidt, A.; Lauge-Pedersen, H.; Rodby-Bousquet, E.; Wagner, P.; Westbom, L. Prevention of dislocation of the hip in children with cerebral palsy: 20-year results of a population-based prevention programme. *Bone Jt. J.* **2014**, *96-B*, 1546–1552. [CrossRef]
10. Valencia, F.G. Management of hip deformities in cerebral palsy. *Orthop. Clin. N. Am.* **2010**, *41*, 549–559. [CrossRef]
11. Czubak, J.; Kowalik, K.; Kawalec, A.; Kwiatkowska, M. Dega pelvic osteotomy: Indications, results and complications. *J. Child Orthop.* **2018**, *12*, 342–348. [CrossRef] [PubMed]
12. Cho, Y.; Park, E.S.; Park, H.K.; Park, J.E.; Rha, D.W. Determinants of Hip and Femoral Deformities in Children With Spastic Cerebral Palsy. *Ann. Rehabil. Med.* **2018**, *42*, 277–285. [CrossRef] [PubMed]
13. Onimus, M.; Manzone, P.; Allamel, G. Prevention of hip dislocation in children with cerebral palsy by early tenotomy of the adductor and psoas muscles. *Ann. Pediatr.* **1993**, *40*, 211–216.
14. Braatz, F.; Eidemuller, A.; Klotz, M.C.; Beckmann, N.A.; Wolf, S.I.; Dreher, T. Hip reconstruction surgery is successful in restoring joint congruity in patients with cerebral palsy: Long-term outcome. *Int. Orthop.* **2014**, *38*, 2237–2243. [CrossRef]
15. Emara, K.; Kersh, M.A.A.; Hayyawi, F.A. Duration of immobilization after developmental dysplasia of the hip and open reduction surgery. *Int. Orthop.* **2019**, *43*, 405–409. [CrossRef]
16. Huh, K.; Rethlefsen, S.A.; Wren, T.A.; Kay, R.M. Surgical management of hip subluxation and dislocation in children with cerebral palsy: Isolated VDRO or combined surgery? *J. Pediatr. Orthop.* **2011**, *31*, 858–863. [CrossRef]
17. Robb, J.E.; Hagglund, G. Hip surveillance and management of the displaced hip in cerebral palsy. *J. Child Orthop.* **2013**, *7*, 407–413. [CrossRef]
18. Kim, S.M.; Sim, E.G.; Lim, S.G.; Park, E.S. Reliability of hip migration index in children with cerebral palsy: The classic and modified methods. *Ann. Rehabil. Med.* **2012**, *36*, 33–38. [CrossRef]
19. Tönnis, D. *Die Angeborene Hüftdysplasie und Hüftluxation im Kindes-und Erwachsenenalter: Grundlagen, Diagnostik, Konservative und Operative Behandlung*; Springer: Berlin/Heidelberg, Germany, 2013.
20. Tönnis, D. Röntgenuntersuchung und arthrographie des hüftgelenks im kleinkindesalter. *Der. Orthopäde* **1997**, *26*, 49–58. [CrossRef]
21. Chiari, K. Medial displacement osteotomy of the pelvis. *Clin. Orthop. Relat. Res.* **1974**, *98*, 55–71. [CrossRef]
22. Salter, R.B. Role of innominate osteotomy in the treatment of congenital dislocation and subluxation of the hip in the older child. *J. Bone Jt. Surg. Am.* **1966**, *48*, 1413–1439. [CrossRef]
23. Pemberton, P.A. Pericapsular Osteotomy of the Ilium for Treatment of Congenital Subluxation and Dislocation of the Hip. *J. Bone Jt. Surg. Am.* **1965**, *47*, 65–86. [CrossRef]
24. Beer, Y.; Smorgick, Y.; Oron, A.; Mirovsky, Y.; Weigl, D.; Agar, G.; Shitrit, R.; Copeliovitch, L. Long-term results of proximal femoral osteotomy in Legg-Calve-Perthes disease. *J. Pediatr. Orthop.* **2008**, *28*, 819–824. [CrossRef]
25. Smith-Petersen, M. A new supra-articular subperiosteal approach to the hip joint. *J. Bone Jt. Surg.* **1917**, *2*, 592–595.
26. Pisecky, L.; Grossbotzl, G.; Gahleitner, M.; Haas, C.; Gotterbarm, T.; Klotz, M.C. Results after spica cast immobilization following hip reconstruction in 95 cases: Is there a need for alternative techniques? *Arch. Orthop. Trauma Surg.* **2021**. [CrossRef]
27. Pisecky, L.; Grossbotzl, G.; Gahleitner, M.; Stevoska, S.; Stadler, C.; Haas, C.; Gotterbarm, T.; Klotz, M.C. Progressive lateralization and constant hip geometry in children with DDH, NDH, and LCPD following hip reconstructive surgery: A cohort study of 73 patients with a mean follow-up of 4.9 years. *Arch. Orthop. Trauma Surg.* **2021**. [CrossRef]
28. Dodwell, E.R.; Pathy, R.; Widmann, R.F.; Green, D.W.; Scher, D.M.; Blanco, J.S.; Doyle, S.M.; Daluiski, A.; Sink, E.L. Reliability of the Modified Clavien-Dindo-Sink Complication Classification System in Pediatric Orthopaedic Surgery. *JBJS Open Access* **2018**, *3*, e0020. [CrossRef]

29. Ruiz Santiago, F.; Santiago Chinchilla, A.; Ansari, A.; Guzman Alvarez, L.; Castellano Garcia Mdel, M.; Martinez Martinez, A.; Tercedor Sanchez, J. Imaging of Hip Pain: From Radiography to Cross-Sectional Imaging Techniques. *Radiol. Res. Pract.* **2016**, *2016*, 6369237. [CrossRef]
30. Reimers, J. The stability of the hip in children. A radiological study of the results of muscle surgery in cerebral palsy. *Acta Orthop. Scand. Suppl.* **1980**, *184*, 1–100. [CrossRef]
31. Park, H.; Abdel-Baki, S.W.; Park, K.B.; Park, B.K.; Rhee, I.; Hong, S.P.; Kim, H.W. Outcome of Femoral Varus Derotational Osteotomy for the Spastic Hip Displacement: Implication for the Indication of Concomitant Pelvic Osteotomy. *J. Clin. Med.* **2020**, *9*, 256. [CrossRef]
32. El-Sayed, M.M.; Hegazy, M.; Abdelatif, N.M.; ElGebeily, M.A.; ElSobky, T.; Nader, S. Dega osteotomy for the management of developmental dysplasia of the hip in children aged 2–8 years: Results of 58 consecutive osteotomies after 13–25 years of follow-up. *J. Child Orthop.* **2015**, *9*, 191–198. [CrossRef] [PubMed]
33. Al-Ghamdi, A.; Rendon, J.S.; Al-Faya, F.; Saran, N.; Benaroch, T.; Hamdy, R.C. Dega osteotomy for the correction of acetabular dysplasia of the hip: A radiographic review of 21 cases. *J. Pediatr. Orthop.* **2012**, *32*, 113–120. [CrossRef] [PubMed]
34. DiFazio, R.; Vessey, J.; Zurakowski, D.; Hresko, M.T.; Matheney, T. Incidence of skin complications and associated charges in children treated with hip spica casts for femur fractures. *J. Pediatr. Orthop.* **2011**, *31*, 17–22. [CrossRef] [PubMed]
35. Kiapekos, N.; Brostrom, E.; Hagglund, G.; Astrand, P. Primary surgery to prevent hip dislocation in children with cerebral palsy in Sweden: A minimum 5-year follow-up by the national surveillance program (CPUP). *Acta Orthop.* **2019**, *90*, 495–500. [CrossRef] [PubMed]

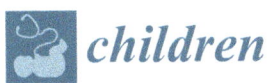

Article

Health-Related Quality of Life after Adolescent Fractures of the Femoral Shaft Stabilized by a Lateral Entry Femoral Nail

Thoralf Randolph Liebs *, Anna Meßling, Milan Milosevic, Steffen Michael Berger and Kai Ziebarth

Inselspital, Department of Paediatric Surgery, University of Bern, 3010 Bern, Switzerland; geppert.anna@gmail.com (A.M.); milan.milosevic@insel.ch (M.M.); steffen.berger@insel.ch (S.M.B.); kai.ziebarth@insel.ch (K.Z.)
* Correspondence: liebs@liebs.eu; Tel.: +41-31-632-2111

Abstract: (1) Background: In adolescents, fractures of the femoral shaft that are not suitable for elastic-stable-intramedullary-nailing (ESIN), are challenging. We aimed to evaluate the health-related quality of life (HRQoL) and complications in adolescents treated with intramedullary rodding using the adolescent lateral trochanteric entry femoral nail (ALFN), and to assess if HRQoL was associated with additional injuries. (2) Methods: We followed-up on 15 adolescents with a diaphyseal femoral fracture who were treated with an ALFN from 2004 to 2017. Patients were asked to fill in a questionnaire that includes the iHOT, Peds-QL, and the Pedi-IKDC. (3) Results: The ALFN was used as a primary method of fixation in 13 patients, and as a fixation for failed ESIN in two cases. All 15 fractures healed radiographically. One distal locking screw broke. After a mean follow-up of 2.8 years, the mean iHOT-12 was 14.0 (SD 15.4), PedsQL-function was 85.7 (SD 19.3), PedsQL-social-score was 86.2 (SD 12.5), and the mean Pedi-IKDC was 77.2 (SD 11.3). In patients where the femoral fracture was an isolated injury, the HRQoL-scores were consistently higher compared with patients who sustained additional injures. (4) Conclusions: Treating diaphyseal fractures in adolescents with an ALFN resulted in good radiographic outcomes in all our cases. HRQoL, as measured by the iHOT, PedsQL, and Pedi-IKDC, was good to excellent; but it was consistently inferior in patients with additional injuries. These results suggest that the ALFN is a good alternative when patients are not suitable for ESIN, and that the HRQoL of adolescents who were treated with an ALFN is mainly influenced by the presence of additional injures, and less by the fracture of the femur itself.

Keywords: fracture; femur; surgery; nail; intramedullary; health-related quality of life

Citation: Liebs, T.R.; Meßling, A.; Milosevic, M.; Berger, S.M.; Ziebarth, K. Health-Related Quality of Life after Adolescent Fractures of the Femoral Shaft Stabilized by a Lateral Entry Femoral Nail. *Children* **2022**, *9*, 327. https://doi.org/10.3390/children9030327

Academic Editors: Axel A. Horsch, Maher A. Ghandour and Matthias Christoph M. Klotz

Received: 28 January 2022
Accepted: 24 February 2022
Published: 1 March 2022

Publisher's Note: MDPI stays neutral with regard to jurisdictional claims in published maps and institutional affiliations.

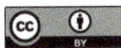

Copyright: © 2022 by the authors. Licensee MDPI, Basel, Switzerland. This article is an open access article distributed under the terms and conditions of the Creative Commons Attribution (CC BY) license (https://creativecommons.org/licenses/by/4.0/).

1. Introduction

Since fractures of the femoral shaft are not too common among children (e.g., 0.89% [1]), many paediatricians and orthopaedic surgeons may have only limited experience in treating these injuries. Nonetheless, given the need for emergency surgery in children 3 years of age and older, every orthopaedic surgeon may be confronted with the need to perform surgery in these children.

The preferred treatment strategy for paediatric femoral fractures is age dependent, ranging from bandage immobilization in new-borns to overhead extension or hip spica cast in children up to about 3 years of age. For older children up to the teenage years, elastic intramedullary nailing (ESIN) is the standard treatment. However, in adolescents the management of diaphyseal femoral fractures is highly debated. Treatment options in that age group include ESIN, external fixation [2], a combination of these two methods, submuscular plating [3], or rigid intramedullary rodding.

Several studies have demonstrated that, due to its flexible nature, elastic intramedullary nailing has an increased risk of complications in heavier or older children. Commonly, a body weight of 50 kg [4,5] or 55 kg [6] is considered as a threshold in that respect. On the other hand, plate fixation involves incisions that might be regarded as unattractive, and plate fixation has been associated with valgus deformity, especially if the plate is not removed [3].

Intramedullary rodding through the piriform fossa, a standard approach known to every orthopaedic surgeon, has been associated with reports of avascular necrosis of the femoral head [7–9] which ultimately may lead to total hip arthroplasty. For this reason, this technique has not been recommended in adolescents.

With advanced knowledge of the blood supply of the femoral head, entry points lateral to the tip of the greater trochanter have been evaluated. These entry points have been reported not to be associated with avascular necrosis. Given these promising reports, Gordon et al. used a rigid intramedullary nail that was designed for fractures of the humerus, and used this humeral nail for the treatment of femoral shaft fractures in 15 children and adolescents [10]. He reported that this technique was "safe, effective and well-tolerated" [10]. Keeler et al. used a rigid interlocking paediatric femoral nail that was based on the design of the modified humeral interlocking nail and which was introduced through the lateral aspect of the greater trochanter. These authors followed 24 fractures and looked at radiographic outcomes. They did not report any avascular necrosis of the femoral head as well [11].

Both these devices were not specifically designed for the treatment of adolescent femoral fractures. Led by the experience gained in adults with helically shaped intramedullary nails, a titanium cannulated adolescent lateral entry femoral nail (ALFN) was developed. Reynolds et al. used this device in 15 patients and reported both a shorter recovery time for patients treated with ALFN in comparison to elastic nailing and a low rate of complications, without major complications [12].

Although these results are promising, rigid nailing with a specially designed paediatric lateral trochanteric entry femoral nail does not appear to be generally accepted for this patient population currently. For example, in the most current guideline of the American Academy of Orthopaedic Surgeons (AAOS) as of December 2020 it was written: "There is currently insufficient literature in specially designed paediatric rigid intramedullary nails . . . for inclusion in the current guideline . . . Limited evidence supports rigid trochanteric entry nailing, submuscular plating, and flexible intramedullary nailing as treatment options for children age eleven years to skeletal maturity diagnosed with diaphyseal femur fractures, but piriformis or near piriformis entry rigid nailing are not treatment options" [13]. In a recent retrospective multicentre study of 16 centres in Germany, in which 53 children with femoral fractures were analysed, only three patients were treated with a lateral trochanteric entry femoral nail [14]. The majority of the other patients were treated with ESIN, of whom eight were revised. Other reported treatments in that report were primary of secondary plates (nine cases), intramedullary nails of adult traumatology, or external fixators [14].

As an additional aspect, none of the studies mentioned above assessed the health-related quality of life (HRQoL) in these patients up to this time.

Therefore, we initiated this study to assess the treatment results of patients that were treated with an ALFN in terms of HRQoL, radiographic healing, and complications. In addition, we aimed to evaluate if HRQoL was associated with additional injuries.

2. Materials and Methods

This is a retrospective analysis of clinical and radiographic results, in which patients, who underwent treatment for a diaphyseal fracture of the femur by an ALFN, were contacted by postal mail.

Several methodological details are identical to sister studies in which the health-related quality of life (HRQoL) after fractures of the lateral third of the clavicle, proximal humerus or supracondylar humerus in children and adolescents was assessed [15–17].

All sequential patients up to 16 years of age, who were treated at our institution with an ALFN for a diaphyseal fracture of the femur during the period January 2004 to

April 2017 were candidates for inclusion in the study. Our institution is one of the leading paediatric trauma centres in the Switzerland, serving more than one million inhabitants.

Patients were identified based on the radiological reports within our Picture Archiving and Communication System (PACS).

For the purpose of this analysis, the inclusion criteria were limited to patients who have sustained a diaphyseal femur fracture. Exclusion criterion was the inability to complete the questionnaires because of cognitive or language difficulties (Figure 1). We did not exclude patients with additional injuries.

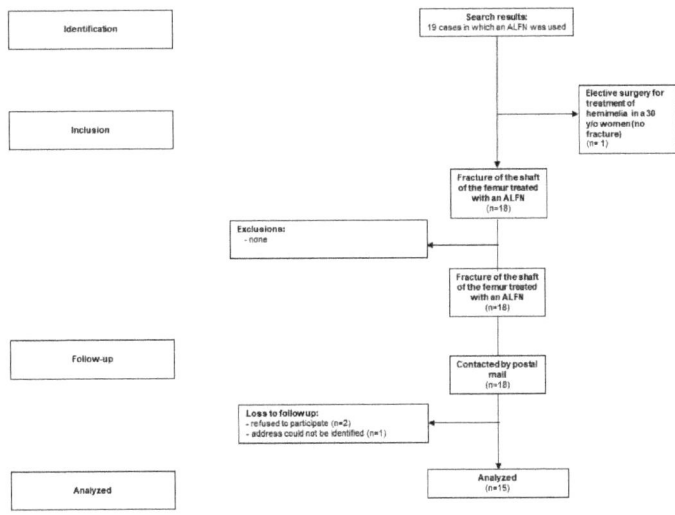

Figure 1. STROBE Participant flow chart.

A radiological analysis was performed to classify the fracture according to the following criteria: AO classification scheme [18], length stability using the Winquist–Hansen classification system [19], open physis of the greater trochanter, fracture healing, avascular necrosis of the femoral head, and growth disturbance of the greater trochanter. The physicians performing the image analysis were not aware of the patient's clinical result, thereby avoiding observer bias.

Beginning in 2016 we sent information about the study, a consent form, and questionnaires to the patients by postal mail (Figure 1). Non-responding participants were reminded three times by mail. Participants still not responding were contacted by phone to determine the reason for non-responding. At that time, it was attempted to administer the questionnaire by phone.

As there are currently no outcome instruments described in the literature to specifically assess the HRQoL after fractures of the femur, we used disease specific outcome measures of the hip and knee instead. For assessing outcomes after injuries around the hip, we chose the International Hip Outcome Tool 12 (iHot-12) [20], which is available in a validated translated version in German. That outcome was reported to provide good validity, reliability, and responsiveness for the evaluation of physically active patients with a hip disorder [20]. There are several other outcome measures regarding hip diseases available; however, none of these were validated in the paediatric population [21]. For assessing the outcome of fractures around the knee, we chose the Pedi-IKDC [22,23], which was reported to have better psychometric properties than the KOOS-Child [24].

As secondary outcomes, we selected the non-disease specific Paediatric Quality of Life Inventory (PedsQL) [25] which is available in a validated translated version. Scores were standardised to 0–100, with higher scores indicating more physical or more social function.

Data on demographics, dates of the injury, the side (right/left), mechanism of the injury, and the treatment course were collected from both the radiological analysis and from the electronic patient chart. In the questionnaire, we included items about concomitant injuries.

Closed reduction and fixation with the ALFN was performed according to the manufacturer's instructions (Synthes, Oberdorf, Switzerland). Special attention was provided to avoid the piriform fossa as an entry point and to use the lateral aspect of the greater trochanter as the entry point instead, typically at the same level as projected to the cranial border of the base of the femoral neck. When selecting the entry point it is important to consider the diameter of the drill (13.0 mm) that will be used for reaming to avoid injury to the femoral circumflex vessels. Postoperatively, patients were allowed weight-bearing as tolerated using crutches. Physiotherapy was used in every patient for instructions on mobilization and for assuring a good range of motion of the ipsilateral hip and knee.

All patients were invited to a routine consultation visit after 4 weeks. At that time, the patients typically were able to walk without crutches and demonstrated a good range of motion of the hip and knee. We usually recommended removal of the implant after 1 year.

After the description of the main outcome measure, we performed a bivariate analysis in which we analysed the HRQoL and other factors in relation to the presence of additional injuries. We used the non-parametric Mann–Whitney U Test for comparisons. All p-values are two-tailed; no corrections were made for multiple comparisons. A statistical analysis was performed using SPSS (SPSS Inc., Chicago, IL, USA).

3. Results

We were able to follow-up on 15 patients (6 girls, 9 boys) who were treated with an ALFN at an average age of 14.0 (SD 1.0) years of age. The mean body weight was 55 kg (SD 7, range from 40 to 68 kg) and the mean body height was 165 cm (SD 8 cm) (Table 1). The ALFN was used as a primary method of fixation in 13 patients, and as a fixation for failed ESIN in two cases (Figures 2 and 3). All 15 fractures healed radiographically. Physis of the greater trochanter were open in eight cases. There were no avascular necrosis of the femoral head and no growth disturbances of the greater trochanter. Complications consisted of a broken distal locking screw in one case, of which a fragment remained in situ during implant removal (Figure 4).

Table 1. Baseline characteristics by additional injury.

	Additional Injury																
	No Additional Injury						With Additional Injury						Total				
	n	Column N %	Mean	SD	Min	Max	n	Column N %	Mean	SD	Min	Max	n	Column N %	Mean	SD	Min	Max
Gender																		
female	3	33%					3	50%					6	40%				
male	6	67%					3	50%					9	60%				
Age at the time of injury [years]	9		13.8	1.0	12.5	15.6	6		14.2	1.0	13.1	15.9	15		14.0	1.0	12.5	15.9
Weight [kg] at time of the injury	9		52	6	40	60	6		59	6	50	68	15		55	7	40	68
Height [cm] at time of the injury	9		164	10	153	178	6		166	5	160	171	15		165	8	153	178
BMI [kg/m^2] at time of the injury	9		19.1	2.0	17.1	23.3	6		21.7	2.2	19.5	25.9	15		20.2	2.4	17.1	25.9
Injured side (right vs. left)																		
right	4	44%					3	50%					7	47%				
left	5	56%					2	33%					7	47%				
bilateral							1	17%					1	7%				
Radiological classification according to the AO																		
32-D/4.1	3	33%					1	17%					4	27%				
32-D/5.1	5	56%					3	50%					8	53%				
32-D/5.2	1	11%					2	33%					3	20%				

Table 1. Cont.

		No Additional Injury						With Additional Injury						Total			
	n	Column N %	Mean	SD	Min	Max	n	Column N %	Mean	SD	Min	Max	n	Column N %	Mean	SD	Min	Max
Winquist and Hansen classification regarding the degree of comminution																		
0: Transverse or short oblique fractures with no comminution	4	44%					1	17%					5	33%				
1: Small butterfly fragment of less than 25% of width of the bone	3	33%					2	33%					5	33%				
2: Butterfly fragment of 50% or less of the width of the bone							2	33%					2	13%				
3: Large butterfly fragment greater than 50% of the width of bone	1	11%											1	7%				
4: Segmental comminution	1	11%					1	17%					2	13%				
ALFN as the primary treatment or as a revision																		
ALFN used for revision of otherwise failed fixation	1	11%					1	17%					2	13%				
ALFN used as primary fixation	8	89%					5	83%					13	87%				
Injury mechanism																		
motor vehicle accident	2	22%					6	100%					8	53%				
sports	4	44%											4	27%				
fall from tree/play	3	33%											3	20%				
Was the skin injured at the time of the injury?																		
No, skin was intact	9	100%					5	83%					14	93%				
Yes, but was just a scratch																		
Yes, a suture was necessary							1	17%					1	7%				

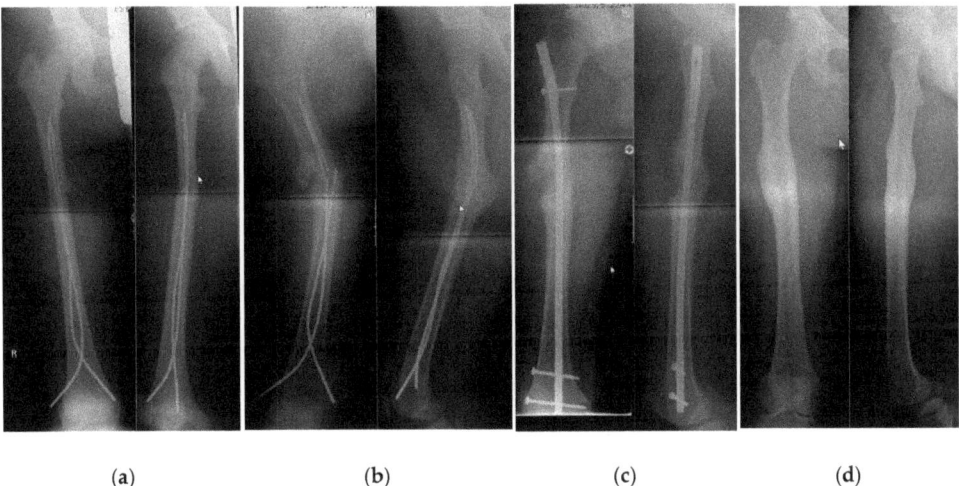

(a)　　　　　(b)　　　　　(c)　　　　　(d)

Figure 2. (**a**) 1 week after ESIN for a femoral fracture. Please note the narrow intramedullary canal, prohibiting the use of nails with a thicker diameter. Although currently we would advance the elastic intramedullary nail further, we do not consider this a reason for the subsequent failure of this fixation. (**b**) Same patient as in Figure 2a, now 9 months after ESIN. There is failure of the elastic nail due to non-union, resulting in a malposition. (**c**) Now 1 week after revision with an ALFN. Note the correction of the malposition. (**d**) After removal of the ALFN: radiographic bony union in correct position.

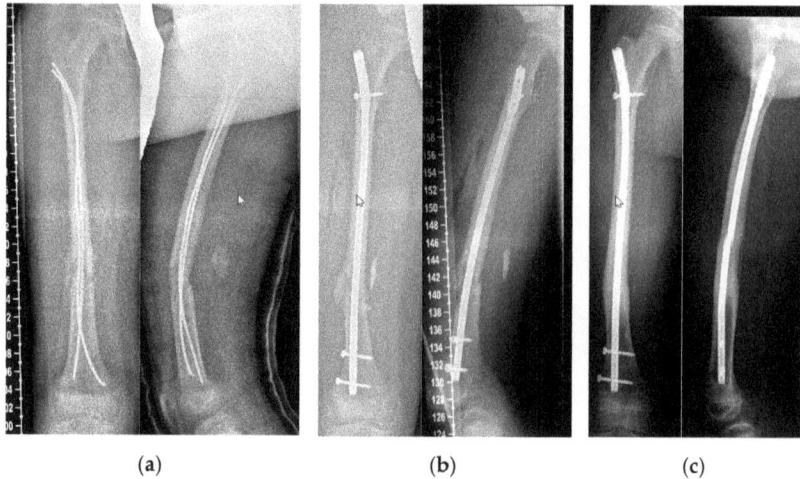

Figure 3. (a) Three days after anterograde ESIN for a femoral fracture. Due to additional injuries an anterograde approach was used. For this reason, it was not possible to achieve as much tension at the level of the fracture as we would have desired. (b) Same patient as in Figure 3a, six weeks after the anterograde ESIN fixation we revised to an ALFN. (c) Now eight months after revision to ALFN, with union in correct position.

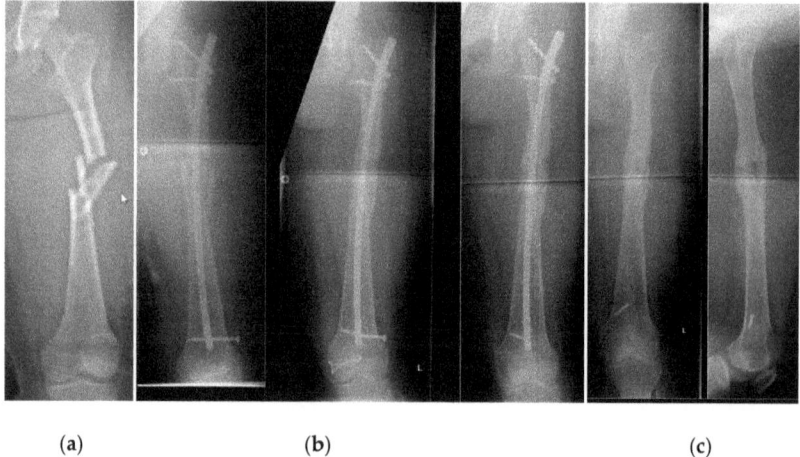

Figure 4. (a) Initial radiograph of a segmental fracture of the femoral shaft without cortical contact. (b) Same patient as in Figure 4a, four weeks after fixation with an ALFN. The position of the femoral neck screw was tolerated as it did not disturb the patient clinically. Only one distal locking screw was used which could have been advanced further. (c) Now after removal of the ALFN. Note the medial fragment of the distal locking screw, which was tolerated.

After a mean follow-up of 2.8 years (SD 2.6, range 0.3 to 7.2 years), the mean iHOT-12 score was 14.0 (SD 15.4), at a scale of 0–100, with lower values representing better HRQoL. The mean function score of the PedsQL was 85.7 (SD 19.3), and the mean social score of the PedsQL was 86.2 (SD 12.5), both at a scale of 0–100, with higher values representing better HRQoL. The mean Pedi-IKDC was 77.2 (SD 11.3) (Table 2).

Table 2. Follow-up data by additional injury.

	Additional Injury																	
	No Additional Injury						With Additional Injury						Total					
	Mean	SD	Min	Max	Count	Column N %	Mean	SD	Min	Max	Count	Column N %	Mean	SD	Min	Max	Count	Column N %
Follow-up duration [years]	2.94	2.91	0.45	7.16	9		2.55	2.29	0.29	5.63	6		2.79	2.6	0.29	7.16	15	
iHOT-12 (0–100)	12.9	14.8			9		15.7	17.4			6		14	15.4			15	
IKDC	80.2	7.54			9		73.1	14.8			6		77.2	11.3			15	
PedsQL physical function	91.8	9.02			9		76.6	27.2			6		85.7	19.3			15	
PedsQL social function	90.8	7.72			9		79.2	15.7			6		86.2	12.5			15	
Are you satisfied with the thigh that was injured?																		
Very satisfied					5	56%					4	67%					9	60%
A little satisfied					3	33%					2	33%					5	33%
A little unsatisfied					1	11%											1	7%
Very unsatisfied																		
Are you satisfied with the treatment that was performed?																		
Very satisfied					5	71%					3	75%					8	73%
A little satisfied					2	29%					1	25%					3	27%
A little unsatisfied																		
Very unsatisfied																		
Now you know the treatment and the results. If you could turn back time, would you choose this treatment again?																		
Yes, definitely					5	71%					3	75%					8	73%
Yes, probably					2	29%					1	25%					3	27%
No, probably not																		
No, not at all																		
How would you describe the pain that you typically experience in your thigh?																		
No pain					2	22%					5	83%					7	47%
Little pain					6	67%											6	40%
Moderate pain					1	11%					1	17%					2	13%
Strong pain																		
When does the pain typically occur?																		
I do not have any pain					4	44%					4	67%					8	53%
Only for the first steps					1	11%					1	17%					2	13%
Only after longer walks (30 min)					4	44%					1	17%					5	33%
When walking																		
Constant pain																		

In patients in whom the femoral fracture was an isolated injury, the HRQoL-scores were consistently higher when compared with patients who sustained additional injures (Table 2). However, provided the low number of patients, that difference was not statistically significant.

4. Discussion

The treatment of fractures of the femoral shaft in adolescents can be challenging. Especially when the intramedullary canal is narrow, it is often not possible to insert elastic intramedullary nails that are strong enough to withstand the forces that act on the femur in teenagers weighing 50 kg or more. This study showed that an adolescent lateral trochanteric entry femoral nail can be used in these cases, for both primary fixation and revision of failed elastic intramedullary fixation, as it led to radiological consolidation of all 15 patients that were analysed in this study. In addition, this study demonstrated that these patients have good health-related quality of life (HRQoL) as measured with the iHOT-12, the IKDC, and the Peds-QL at a mean follow-up of 2.8 years.

Despite these advantages, specifically designed adolescent lateral trochanteric femoral nails, such as den ALFN, are not yet the standard care in all institutions dealing with femoral fractures in adolescents [13,14].

4.1. Limitations

There are several limitations to this study: First, this was a mono-centre study, suggesting limited external validity. However, we are the only hospital treating paediatric trauma in a greater geographical area and all sequential patients were included in our study. This should reduce the probability of a bias in the run-in phase, making a high external validity probable [15]. In addition it has been stated that no single study is capable of providing full external validity, since it has been reported that great variation exists across and within countries for orthopaedic treatments [26]. Second, we had only 15 cases. This might be considered a small case series. However, all other publications on the HRQoL after femoral fractures in this age group treated with intramedullary rodding did not report on more patients than we reported. Third, the examined radiographs were not specifically prepared for this analysis, but were made routinely. Therefore the quality of these radiographs is comparable to the situation of the clinician [15]. Moreover, the physician classifying the fractures was not aware of the clinical result of the patient, thereby the radiological assessment could be regarded as blinded [15]. Fourth, as this study has a retrospective design it suffers from typical methodological weaknesses, such as no intermediate data points and missing data on the HRQoL prior to the injury. While the latter is considered a methodological weakness in studies analysing adult fractures, this does not necessarily apply to adolescent fractures, as adolescents usually have no physical limitations before the injury. Therefore it can be assumed that limitations of the disease-specific outcome measure are in fact attributable to the injury [15]. Fifth, there is no disease-specific outcome instrument for assessing the HRQoL after fractures of the femur. Therefore, we used accepted disease-specific outcome instruments for the adjacent hip and knee joint. Unfortunately, this limits the number of comparable literature considerably. Sixth, our follow-up rate was 83%. This rate is above the recommended 80% that is commonly used as a threshold and most other studies we are aware of have a lower rate of follow-up, if the follow-up is reported at all. In addition, we were not able to identify another study that assessed the HRQoL in a comparable patient group. Seventh, we do not know how the ALFN compares to other treatment options in terms of HRQoL. As we do not have a comparison group in our study and we are not aware of comparable publications in the literature, that question will be subject of further studies. Eighth, we did not exclude patients with additional injuries, as we wanted to report the results of this procedure on all subsequent patients in whom we used this device. Therefore, we stratified the results according to additional injures in the tables so that readers who are interested in the results of patients who did not sustain additional injuries can be referred to the tables.

4.2. Demographics, Radiographic Analysis and Complications

As can be seen in Table 1, the average patient who was treated with an ALFN in this study was 14 years old of age, had a body height of 165 cm, and had a body weight of 55 kg. These demographics are comparable to the literature [27]. All fractures healed radiographically and there was no evidence of avascular necrosis of the femoral head or growth disturbances of the greater trochanter. These results are compatible with Keeler [11], who also did not report such complications in her innovative study when she used humeral nails for femoral fractures. Apart from one screw breakage during implant removal, which can be attributed to the fact that only one instead of two locking screws was used, there were no complications. A fragment of that screw remained in the intramedullary canal (Figure 4).

4.3. Health-Related Quality of Life and AO Classification

The HRQoL in this study as assessed by the iHOT-12, the IKDC, and the Peds-QL was good, but not perfect. This was true for both the disease-specific and the non-disease-specific outcome measures. This indicates that there could be a limitation in HRQoL after these injuries. This is compatible with the literature, as other authors have also described that there may be significant reduction in HRQoL after fractures of the lower limb. For example, in a study with 162 children, of which 54.8% had femoral fractures, there were physical function scores that were lower than age-matched norms at 6 months after the injury [28].

4.4. HRQoL and Other Injuries

The HRQoL scores were consistently better in the group without additional injuries compared with the adolescents who sustained additional injuries. This indicates that the HRQoL of adolescents who were treated with an ALFN is mainly influenced by the presence of additional injures, and less by the fracture of the femur itself.

5. Conclusions

The ALFN is a feasible treatment option in the adolescent population for the treatment of femoral shaft fractures, especially when patients are overweight or have a narrow intramedullary canal. Our study showed excellent health-related quality of life and low rates of adverse events, there were no cases of AVN or disturbance of trochanteric growth. Given further advantages of the ALFN, such as less soft tissue injury compared with plate fixation, the possibility of immediate full weight-bearing, low risk of non-union, and the avoidance of an external fixator, we prefer the ALFN for the treatment of femoral shaft fractures in cases when ESIN is not suitable.

Author Contributions: Conceptualization, T.R.L.; methodology, T.R.L.; validation, M.M., S.M.B. and K.Z.; formal analysis, T.R.L.; investigation, A.M.; resources, T.R.L., M.M., K.Z., S.M.B.; data curation, A.M.; writing—original draft preparation, T.R.L.; writing—review and editing, T.R.L., A.M., M.M., S.M.B., K.Z.; visualization, T.R.L.; supervision, T.R.L.; project administration, S.M.B., M.M., K.Z. All authors have read and agreed to the published version of the manuscript.

Funding: This research received no external funding.

Institutional Review Board Statement: The study was conducted in accordance with the Declaration of Helsinki, and approved by both the Institutional Review Board of the Paediatric Clinics of Inselspital, University of Bern, and the Ethics Commission of the Canton of Bern (Basec-Nr: 2016-00011, date of approval: 3 May 2016), both in Switzerland.

Informed Consent Statement: Informed consent was obtained from all subjects or their parents involved in the study.

Conflicts of Interest: The authors declare no conflict of interest.

References

1. Lyons, R.A.; Delahunty, A.M.; Kraus, D.; Heaven, M.; McCabe, M.; Allen, H.; Nash, P. Children's fractures: A population based study. *Inj. Prev.* **1999**, *5*, 129–132. [CrossRef] [PubMed]
2. Bennek, J.; Bühligen, U.; Rothe, K.; Müller, W.; Rolle, U.; Gioc, T.; Bennek, C. Fracture treatment in children—data analysis and follow-up results of a prospective study. *Injury* **2001**, *32*, 26–29. [CrossRef]
3. Kelly, B.; Heyworth, B.; Yen, Y.-M.; Hedequist, D. Adverse Sequelae Due to Plate Retention Following Submuscular Plating for Pediatric Femur Fractures. *J. Orthop. Trauma* **2013**, *27*, 726–729. [CrossRef]
4. Moroz, L.A.; Launay, F.; Kocher, M.S.; Newton, P.O.; Frick, S.L.; Sponseller, P.D.; Flynn, J.M. Titanium elastic nailing of fractures of the femur in children. *J. Bone Jt. Surgery. Br. Vol.* **2006**, *88*, 1361–1366. [CrossRef] [PubMed]
5. Weiss, J.M.; Choi, P.; Ghatan, C.; Skaggs, D.L.; Kay, R.M. Complications with flexible nailing of femur fractures more than double with child obesity and weight > 50 kg. *J. Child. Orthop.* **2009**, *3*, 53–58. [CrossRef] [PubMed]

6. Canavese, F.; Marengo, L.; Andreacchio, A.; Mansour, M.; Paonessa, M.; Rousset, M.; Samba, A.; Dimeglio, A. Complications of elastic stable intramedullary nailing of femoral shaft fractures in children weighing fifty kilograms (one hundred and ten pounds) and more. *Int. Orthop.* **2016**, *40*, 2627–2634. [CrossRef]
7. Stans, A.A.; Morrissy, R.T.; Renwick, S.E. Femoral shaft fracture treatment in patients age 6 to 16 years. *J. Pediatr. Orthop.* **1999**, *19*, 222–228. [CrossRef]
8. Mileski, R.A.; Garvin, K.L.; Crosby, L.A. Avascular necrosis of the femoral head in an adolescent following intramedullary nailing of the femur. A case report. *J. Bone Joint Surg. Am.* **1994**, *76*, 1706–1708. [CrossRef]
9. O'malley, D.E.; Mazur, J.M.; Cummings, R.J. Femoral Head Avascular Necrosis Associated with Intramedullary Nailing in an Adolescent. *J. Pediatr. Orthop.* **1995**, *15*, 21–23. [CrossRef]
10. Gordon, J.E.; Khanna, N.; Luhmann, S.J.; Dobbs, M.B.; Ortman, M.R.; Schoenecker, P.L. Intramedullary nailing of femoral fractures in children through the lateral aspect of the greater trochanter using a modified rigid humeral intramedullary nail: Preliminary results of a new technique in 15 children. *J. Orthop. Trauma* **2004**, *18*, 416–422. [CrossRef]
11. Keeler, K.A.; Dart, B.; Luhmann, S.J.; Schoenecker, P.L.; Ortman, M.R.; Dobbs, M.B.; Gordon, J.E. Antegrade Intramedullary Nailing of Pediatric Femoral Fractures Using an Interlocking Pediatric Femoral Nail and a Lateral Trochanteric Entry Point. *J. Pediatr. Orthop.* **2009**, *29*, 345–351. [CrossRef] [PubMed]
12. Reynolds, R.A.K.; Legakis, J.E.; Thomas, R.; Slongo, T.F.; Hunter, J.B.; Clavert, J.-M. Intramedullary nails for pediatric diaphyseal femur fractures in older, heavier children: Early results. *J. Child. Orthop.* **2012**, *6*, 181–188. [CrossRef] [PubMed]
13. American Academy of Orthopaedic Surgeons. *Treatment of Pediatric Diaphyseal Femur Fractures Evidence-Based Clinical Practice Guideline*; American Academy of Orthopaedic Surgeons: Rosemont, IL, USA, 2020.
14. Rapp, M.; Kraus, R.; Illing, P.; Sommerfeldt, D.W.; Kaiser, M.M. Treatment of femoral shaft fractures in children and adolescents >/=50 kg: A retrospective multicenter trial. *Unfallchirurg* **2018**, *121*, 47–57. [CrossRef] [PubMed]
15. Liebs, T.; Ryser, B.; Kaiser, N.; Slongo, T.; Berger, S.; Ziebarth, K. Health-related Quality of Life After Fractures of the Lateral Third of the Clavicle in Children and Adolescents. *J. Pediatr. Orthop.* **2019**, *39*, e542–e547. [CrossRef] [PubMed]
16. Liebs, T.R.; Burgard, M.; Kaiser, N.; Slongo, T.; Berger, S.; Ryser, B.; Ziebarth, K. Health-related quality of life after paediatric supracondylar humeral fractures. *Bone Jt. J.* **2020**, *102-B*, 755–765. [CrossRef] [PubMed]
17. Liebs, T.R.; Rompen, I.; Berger, S.M.; Ziebarth, K. Health-related quality of life after conservatively and surgically-treated paediatric proximal humeral fractures. *J. Child. Orthop.* **2021**, *15*, 204–214. [CrossRef]
18. Slongo, T.; Audige, L. AO Paediatric Classification Group. Distal metaphyseal fractures (13-M). In *AO Paediatric Comprehensive Classification of Long-Bone Fractures (PCCF)*; Slongo, T., Audige, L., AO Paediatric Classification Group, Eds.; AO Foundation: Davos, Switzerland, 2007; p. 15.
19. Winquist, R.A.; Hansen, S.T., Jr.; Clawson, D.K. Closed intramedullary nailing of femoral fractures. A report of five hundred and twenty cases. *J. Bone Joint Surg. Am.* **1984**, *66*, 529–539. [CrossRef]
20. Baumann, F.; Popp, D.; Müller, K.; Müller, M.; Schmitz, P.; Nerlich, M.; Fickert, S. Validation of a German version of the International Hip Outcome Tool 12 (iHOT12) according to the COSMIN checklist. *Heallth Qual. Life Outcomes* **2016**, *14*, 52. [CrossRef]
21. d'Entremont, A.G.; Cooper, A.P.; Johari, A.; Mulpuri, K. What clinimetric evidence exists for using hip-specific patient-reported outcome measures in pediatric hip impingement? *Clin. Orthop. Relat. Res.* **2015**, *473*, 1361–1367. [CrossRef]
22. Kocher, M.S.; Smith, J.T.; Iversen, M.D.; Brustowicz, K.; Ogunwole, O.; Andersen, J.; Yoo, W.J.; Mcfeely, E.D.; Anderson, A.F.; Zurakowski, D. Reliability, Validity, and Responsiveness of a Modified International Knee Documentation Committee Subjective Knee Form (Pedi-IKDC) in Children with Knee Disorders. *Am. J. Sports Med.* **2010**, *39*, 933–939. [CrossRef]
23. Nasreddine, A.Y.; Connell, P.L.; Kalish, L.A.; Nelson, S.; Iversen, M.D.; Anderson, A.F.; Kocher, M.S. The Pediatric International Knee Documentation Committee (Pedi-IKDC) Subjective Knee Evaluation Form: Normative Data. *Am. J. Sports Med.* **2017**, *45*, 527–534. [CrossRef] [PubMed]
24. van der Velden, C.A.; van der Steen, M.C.; Leenders, J.; van Douveren, F.Q.M.P.; Janssen, R.P.A.; Reijman, M. Pedi-IKDC or KOOS-child: Which questionnaire should be used in children with knee disorders? *BMC Musculoskelet. Disord.* **2019**, *20*, 240. [CrossRef] [PubMed]
25. Mahan, S.T.; Kalish, L.A.; Connell, P.L.; Harris, M.; Abdul-Rahim, Z.; Waters, P. PedsQL Correlates to PODCI in Pediatric Orthopaedic Outpatient Clinic. *J. Pediatr. Orthop.* **2014**, *34*, e22–e26. [CrossRef] [PubMed]
26. Ackerman, I.N.; Dieppe, P.A.; March, L.M.; Roos, E.M.; Nilsdotter, A.K.; Brown, G.C.; Sloan, K.E.; Osborne, R.H. Variation in age and physical status prior to total knee and hip replacement surgery: A comparison of centers in Australia and Europe. *Arthritis Care Res.* **2009**, *61*, 166–173. [CrossRef] [PubMed]
27. Gordon, J.E.; Mehlman, C.T. The Community Orthopaedic Surgeon Taking Trauma Call: Pediatric Femoral Shaft Fracture Pearls and Pitfalls. *J. Orthop. Trauma* **2017**, *31*, S16–S21. [CrossRef]
28. Winthrop, A.L.; Brasel, K.J.; Stahovic, L.; Paulson, J.; Schneeberger, B.; Kuhn, E.M. Quality of life and functional outcome after pediatric trauma. *J. Trauma* **2005**, *58*, 468–473. [CrossRef]

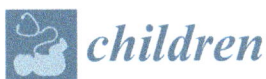

Article

Supracondylar Fractures of the Humerus: Association of Neurovascular Lesions with Degree of Fracture Displacement in Children—A Retrospective Study

Ryszard Tomaszewski [1,2], Karol Pethe [1], Jacek Kler [1], Erich Rutz [3,4], Johannes Mayr [5,*] and Jerzy Dajka [6,7]

[1] Department of Pediatric Traumatology and Orthopedics, Upper Silesian Child Centre, 40-752 Katowice, Poland; tomaszewskir@gmail.com (R.T.); karol.pethe@gmail.com (K.P.); jacek.kler@gmail.com (J.K.)
[2] Institute of Biomedical Engineering, Faculty of Science and Technology, University of Silesia, 40-007 Katowice, Poland
[3] Department of Orthopaedics, The Royal Children's Hospital Melbourne, Melbourne, VIC 3052, Australia; erich_rutz@hotmail.com
[4] Murdoch Children's Research Institute, MCRI, Melbourne, VIC 3052, Australia
[5] Department of Pediatric Surgery, University Children's Hospital Basel, University of Basel, 4031 Basel, Switzerland
[6] Institute of Physics, Faculty of Science and Technology, University of Silesia, 40-007 Katowice, Poland; jerzy.dajka@us.edu.pl
[7] Silesian Center for Education and Interdisciplinary Research, University of Silesia, 40-007 Katowice, Poland
* Correspondence: johannes.mayr@ukbb.ch; Tel.: +41-61-704-2811

Citation: Tomaszewski, R.; Pethe, K.; Kler, J.; Rutz, E.; Mayr, J.; Dajka, J. Supracondylar Fractures of the Humerus: Association of Neurovascular Lesions with Degree of Fracture Displacement in Children—A Retrospective Study. *Children* **2022**, *9*, 308. https://doi.org/10.3390/children9030308

Academic Editors: Axel A. Horsch, Maher A. Ghandour and Matthias Christoph M. Klotz

Received: 22 January 2022
Accepted: 21 February 2022
Published: 24 February 2022

Publisher's Note: MDPI stays neutral with regard to jurisdictional claims in published maps and institutional affiliations.

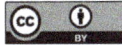

Copyright: © 2022 by the authors. Licensee MDPI, Basel, Switzerland. This article is an open access article distributed under the terms and conditions of the Creative Commons Attribution (CC BY) license (https://creativecommons.org/licenses/by/4.0/).

Abstract: Supracondylar humerus fractures (ScHF) account for 60% of fractures of the elbow region in children. We assessed the relationship between neurovascular complications and the degree of fracture displacement as rated on the basis of modified Gartland classification. Moreover, we aimed to evaluate predisposing factors, e.g., age and gender, and outcomes of neurovascular complications in ScHF. Between 2004 and 2019, we treated 329 patients with ScHF at the Department of Traumatology and Orthopedics of the Upper Silesian Child Centre, Katowice, Poland. Mean age of patients (189 boys and 140 girls) was 7.2 years (Confidence interval: 6.89, 7.45). Undisplaced fractures were treated conservatively with a cast. Displaced fractures were managed by closed reduction and percutaneous Kirschner wire fixation using two pins inserted laterally. We retrospectively assessed the number of neurovascular lesions at baseline and recorded any iatrogenic injury resulting from the surgical intervention. Acute neurovascular lesions occurred in 44 of 329 ScHF patients (13.4%). The incidence of accompanying neurovascular injuries was positively associated with the severity of fracture displacement characterized by Gartland score. Vascular injuries occurred mainly in Gartland type IV ScHF, while nerve lesions occurred in both Gartland type III and IV ScHF. We noted a significantly higher mean Gartland score and mean age at injury in the group of children suffering from neurovascular injuries when compared to those in the group without such injuries ($p = 0.045$ and $p = 0.04$, respectively). We observed no secondary nerve lesions after surgical treatment. For the treatment of ScHF in children, we recommend closed reduction and stabilization of displaced fractures with K-wires inserted percutaneously from the lateral aspect of the upper arm. We advocate vessel exploration in case of absent distal pulses after closed reduction but do not consider primary nerve exploration necessary, unless a complete primary sensomotoric nerve lesion is present.

Keywords: supracondylar humerus fractures; treatment; children; vascular injury; neurologic injury

1. Introduction

Supracondylar humerus fracture (ScHF) represents a common bone injury in children, accounting for 60% of elbow fractures in the pediatric population [1]. ScHF mainly affects children below the age of seven years [2]. After the age of seven years, ScHF represents the second most frequent fracture [3]. Male predominance is typical, with a male-to-female ratio of 3:2 [4].

Extension-type ScHF caused by falling onto an extended elbow account for 97% to 99% of ScHF [2,5,6]. Left or non-dominant limbs are most often affected [4]. Fractures are typically classified according to Gartland [7]. Four types are distinguished, i.e., type I (non-displaced), type II (displaced, but with the intact posterior cortex), type III (completely displaced, with either posteromedial or posterolateral displacement), and type IV (displaced with multidirectional instability due to circumferential periosteal disruption) [8].

Fractures of Gartland types II, III, and IV are usually managed by closed reduction and surgical stabilization. The preferred surgical technique to stabilize ScHF is K-wire fixation, most commonly by inserting two parallel or diverging K-wires from the lateral side of the humerus [9].

The most frequently observed complications after ScHF comprise axial malalignment (e.g., cubitus varus in a frontal plane and residual hyperextension malalignment in a lateral plane), paresthesia, and superficial pin infections [10].

Terpstra et al. found that the incidence of paresthesia complicating ScHF treated between 9 p.m. and 2 a.m. was higher when compared to the incidence of nerve injuries observed in ScHF treated during office hours [11]. According to their literature review, it appears safe to postpone surgery to office hours, if circumstances are not optimal for acute surgery at nighttime and if there is no medical contraindication [11].

Pavone et al. compared the outcomes of ScHF in a group of children treated with crossed pins to the outcomes in a group of children stabilized by lateral pin constructs. They found a satisfactory outcome with similar results regarding joint function recovery and postoperative complications [10].

Severe complications related to ScHF, including nerve and vessel lesions, can be primary, i.e., originating from the initial injury, or secondary as an iatrogenic injury resulting from fracture treatment [3,12,13]. Nerve lesions occur in 5.8% to 14% of children suffering from ScHF [5,6,14,15], and the incidence of vascular injuries ranges from 3.2% to 14.3% [6,16–19]. For ScHF complicated by neurovascular injuries, urgent reduction and stable fixation are recommended [20]. These fractures should be managed by the close collaboration of pediatric surgeons, neurosurgeons, and vascular surgeons [20,21].

We aimed to determine whether there is an association between the degree of fracture displacement and incidence as well as outcome of accompanying neurovascular lesions. We hypothesized that the incidence of primary neurovascular injuries complicating ScHF in children is unrelated to the degree of fracture displacement as classified by Gartland. Moreover, we aimed to evaluate predisposing factors and outcome of nerve and vessel injuries in ScHF.

2. Patients and Methods

2.1. Demographic and Baseline Assessments

We retrospectively evaluated 329 patients with ScHF who were treated at our department between January 2004 and July 2019.

We included children younger than 17 years who suffered acute ScHF and were initially referred to the Department of Pediatric Traumatology and Orthopedics, Upper Silesian Child Centre, Katowice, Poland.

The exclusion criteria comprised patients older than 16 years at the time of injury, polytraumatized patients, patients suffering from pathological fractures or recurrent fractures of the elbow region, and patients suffering from psychomotor dysfunctions or neuromuscular disorders. We also excluded patients with incomplete medical records or loss to follow-up.

We analyzed patient demographics, i.e., age and sex, and baseline characteristics, i.e., type of fracture according to Gartland, presence of accompanying nerve lesions and/or vascular injuries, and laterality of injury.

2.2. Clinical and Radiographic Assessments

Every ScHF patient admitted to the hospital for fracture treatment was assessed clinically and radiographically at the Accident and Emergency department. Fractures were categorized according to the modified Gartland classification based on X-ray images in anteroposterior (AP) and lateral projections [7]. All patients underwent evaluations of radial and ulnar pulse and capillary refill time as well as forearm and hand innervation.

We used the protocol by Marsh et al. [22] to improve the assessment and documentation of the neurologic status in children with arm fractures. The protocol by Marsh et al. does, however, not include any sensory or vascular assessment and does not document posterior interosseous nerve function [22]. A simple finger play for children was used to guide physicians' assessments of motor function of median, radial, ulnar, and anterior interosseous nerves.

We grouped patients into those with neurovascular complications (group 1) and those without neurovascular lesions (group 2).

2.3. Treatments

Non-displaced fractures (Gartland type I) were treated conservatively. Displaced fractures were managed by closed reduction and K-wire fixation. Twelve of 329 patients (3.6%) underwent open reduction, because closed reduction failed. Overall, 12 of 329 patients (3.6%) required subsequent surgery, i.e., 10 patients (3.0%) because of unsatisfactory repositioning and 2 patients (0.6%) due to neurovascular complications. The mean time from hospital admission to surgery was 6.5 h (range: 0.5 h to 27.0 h).

Closed or open reduction of ScHF was performed under general anesthesia with the patients placed in the supine position. This was followed by fracture fixation by diverging K-wires inserted from the lateral aspect of the distal humerus. Subsequently, each patient received a long-arm plaster cast.

2.4. Ethical Approval

Ethical approval (PCN/022/KB/11/21) was waived by the local Ethics Committee of the Silesian Medical University of Katowice, Poland, because of the retrospective nature of the study and the fact that the procedures were part of routine care.

2.5. Statistical Analysis

We analyzed the data using R (version 3.6.1 operating on x86_64, linux-gnu platform). Differences between groups were assessed using multi-way ANOVA verified by non-parametric Kruskal–Wallis and adonis tests form the vegan R-package. All predictions of ANOVA were in agreement with non-parametric results, thus confirming the robustness of parametric methods. A p-value of <0.05 was considered statistically significant.

3. Results

3.1. Patient Demographics and Number of Patients per Gartland Type at Baseline

We included 329 patients (140 girls and 189 boys) in this analysis. The mean age of the children was 7.2 years (CI: 6.89, 7.45), and the mean Gartland score amounted to 2.86 (CI: 2.75, 2.97).

The catchment area of the Department of Pediatric Traumatology and Orthopedics, Upper Silesian Child Centre, Katowice, comprised the population of the Silesian county (4.5 mill. inhabitants) with 16.8% of the population younger than 18 years of age. Table 1 shows the patients' demographics.

Table 1. Patients' demographics (n = 329).

Gender (female/male; %)	140 (42.6%)/189 (57.4%)
Age (years; CI)	7.2 (CI: 6.89, 7.45)
Ethnicity (n; %)	Caucasian (326; 99.1%); Asian (2; 0.61%); African (1; 0.3%)

Table 2 demonstrates the mean and variation of Gartland scores and patients' ages for the total study population.

Table 2. Mean values and variation of Gartland scores and patients' ages at baseline.

All Patients (*n* = 329)	Mean and CI	Variation and CI
Gartland score	2.86 CI = 2.75–2.97	0.95 CI = 0.82–1.11
Age (years)	7.2 CI = 6.89–7.45	6.76 CI = 5.84–7.93

The mean age of girls (*n* = 140) amounted to 6.9 years (range: 1.5 years—14 years). Boys (*n* = 189) were 7.4 years old on average (range: 6 months—16 years). The mean ages of girls and boys did not differ significantly.

Figure 1 shows the total number of male and female patients per Gartland type (I to IV) at baseline. The mean Gartland score was 2.9 for both girls and boys. Thus, the mean Gartland score was not influenced by gender.

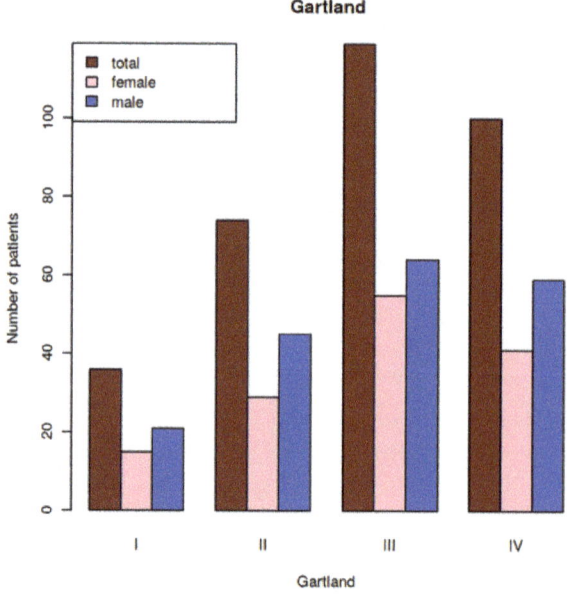

Figure 1. Number of patients (total, male, and female) by Gartland type.

3.2. Relationship between the Incidence of Neurovascular Lesions and the Gartland Score

Overall, 44 of the 329 patients (13.4%) exhibited neurovascular lesions (group 1) at baseline. Group 2 consisted of 285 patients (86.6% of the 329 patients) without neurovascular lesions (Table 3). Table 3 shows the numbers of patients with and without neurovascular lesions by Gartland type.

Table 3. Numbers of patients with and without neurovascular lesions per Gartland type.

Number of Patients	Gartland Type			
	I	II	III	IV
Total (*n* = 329)	36	74	119	100
With neurovascular lesions (group 1; *n* = 44)	1	2	14	27
Without neurovascular lesions (group 2; *n* = 285)	35	72	105	73

Notably, no patient developed late-presenting neurovascular complications or compartment syndrome during the 24 h in-patient observation period.

The mean Gartland scores were higher in the group of patients with neurovascular lesions (group 1) than in those without neurovascular lesions (group 2). Thus, there was a positive association between the incidence of neurovascular lesions and the Gartland score at baseline ($p = 0.045$; Table 4).

Table 4. Mean Gartland scores and variations and mean patients' ages for the patients with and without neurovascular lesions.

	Patients with Neurovascular Lesions (Group 1, $n = 44$)		Patients without Neurovascular Lesions (Group 2, $n = 285$)		p-Value
	Mean and CI	Variation and CI	Mean and CI	Variation and CI	
Gartland score	3.52 CI = 3.31–3.73	0.48 CI = 0.33–0.78	2.75 CI = 2.64–2.87	0.94 CI = 0.81–1.12	0.045
Age (years)	8.2 CI = 7.32–9.02	7.81 CI = 5.33–12.54	7.0 CI = 6.72–7.31	6.45 CI = 5.51–7.66	0.04

Fractures of low Gartland types were associated with fewer neurovascular lesions. In the patient group with neurovascular lesions (group 1), only one patient with Gartland type I fracture and two patients with Gartland type II fractures suffered accompanying nerve injuries (Table 5). The incidence of vascular injuries peaked in patients with Gartland type IV fractures, while nerve lesions occurred most frequently in patients with Gartland type III and IV fractures (Table 5).

Table 5. Number of patients with neurovascular lesions per Gartland type.

Number of Patients with Neurovascular Lesions	Gartland Type			
	I	II	III	IV
Total ($n = 44$)	1	2	14	27
Nerve lesions ($n = 24$)	1	2	11	10
Vascular lesions ($n = 12$)	0	0	1	11
Combined neurovascular injuries ($n = 8$)	0	0	2	6

Types of Nerve Injuries Associated with ScHF

Nerve lesions without accompanying vascular injuries occurred in 32 of 329 patients (9.7%) (Table 6).

Table 6. Types of nerve lesion and Gartland types of nerve injuries not accompanied by vascular lesions.

Type of Predominant Nerve Lesion	Gartland Type			
	I	II	III	IV
Median nerve lesion	1	2	6	9
Anterior interosseous nerve lesion	0	0	3	4
Ulnar nerve lesion	0	0	3	3
Radial nerve lesion	0	0	1	0

Eight children (2.4%) exhibited combined neurovascular injuries (Table 5). Among these, one child suffered anterior interosseous nerve injury and brachial artery thrombosis, which required surgical treatment. Another two children presented with anterior interosseous nerve injury combined with brachial artery injury, and five patients suffered median nerve injury accompanied by brachial artery injury.

We did not observe any posttraumatic compartment syndrome or posttraumatic osteomyelitis.

3.3. Relationship of the Patient Age and the Presence of Neurovascular Lesions

The mean age of ScHF patients with neurovascular lesions (group 1; n = 44) was 8.2 years (CI: 7.32, 9.02). In patients who did not suffer any neurovascular complications (group 2; n = 285), the mean age was 7.0 years (CI: 6.72, 7.31). Thus, patients without neurovascular lesions were significantly younger than those who suffered neurovascular lesions (p = 0.04; Table 4, Figure 2).

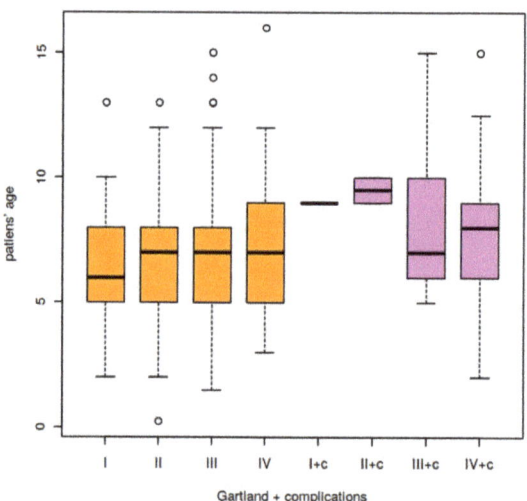

Figure 2. Ages of patients without (orange) and with (purple) neurovascular lesions by Gartland type. c, complications.

The mean age of patients increased with the increasing Gartland type (Table 7).

Table 7. Mean value and variation of patients' ages per Gartland type.

| All Patients | Gartland Type | | | |
(n = 329)	I	II	III	IV
Mean age and CI (years)	6.4 CI = 5.63–7.26	6.9 CI = 6.39–7.5	7.4 CI = 6.87–7.85	7.4 CI = 6.86–7.91
Variation	5.74 CI = 3.78–9.77	5.73 CI = 4.25–8.16	7.31 CI = 5.76–9.61	7.12 CI = 5.49–9.6

3.4. Relationship of Neurovascular Lesions, Gartland Type, and Patient Gender

The mean age of the girls with neurovascular complications amounted to 7.6 years (range: 2–14 years), and their mean Gartland score was 3.6. The mean age of the girls without neurovascular complications was 6.8 years (range: 1.5–14 years), with a mean Gartland score of 2.8. In the group of boys with neurovascular complications, the mean age was 8.5 years (range: 3–15 years), and the mean Gartland score reached 3.4. The mean age of the boys without neurovascular complications was 7.2 years (range: 6 months–16 years), and their mean Gartland score reached 2.8. There was no significant influence of gender on the incidence of neurovascular lesions in children with ScHF.

3.5. Relationship of Fracture Laterality (Right or Left) on the Gartland Score

Extension-type fractures constituted 99% of all fractures. The left upper extremity was affected in 218 of 329 patients (66.3%; Figure 3). The mean Gartland score of fractures of the left humerus was 2.9, and the mean age of the affected children was 7.3 years (range: 1.5–15 years). The mean Gartland score of fractures of the right humerus was 2.8, and the patients' mean age was 7.0 years (range: 6 months–16 years). Thus, the laterality of the fracture did not influence the Gartland score, nor was there any significant age difference between patients with left-sided or right-sided humerus fractures (Figure 3).

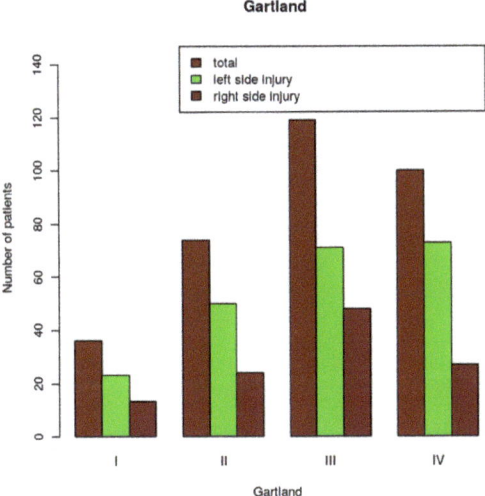

Figure 3. Number of patients per fracture laterality and Gartland type.

3.6. Outcome of Nerve Lesions and Vascular Injuries

In 30 of the 32 children (93.8%) with nerve injuries at baseline, nerve lesions resolved spontaneously within four weeks after the reduction and stable fixation of ScHF. In one patient suffering from Gartland type III ScHF, open reduction was conducted initially. The surgical release of the ulnar nerve was performed two months after the injury, because ulnar nerve function did not improve. In an additional patient with Gartland type IV ScHF, we undertook the surgical release of the median nerve after four weeks due to missing signs of nerve recovery. In these two patients, nerve function recovered after the averages of 100 and 146 days, respectively.

The 20 children who presented with absent forearm pulses and the diminished oxygen saturation of the ipsilateral hand (Table 5) underwent closed fracture reduction. After the reduction and stabilization of the fracture, we re-evaluated forearm pulses and the oxygen saturation of the hand and conducted the Doppler sonography of the ipsilateral hand and forearm arteries. In 17 of these patients, perfusion improved after closed reduction, while the surgical revision of the brachial artery to treat thrombosis was necessary in three patients. One of these children sustained an open supracondylar fracture (Gustilo-Anderson grade IIIc).

At follow-up at least one year after the injury, we noted no differences in limb growth. One child complained of intolerance to cold temperatures. The duplex sonography revealed a reduced flow (<50%) of the ipsilateral forearm arteries in three of the 20 children who initially presented with absent forearm pulses.

4. Discussion

In our study, in pediatric patients, the incidence of neurovascular complications was related to the severity of ScHF displacement as rated by the modified Gartland classification [2]. However, nerve injuries occurred predominantly in Gartland types III and IV fractures, while acute vascular injuries were seen mainly in Gartland type IV fractures. We found a higher prevalence of Gartland type I fractures in younger children and a higher incidence of neurovascular complications in older children. The gender and laterality of fractures did not affect the incidence of neurovascular complications.

Vallila et al. reported that 63% of compensation claims for complications in pediatric fractures in Finland between 1990 and 2010 were related to the treatment of ScHF [23].

Early complications including vessel and nerve damage, muscle destruction, and acute compartment syndrome usually appear immediately after suffering ScHF. Varus and, less frequently, valgus deformity, hyperextension malalignment, and restriction of elbow range of motion represent the most common late complications of displaced ScHF in children [2,24].

We observed a mean time from admission to surgery of 6.5 h which is similar to the time interval proposed by Pavone et al. (<8 h) [25]. However, Schmid et al. showed that postponing surgery does not influence the rate of open reductions, incidence of postoperative complications, and overall outcome [26].

We performed closed reduction and percutaneous lateral pin fixation in the supine position of the patient. Pavone et al. demonstrated good radiographic outcomes and similar complication rates after closed reduction and percutaneous pinning in Gartland type III fractures treated in either the supine or the prone position of the patient [25].

4.1. Incidence of Nerve Lesions

According to the literature, ScHF is complicated by nerve injuries in 5.8% to 14% of pediatric patients [5,6,12,13]. Most nerve lesions associated with ScHF are caused by nerves entrapped within the fracture rather than by sharp bone fragments or K-wires [27]. In our study, the incidence of nerve lesions was related to the degree of fracture displacement and amounted to 9.7% in total. This figure is in line with previously published incidences of nerve injuries in ScHF [5,6,12,13].

In the study reported by Valencia et al. [12], neurovascular complications occurred exclusively in Gartland type III injuries. In our study population, we did, however, observe a small number of neurologic lesions even in Gartland type I ($n = 1$) and type II ($n = 2$) fractures, although the incidence peaked in Gartland type III and type IV fractures.

4.1.1. Types of Nerve Injuries Associated with ScHF

In our study, most neurologic injuries involved the median nerve and anterior interosseous nerve (Table 6). The type of nerve injury is influenced by the fracture type and direction of fracture displacement [28].

The median nerve tends to be affected in case of posterolateral displacement [29]. In the literature, the most common neurologic deficit associated with ScHF in children is reported to be neurapraxia which usually resolves spontaneously within two to three months but can take up to six months [12,30]. In accordance with Omid et al., we noted that the most frequent nerve complications related to ScHF in children were median and anterior interosseous nerve injuries [2].

4.1.2. Assessment of Neurologic Function

Technically, it is possible to differentiate between anterior interosseous nerve and median nerve palsies by assessing motor function, based on the flexion of the middle-finger proximal interphalangeal joint [30]. However, the assessment of neurologic function before and after surgical treatment in young children may be challenging or even impossible due to the children's cooperation [6,13,31].

There is no significant association between the timing of the surgical procedure and partial or complete nerve recovery [32]. In our study, the recovery of impaired nerve function took an average of four weeks in 93.8% of patients who initially presented nerve injuries.

4.2. Iatrogenic Nerve Injuries

Current studies report an incidence of iatrogenic nerve injury between 3% and 4% [12,13]. It is noteworthy that we did not observe any iatrogenic nerve injuries in our study population. We used the lateral pinning technique that permits the safe and reliable stabilization of Gartland type II, III, and IV ScHF [33]. Pesenti et al. demonstrated that crossed pin constructs are more prone to ulnar nerve injury than lateral pin constructs [34]. Minimal incision over the medial epicondyle in order to identify the bony prominence of the medial epicondyle in case of massive soft tissue swelling can help to reduce the rate of ulnar nerve injuries in crossed pin constructs [34]. Larson et al. reported that crossed pinning is biomechanically more stable than lateral pin constructs but carries a higher risk of ulnar nerve injury during the insertion of the medial pin [35]. Afaque et al. and Pavone et al. demonstrated that there is no significant difference between lateral pinning and crossed pinning in terms of functional outcome, biomechanical stability, and incidence of complications [10,36].

4.3. Incidence of Non-Iatrogenic Vascular Injuries

Traumatic, non-iatrogenic vascular injuries in children are rare and mainly involve the brachial artery.

Surprisingly, a single patient in our subgroup of patients with Gartland type III fractures experienced isolated arterial injury, while two patients in this subgroup presented with combined nerve and arterial lesions. In our study, most isolated arterial lesions occurred in patients with Gartland type IV fractures ($n = 11$), while six patients in this subgroup exhibited combined neural and arterial injuries. Our findings are in accordance with the observation of Garbuz et al. who described that the incidence of concomitant nerve lesions in patients suffering from ScHF complicated by absent radial pulse is 60% [37].

4.4. Combined Vascular and Neurologic Lesions

Louahem et al. [38] noted the possibility of combined neurovascular complications in patients with ScHF. The therapeutic approaches in these patients were the same as in isolated nerve or vessel injuries. In our patients with ScHF, we observed neurovascular complications mainly in Gartland type IV (six patients) and type III (two patients) ScHF, confirming our previous observation of a higher incidence of neurovascular complications in ScHF with significant displacement and instability.

4.5. Study Limitations and Strengths

4.5.1. Study Limitations

The main study limitation was the retrospective study design and lack of standardization of evaluations. Furthermore, various medical teams attended to our patients because of the prolonged study period (2004–2019), and diagnostic procedures may have changed in the course of the 15-year period.

4.5.2. Study Strengths

Our study describes the functional outcomes of a large number of pediatric ScHF patients who were treated by surgical stabilization. Operations were performed by different surgeons, and therefore, our results may be generalized. We were able to confirm the association between the more marked fracture displacement (i.e., higher Gartland type) and the incidence of neurovascular complications.

We demonstrated a good recovery of impaired neurovascular function after closed reduction and stable retention by K-wires inserted from the lateral aspect of the upper arm.

5. Conclusions

1. The incidence of neurovascular complications was related to the degree of ScHF displacement as classified according to Gartland. Vascular complications mainly accompanied Gartland type IV ScHF, whereas nerve lesions occurred in Gartland type III and IV ScHF.
2. For the treatment of displaced ScHF, we recommend closed reduction and stabilization by K-wires inserted percutaneously from the lateral aspect of the distal humerus. If the

impaired perfusion of the forearm persists after fracture reduction and stabilization or if complete nerve paralysis or iatrogenic nerve lesion develops, surgical treatments of these neurovascular complications should be considered.

Author Contributions: R.T.: conceptualization, investigation, data curation, writing—original draft, and project administration; K.P.: data curation and writing—original draft; J.K.: data curation and writing—original draft; E.R.: writing—review and editing; J.M.: writing—review and editing and supervision; J.D.: methodology, software, formal analysis, visualization, and validation. All authors have read and agreed to the published version of the manuscript.

Funding: No funding was obtained for this study.

Institutional Review Board Statement: Ethical approval (PCN/022/KB/11/21) was waived by the local Ethics Committee of the Silesian Medical University of Katowice, Poland, because of the retrospective nature of the study and the fact that the procedures were part of routine care. The study was conducted in accordance with the Declaration of Helsinki.

Informed Consent Statement: Informed Consent statement was waived due to the retrospective nature of the study and the fact that the procedures were part of routine care.

Data Availability Statement: The data presented in this study are available on request from the first author. The data are not publicly available due to hospital guidelines.

Acknowledgments: We gratefully acknowledge the writing and editing assistance by Silvia Rogers, Director of MediWrite, Basel, Switzerland.

Conflicts of Interest: The authors declare no conflict of interest.

Abbreviations

ScHF   supracondylar humerus fracture
AP   anteroposterior

References

1. Houshian, S.; Mehdi, B.; Larsen, M.S. The epidemiology of elbow fracture in children: Analysis of 355fractures, with special reference to supracondylar humerus fractures. *J. Orthop. Sci.* **2001**, *6*, 312–315. [CrossRef] [PubMed]
2. Omid, R.; Choi, P.D.; Skaggs, D.L. Supracondylar humeral fractures in children. *J. Bone Jt. Surg.* **2008**, *90*, 1121–1132. [CrossRef] [PubMed]
3. Cheng, J.C.Y.; Lam, T.P.; Shen, W.Y. Closed Reduction and Percutaneous Pinning for Type III Displaced Supracondylar Fractures of the Humerus in Children. *J. Orthop. Trauma* **1995**, *9*, 511–515. [CrossRef] [PubMed]
4. Cheng, J.C.; Lam, T.P.; Maffulli, N. Epidemiological features of supracondylar fractures of the humerus in Chinese children. *J. Pediatr. Orthop.* **2001**, *10*, 63–67.
5. Mazzini, J.P.; Rodriguez-Martin, J.; Andres-Esteban, E.M. Does open reduction and pinning affect outcome in severely displaced supracondylar humeral fractures in children? A systematic review. *Strat. Trauma Limb Reconstr.* **2010**, *5*, 57–64. [CrossRef]
6. Farnsworth, C.L.; Silva, P.D.; Mubarak, S.J. Etiology of Supracondylar Humerus Fractures. *J. Pediatr. Orthop.* **1998**, *18*, 38–42. [CrossRef]
7. Gartland, J.J. Management of supracondylar fractures of the humerus in children. *Surg. Gynecol. Obstet.* **1959**, *109*, 145–154.
8. Rockwood, C.A.; Beaty, J.H.; Kasser, J.R. *Rockwood and Wilkins' Fractures in Children*; Lippincott Williams & Wilkins: Philadelphia, PA, USA, 2010.
9. Agus, H.; Kalenderer, Ö.; Kayali, C. Closed reduction and percutaneous pinning results in children with supracondylar humerus fractures. *Acta Orthop. Traumatol. Turc.* **1999**, *33*, 18–22.
10. Pavone, V.; Riccioli, M.; Testa, G.; Lucenti, L.; De Cristo, C.; Condorelli, G.; Avondo, S.; Sessa, G. Surgical Treatment of Displaced Supracondylar Pediatric Humerus Fractures: Comparison of Two Pinning Techniques. *J. Funct. Morphol. Kinesiol.* **2016**, *1*, 39–47. [CrossRef]
11. Terpstra, S.E.S.; Burgers, P.T.B.W.; Huub, J.L.; van der Heide, H.J.L.; Bas de Witte, P. Pediatric Supracondylar Humerus Fractures: Should We Avoid Surgery during After-Hours? *Children* **2022**, *9*, 189. [CrossRef]
12. Cramer, K.E.; Green, N.E.; Devito, D.P. Incidence of Anterior Interosseous Nerve Palsy in Supracondylar Humerus Fractures in Children. *J. Pediatr. Orthop.* **1993**, *13*, 502–505. [CrossRef] [PubMed]
13. Joiner, E.R.; Skaggs, D.L.; Arkader, A.; Andras, L.M.; Lightdale-Miric, N.R.; Pace, J.L.; Ryan, D.D. Iatrogenic nerve injuries in the treatment of supracondylar humerus fractures: Are we really just missing nerve injuries on preoperative examination? *J. Pediatr. Orthop.* **2014**, *34*, 388–392. [CrossRef] [PubMed]

14. Valencia, M.; Moraleda, L.; Díez-Sebastián, J. Long-term Functional Results of Neurological Complications of Pediatric Humeral Supracondylar Fractures. *J. Pediatr. Orthop.* **2015**, *35*, 606–610. [CrossRef] [PubMed]
15. Brown, I.C.; Zinar, D.M. Traumatic and Iatrogenic Neurological Complications After Supracondylar Humerus Fractures in Children. *J. Pediatr. Orthop.* **1995**, *15*, 440–443. [CrossRef]
16. McGraw, J.J.; Akbarnia, B.A.; Hanel, D.P.; Keppler, L.; Burdge, R.E. Neurological Complications Resulting from Supracondylar Fractures of the Humerus in Children. *J. Pediatr. Orthop.* **1986**, *6*, 647–650. [CrossRef]
17. Brahmamdam, P.; Plummer, M.; Modrall, J.G.; Megison, S.M.; Clagett, G.P.; Valentine, R.J. Hand ischemia associated with elbow trauma in children. *J. Vasc. Surg.* **2011**, *54*, 773–778. [CrossRef] [PubMed]
18. Sabharwal, S.; Tredwell, S.J.; Beauchamp, R.D.; Mackenzie, W.G.; Jakubec, D.M.; Cairns, R.; LeBlanc, J.G. Management of Pulseless Pink Hand in Pediatric Supracondylar Fractures of Humerus. *J. Pediatr. Orthop.* **1997**, *17*, 303–310. [CrossRef]
19. Noaman, H.H. Microsurgical reconstruction of brachial artery injuries in displaced supracondylar fracture humerus in children. *Microsurgery* **2006**, *26*, 498–505. [CrossRef]
20. Wegmann, H.; Eberl, R.; Kraus, T.; Till, H.; Eder, C.; Singer, G. The impact of arterial vessel injuries associated with pediatric supracondylar humeral fractures. *J. Trauma Acute Care Surg.* **2014**, *77*, 381–385. [CrossRef]
21. Wang, J.H.; Morris, W.Z.; Bafus, B.T.; Liu, R.W. Pediatric Supracondylar Humerus Fractures: AAOS Appropriate Use Criteria Versus Actual Management at a Pediatric Level 1 Trauma Center. *J. Pediatr. Orthop.* **2019**, *39*, e578–e585. [CrossRef] [PubMed]
22. Marsh, A.G.; Robertson, J.S.; Godman, A.; Boyle, J.; Huntley, J.S. Introduction of a simple guideline to improve neurological assessment in paediatric patients presenting with upper limb fractures. *Emerg. Med. J.* **2016**, *33*, 273–277. [CrossRef] [PubMed]
23. Vallila, N.; Sommarhem, A.; Paavola, M.; Nietosvaara, Y. Pediatric distal humeral fractures and complications of treatment in Finland: A review of compensation claims from 1990 through 2010. *J. Bone Jt. Surg. Am.* **2015**, *97*, 494–499. [CrossRef] [PubMed]
24. Shenoy, P.; Islam, A.; Puri, R. Current Management of Paediatric Supracondylar Fractures of the Humerus. *Cureus* **2020**, *12*, e8137. [CrossRef]
25. Pavone, V.; Vescio, A.; Riccioli, M.; Culmone, A.; Cosentino, P.; Caponnetto, M.; Dimartino, S.; Testa, G. Is Supine Position Superior to Prone Position in the Surgical Pinning of Supracondylar Humerus Fracture in Children? *J. Funct. Morphol. Kinesiol.* **2020**, *5*, 57. [CrossRef]
26. Schmid, T.G.J.; Joeris, A.; Slongo, T.; Ahmad, S.S.; Ziebarth, K. Displaced supracondylar humeral fractures: Influence of delay of surgery on the incidence of open reduction, complications and outcome. *Arch. Orthop. Trauma Surg.* **2015**, *135*, 963–969. [CrossRef] [PubMed]
27. Leversedge, F.J.; Moore, T.J.; Peterson, B.C.; Seiler, J.G., III. Compartment syndrome of the upper extremity. *J. Hand Surg.* **2011**, *36*, 544–560. [CrossRef]
28. Babal, J.C.; Mehlman, C.T.; Klein, G. Nerve Injuries Associated with Pediatric Supracondylar Humeral Fractures: A Meta-analysis. *J. Pediatr. Orthop.* **2010**, *30*, 253–263. [CrossRef]
29. Ristic, S.; Strauch, R.J.; Rosenwasser, M.P. The Assessment and Treatment of Nerve Dysfunction After Trauma Around the Elbow. *Clin. Orthop. Relat. Res.* **2000**, *370*, 138–153. [CrossRef]
30. Culp, R.W.; Osterman, A.L.; Davidson, R.S.; Skirven, T.; Bora, F.W. Neural injuries associated with supracondylar fractures of the humerus in children. *J. Bone Jt. Surg.* **1990**, *72*, 1211–1215. [CrossRef]
31. Harris, N.; Ali, F. (Eds.) *Examination Techniques in Orthopaedics*, 2nd ed.; Cambridge University Press: Cambridge, UK, 2014.
32. Barrett, K.K.; Skaggs, D.L.; Sawyer, J.R.; Andras, L.; Moisan, A.; Goodbody, C.; Flynn, J.M. Supracondylar Humeral Fractures with Isolated Anterior Interosseous Nerve Injuries: Is Urgent Treatment Necessary? *J. Bone Jt. Surg.* **2014**, *96*, 1793–1797. [CrossRef]
33. Begovic, N.; Paunovic, Z.; Djuraskovic, Z.; Lazovic, L.; Mijovic, T.; Babic, S. Lateral pinning versus others procedures in the treatment of supracondylar humerus fractures in children. *Acta Orthop. Belg.* **2016**, *82*, 866–871. [PubMed]
34. Pesenti, S.; Ecalle, A.; Gaubert, L.; Peltier, E.; Choufani, E.; Viehweger, E.; Jouve, J.-L.; Launay, F. Operative management of supracondylar humeral fractures in children: Comparison of five fixation methods. *Orthop. Traumatol. Surg. Res.* **2017**, *103*, 771–775. [CrossRef] [PubMed]
35. Larson, L.; Firoozbakhsh, K.; Passarelli, R.; Bosch, P. Biomechanical Analysis of Pinning Techniques for Pediatric Supracondylar Humerus Fractures. *J. Pediatr. Orthop.* **2006**, *26*, 573–578. [CrossRef]
36. Afaque, S.F.; Singh, A.; Maharjan, R.; Ranjan, R.; Panda, A.K.; Mishra, A. Comparison of clinic-radiological outcome of cross pinning versus lateral pinning for displaced supracondylar fracture of humerus in children: A randomized controlled trial. *J. Clin. Orthop. Trauma* **2020**, *11*, 259–263. [CrossRef] [PubMed]
37. Garbuz, D.S.; Leitch, K.; Wright, J.G. The treatment of supracondylar fractures in children with an absent radial pulse. *J. Pediatr. Orthop.* **1996**, *16*, 594–596. [CrossRef] [PubMed]
38. Louahem, D.M.; Nebunescu, A.; Canavese, F.; Dimeglio, A. Neurovascular complications and severe displacement in supracondylar humerus fractures in children: Defensive or offensive strategy? *J. Pediatr. Orthop. B* **2006**, *15*, 51–57. [CrossRef] [PubMed]

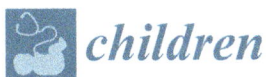

Article

Foam Splint versus Spica Cast—Early Mobilization after Hip Reconstructive Surgery in Children—Preliminary Data from a Prospective Randomized Clinical Trial

Lorenz Pisecky [1,*], Gerhard Großbötzl [1], Manuel Gahleitner [1], Christian Stadler [1], Stella Stevoska [1], Christina Haas [1], Tobias Gotterbarm [1] and Matthias Christoph Michael Klotz [2]

[1] Department for Orthopaedics and Traumatology, Johannes Kepler University Linz, Kepler University Hospital GmbH, Altenberger Strasse 96, 4040 Linz and Krankenhausstraße 9, 4020 Linz, Austria; gerhard.grossboetzl@kepleruniklinikum.at (G.G.); manuel.gahleitner@kepleruniklinikum.at (M.G.); christian.stadler@kepleruniklinikum.at (C.S.); stella.stevoska@kepleruniklinikum.at (S.S.); christina.haas@kepleruniklinikum.at (C.H.); tobias.gotterbarm@kepleruniklinikum.at (T.G.)
[2] Department for Orthopaedics and Traumatology, Marienkrankenhaus Soest GmbH, Widumgasse 5, 59494 Soest, Germany; mcmklotz@gmx.net
* Correspondence: Lorenz.pisecky@kepleruniklinikum.at

Abstract: Background: Surgical hip joint reconstruction may be the method of choice for children and adolescents with developmental dysplasia of the hip (DDH), as well as neurogenic dislocation of the hip (NDH) and Legg–Calvé–Perthes disease (LCPD). Following pelvic surgery, immobilization using a spica cast is considered to be the gold standard, despite the fact that casting may cause complications, such as hygienic problems, skin lesions, neurological deficits, and rigidity of the adjacent joints. An alternative for postoperative immobilization is a foam splint. The purpose of this randomized controlled trial was to compare spica cast and foam splint immobilization after hip reconstruction in children and adolescents with DDH, NDH, and LCPD. Methods: In a prospective randomized clinical trial, children and adolescents (age: 4–14 years), who received hip reconstructive surgery (osteotomy of the ilium and proximal femur, open reduction, soft tissue techniques) for DDH, NDH, and LCPD were included. Patient recruitment, group allocation, surgery, and aftercare were carried out in a department for orthopaedic surgery in Central Europe. Standardized questionnaires SF-36 (Short Form-36), EQ-5D (Euro Quality of Life 5D and CPCHILD (Caregiver Priorities and Child Health Index of Life with Disabilities) were gathered before, six, and twelve weeks after surgery from each patient. Group one received a spica cast and group two a foam splint for a period of six weeks postoperatively. There was no difference in surgical treatment. Results: Twenty-one out of thirty planned patients were enrolled in the study. One patient had to be excluded because of a lack of compliance. All quality of life (QOL) scores showed a significant reduction at the 6-week follow-up compared to the preoperative assessment. After twelve weeks, the scores came back close to the preoperative values. A significant reduction was seen in the spica cast group pre- vs. postoperatively for the variables CPCHILD (81% vs. 64%, $p = 0.001$), EQ-5d (65% vs. 45%, $p = 0.014$), and SF-36 (85% vs. 74%, $p = 0.004$). The corresponding values for the foam splint group also presented a reduction for all scores, but without statistical significance. Complications occurred in five cases. Conclusions: Recent retrospective studies suggest that foam splint immobilization after hip reconstruction surgery is a safe and feasible method, promising fewer complications compared to spica casting. The preliminary results of this prospective randomized clinical trial show an improvement of the scores when using a foam splint compared to the conventionally used spica cast. Benefits for the patients may be fewer adverse events and no need to undergo a second round of anaesthesia for recasting. Data suggest higher patient and caretaker satisfaction in the foam splint group.

Keywords: dysplasia of the hip; hip reconstructive surgery; spica cast; foam splint; complications; quality of life; prospective randomized clinical trial

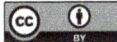

Citation: Pisecky, L.; Großbötzl, G.; Gahleitner, M.; Stadler, C.; Stevoska, S.; Haas, C.; Gotterbarm, T.; Klotz, M.C.M. Foam Splint versus Spica Cast—Early Mobilization after Hip Reconstructive Surgery in Children—Preliminary Data from a Prospective Randomized Clinical Trial. *Children* **2022**, *9*, 288. https://doi.org/10.3390/children9020288

Academic Editor: Angelo Gabriele Aulisa

Received: 21 December 2021
Accepted: 16 February 2022
Published: 18 February 2022

Publisher's Note: MDPI stays neutral with regard to jurisdictional claims in published maps and institutional affiliations.

Copyright: © 2022 by the authors. Licensee MDPI, Basel, Switzerland. This article is an open access article distributed under the terms and conditions of the Creative Commons Attribution (CC BY) license (https://creativecommons.org/licenses/by/4.0/).

1. Introduction

Developmental dysplasia of the hip joint (DDH) and deformations of the proximal femur may occur congenitally. Other diseases, such as cerebral palsy (CP) or myelomeningocele (MMC), can result in neuromuscular dysplasia of the hip (NDH) and/or dislocation of the hip [1]. Consequences may be pain when walking/standing/sitting, as well as difficulty in ambulating or even the inability to stand.

In early childhood, DDH or dislocation of the hip may be treated by casting or splinting. In case of failed conservative treatment, surgical reposition and reconstruction of the hip is needed.

Children with neuromuscular disorders show a high incidence of hip dislocations and failed conservative treatment due to NDH [2]. In CP, different authors found that hip dislocation occurred in 18–60% of their patients [3].

Besides DDH and NDH, young patients with Legg–Calvé–Perthes disease (LCPD) benefit from pelvic reconstruction, with the aim of improving the hip containment to prevent further lateralization or to support the rebuilding of the femoral head [4–6].

Especially in older ambulating children, tight soft tissue makes the procedure challenging. A combination of soft tissue and bony procedures may be necessary to achieve a reduction of the joint [7,8].

Postoperative immobilization is usually performed by spica casting for six weeks, followed by physiotherapy [9]. Most surgeons prefer casting to avoid secondary dislocation, especially in patients with spasticity.

A broad variety of complications is known: hygienic problems, skin lesions, neurological complications, and rigidity of the joints after casting. In some institutions, a change of the spica cast is performed in a second short round of general anaesthesia two weeks after surgery.

An alternative for postoperative immobilization is a foam splint. It protects the surgically treated hip from dislocation, provides access to the wound, and allows physiotherapy of the adjacent joints.

Retrospective studies showed the safety of the foam splint concerning the healing of the bone and promised fewer complications. Gather et al. showed in 2018 that foam splinting is not inferior to spica casting with regard to major complications such as the dislocation of the bone wedge, avascular necrosis of the acetabulum or femur, events of osseous non-union, or nerve injury [10].

Despite this retrospective data, there is no final consensus on the best means of postoperative immobilization in the treatment of DDH. It is assumed that foam splinting leads to a smaller number of complications and higher patient and caregiver satisfaction.

In a prospective randomized clinical trial, the study group now aims to test the hypothesis that the foam splint leads to a higher satisfaction of the patient and the caretaker by measuring well-established quality of life (QOL) scores pre- and postoperatively.

Furthermore, a lower number of complications is expected. Benefits for the patients may be fewer unplanned outpatient contacts, a higher quality of life during the aftercare process, and no need to undergo a second round of anaesthesia for recasting. Up to now, a comparable study does not exist, as trials dealing with foam splinting after pelvic reconstruction were performed in most cases retrospectively and/or were non-randomized [10–12].

2. Materials and Methods

The study group of a Central European department for orthopaedic surgery designed a non-blinded, prospective randomized clinical trial to test the following hypothesis: foam splinting leads to a higher postoperative satisfaction of patients and their caretakers in cases of pelvic reconstruction.

Ethical approvement was obtained prior to the conduction of the clinical trial (Ethikkommission des Landes Oberösterreich EK Nr: 1183/2018), and a scientific grant by the Medical

Society of Upper Austria funds the research. The clinical trial was registered at the German Clinical Trials Register after ethical approval (DRKS-ID: DRKS00016861).

Patients were recruited in the outpatient clinic for paediatric orthopaedics and neuro-orthopaedics at the study site. Recruitment was performed by a single paediatric orthopaedic surgeon with more than 20 years of clinical experience.

Included patients were children and adolescents from 4 to 14 years of age with the diagnoses 'congenital dysplasia of the hip', 'neuromuscular dysplasia of the hip', and 'Legg–Calvé–Perthes disease', with indication for hip reconstructive surgery. Indications for surgery were a Reimers migration index of 40% or higher or 25–40% with progression, Tönnis classification II or higher, or an AC-Index above the Tönnis standard and head-at-risk signs in cases of LCPD.

The standardized questionnaires (SF-36, EQ-5D, and CPCHILD) were completed before surgery and after 6 and 12 weeks, and participation was mandatory. Post-trial care was performed within a standardized yearly routine check-up and did not differ in the two groups. All planned postoperative follow-up checks were conducted at the outpatient clinic for paediatric orthopaedics and neuro-orthopaedics at the study site by one senior and one junior paediatric orthopaedic surgeon. The algorithm of the recruitment process is shown in Figure 1.

Obtained informed consent from the patient and legal guardian was mandatory and collected by the surgeon prior to the procedure.

Two groups with differing immobilization protocols were formed.

Group one, the control group, was treated using a standardized spica cast with slight flexion of the hip of about 10–15 degrees, 10 degrees inward rotation of the hip and 30 degrees of abduction of the hip (Figure 2). Two weeks after surgery, a second short general round of anaesthesia for the removal of the skin suture and to change the cast was necessary.

Group two, the intervention group, was treated using immobilization with a foam splint for six weeks with slight flexion of the hip of about 10–15 degrees, 10 degrees inward rotation of the hip and 30 degrees of abduction of the hip (Figure 3). No second round of anaesthesia for recasting in the operating room was needed in group two. During the period of immobilization in group two, physiotherapy of the lower extremity was performed considering the patient's needs by experienced neuro-paediatric physiotherapists.

The assignment process to the two groups was random, using a coin toss four to six weeks prior to surgery. The randomization process was performed by a junior paediatric orthopaedic surgeon, and observed by a senior paediatric orthopaedic surgeon in awareness of the possibility of unintentional unbalanced results [14]. The randomization process was chosen as the simplest method and to avoid manipulation by the change of chronological order, as would be possible in a fixed randomization sequence.

There was no difference in the surgical technique between both groups. Included surgical techniques were derotating varisation osteotomy of the femur (DVO), Pemberton acetabuloplasty, and Salter and Chiari osteotomy. Soft tissue techniques were tenotomy of the psoas muscle, of the adductor muscles, of the knee flexors, and the lengthening of quadriceps tendon.

Standardized questionnaires were used to measure the quality of life and the quality of aftertreatment 6 and 12 weeks after surgery (Table 1). The questionnaires used were the 'Caregiver Priorities and Child Health Index of Life with Disabilities' (CPCHILD), the 'Short Form 36' (SF-36), and the 'Euro Quality of Life 5D' (EQ-5D) [15–17]. The evaluation of the questionnaires was performed by a junior paediatric orthopaedic surgeon. Mobility was measured using the 'Gross Motorfunction Classification System' (GMFCS) scale [18].

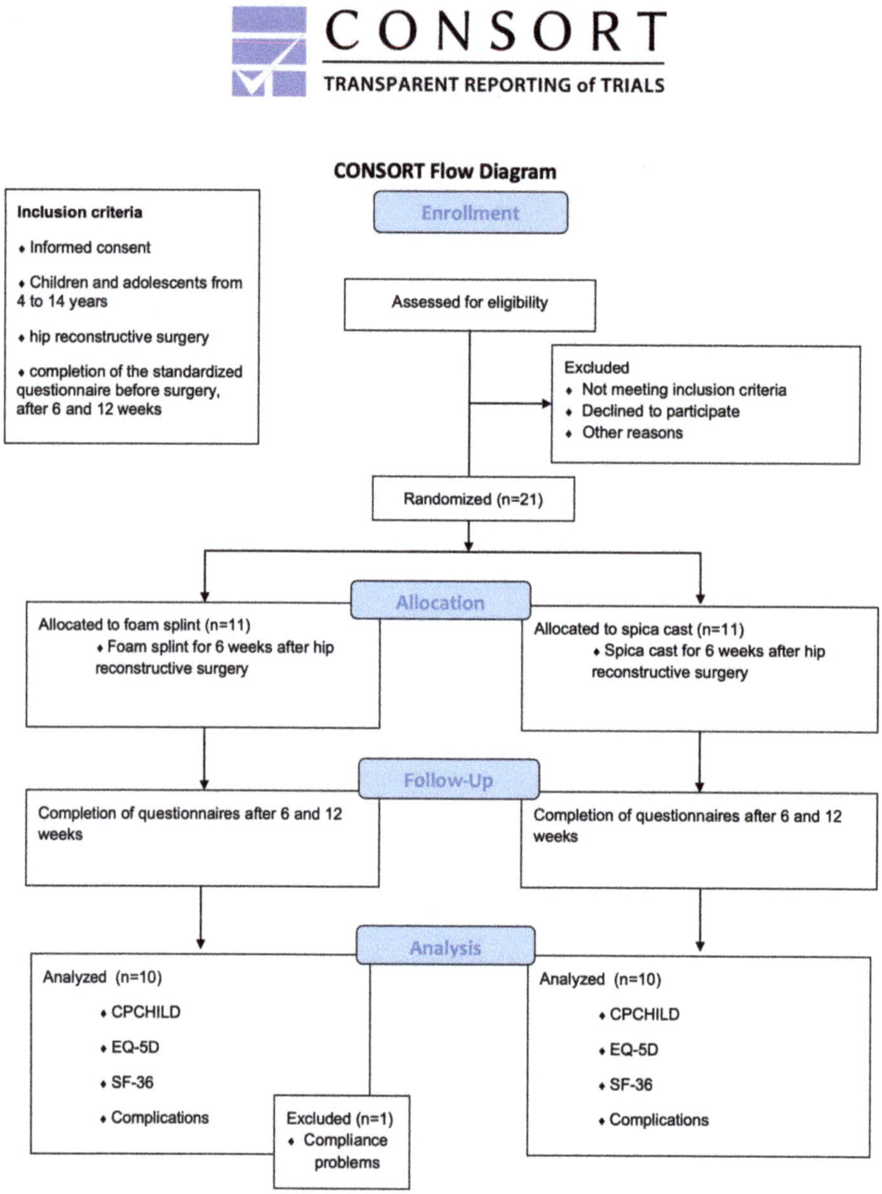

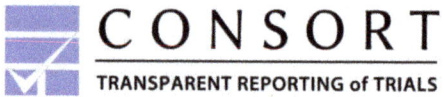

Figure 1. The algorithm of the trial; CONSORT diagram adapted from [13].

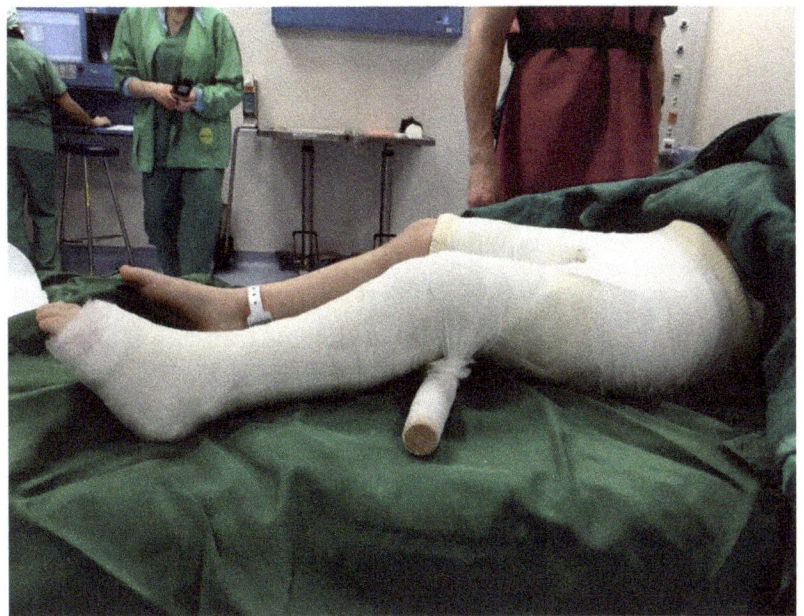
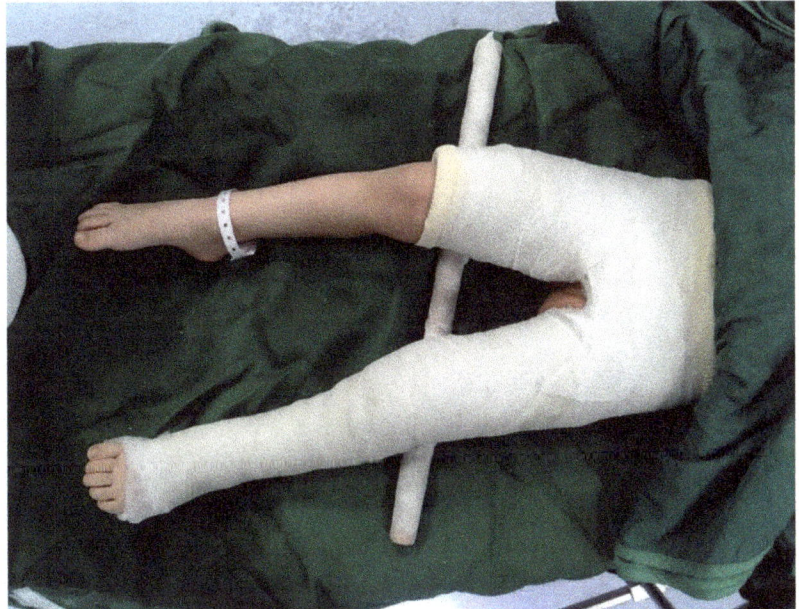

Figure 2. Postoperative spica cast.

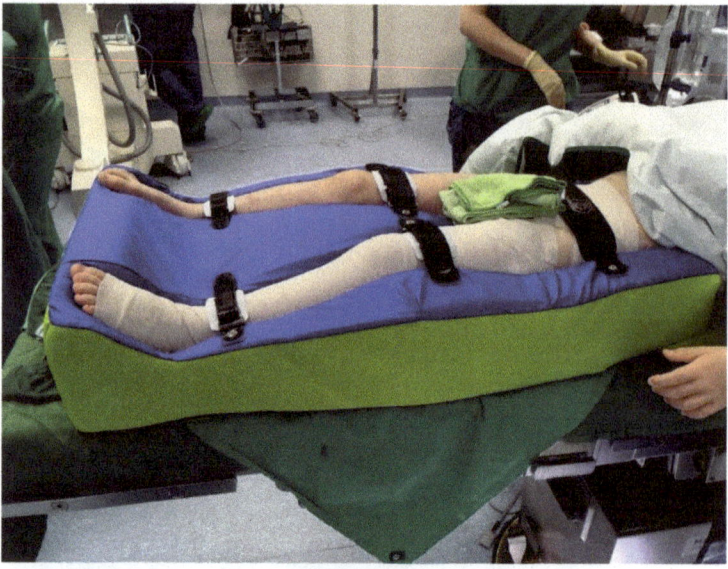

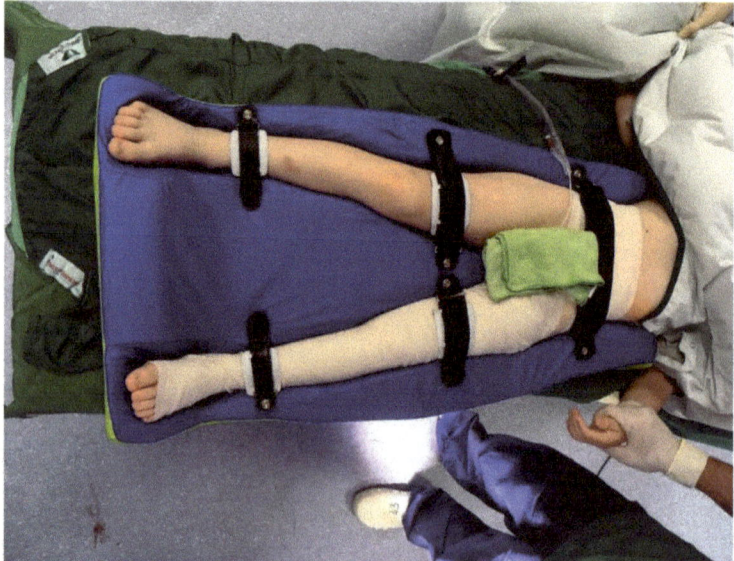

Figure 3. Postoperative foam splint.

The main hypothesis to test was: foam splinting for immobilization after hip reconstructive surgery leads to a higher satisfaction of the patients and a higher quality of care than spica casting, measured with the parameter 'Caregiver Priorities and Child Health Index of Life with Disabilities' (CPCHILD) [15,19].

The side issue was: are there fewer complications, such as hygienic problems, skin lesions, and neurological complications?

The clinical endpoint of the study was the completion of the 12-week postoperative questionnaire. Only patients with full completion of the questionnaires were included in the further statistical analysis. Criteria for exclusion were a lack of consent and cooperation.

Data storage and analysis were performed pseudonymized, and only study authors have access to the full datasets.

Statistical methods included a detailed epidemiological description with mean and standard deviation, minimum, maximum, and median for continuous data and scores, and relative frequency for all variables. The main characteristics were analysed with a t-test or chi-square test. Values for p are given and values <0.05 are considered to be statistically significant. When appropriate, graphical methods for visualisation are used.

The calculation of sample size used a two-sided t-test (difference between two independent means), effect of Cohen's d 1.1, alpha = 0.05, 1-beta = 0.80, and allocation ratio 1:1, and this resulted in a number of 15 patients per group (Software G*Power 3.1). Statistical analysis was planned in accordance with the local institute for biomedical statistics.

Table 1. Schedule of enrolment, interventions, and assessments.

	STUDY PERIOD				
	Enrolment	Allocation	Post-Allocation		Close-Out
TIMEPOINT	−t1	0	t1	t2	t3
ENROLMENT:	X				
Eligibility screen	X				
Informed consent	X				
Allocation		X			
INTERVENTIONS:					
Spica Cast			←——————→		
Foam Splint			←——————→		
ASSESSMENTS:	X		X	X	X
CPCHILD	X			X	X
SF-36	X			X	X
EQ-5D	X			X	X
Complications screen			X	X	X

t1 = surgery, t2 = 6 weeks after surgery, t3 = 12 weeks after surgery. X = action; ←——→ = interventional process.

Patient and Public Involvement

The planning study was supported by the local ethical review committee, including the representative for disabled patients, which provides professional ethical and legal advice. The ethical review committee reviewed the study protocol during the planning of the clinical trial and gave advice on ethical and legal topics, as well as statistical issues. The committee partnered with the study group for the design of the study, the informational material to support the intervention, and the burden of the intervention from the patient's perspective.

3. Results

Twenty-one out of thirty planned patients were involved (Table 2) until the end of 2021. One patient had to be excluded from further analysis due to parental compliance problems using the foam splint. This patient had to be casted two weeks postoperatively and further postoperative regime was unremarkable.

A complete dataset is available for 20 patients, wherein 10 received a spica cast and 10 a foam splint.

Of 15 patients with NDH, 0 were GMFCS type I, 1 was type II, 3 were type III, 2 were type IV, and 9 were type V. Eight of these patients received a spica cast, showing the efficiency of the randomization process.

Complications occurred in five patients. In the foam splint group, two patients suffered from superficial skin lesions on their medial malleolus. Both cases were seen in children with spasticity of the lower extremity. Analysing those cases revealed that the foam splint was too tight around the ankles. The design of the foam splint had to be adapted for the following cases by the orthopaedic technician. The superficial skin lesions were draped with foam patches and healed within one week. One patient of the foam splint group suffered from a deep wound infection of the proximal lateral femur 4 days postoperatively. The wound had to be revised surgically on the fifth postoperative day and healed under antibiotic treatment within two weeks.

Table 2. Epidemiologic data and procedures.

	DDH	NDH	LCPD
N (hips)	4	15	2
age at surgery	5.4y ± 3.6	8.0y ± 3.0	6.5y ± 0.6
m:f	2:2	8:7	2:0
right:left	2:2	8:7	0:2
bilateral	0	0	0
Surgical procedure in detail			
Femoral osteotomy	4	15	2
Osteotomy of ilium	4	15	2
Salter osteotomy	0	0	2
Chiari osteotomy	0	1	0
Pemberton osteotomy	4	14	0
Psoas tenotomy	0	3	0
Adductor tenotomy	0	4	0
Open reduction	2	6	0
Hamstring lengthening	0	2	0
Lengthening of extension mechanism	0	1	0

In the spica cast group, one patient showed a superficial skin lesion on the heel caused by the cast. This was seen two weeks postoperatively during the planned recasting. The second cast ended just above the ankle, the heel was covered with foam patches and healed within two weeks. One patient of the spica cast group suffered from a deep wound infection of the groin five days postoperatively and had to be revised surgically on the sixth day postoperatively. The wound healed under antibiotic treatment within two weeks. In none of the patients did the osteosynthesis material have to be revised.

The quality of life (QOL) scores showed a significant reduction at the 6-week follow-up compared to the preoperative assessment. The scores came back close to the preoperative values until the second postoperative assessment after twelve weeks (Table 3).

Table 3. Comparison of QOL scores at the three assessments.

	CPpre	Low–High	SD	EQ-5Dpre	Low–High	SD	SF-36pre	Low–High	SD
Total	77%	50–100	20	62%	24–100	25	82%	63–99	10
Foam splint	74%	50–100	22	60%	24–100	26	80%	63–99	11
Spica cast	81%	52–100	16	65%	37–94	24	85%	72–97	9
diff		7%	10		5%	12		5%	5
p		0.595			0.803			0.360	
	CPpost1	low–high	SD	EQ-5Dpost1	low–high	SD	SF-36post1	low–high	SD
Total	69%	36–89	14	49%	35–81	13	76%	66–87	5
Foam splint	73%	58–89	13	53%	38–81	15	78%	73–87	5
Spica cast	64%	36–78	14	45%	35–68	10	74%	66–80	5
diff		9%	7		8%	6		4%	2
p		0.147			0.253			0.087	
	CPpost2	low–high	SD	EQ-5Dpost2	low–high	SD	SF-36post2	low–high	SD
Total	69%	36–99	15	66%	34–98	19	84%	72–97	7
Foam splint	79%	60–99	15	65%	41–98	15	87%	78–97	5
Spica cast	74%	36–78	14	66%	34–68	17	82%	72–91	7
diff		5%	6		1%	9		5%	3
p		0.385			0.873			0.110	

A significant reduction of all QOL scores was seen in the spica cast group pre- vs. postoperatively for the variables CPCHILD (81% vs. 64%, $p = 0.001$), EQ-5d (65% vs. 45%, $p = 0.014$), and SF-36 (85% vs. 74%, $p = 0.004$).

Furthermore, the values for the foam splint group also presented a reduction but did not show statistical significance. (Table 4).

Table 4. Comparison of pre- and postoperative QOL scores, split up by mode of immobilization.

	CP	Low–High	SD	EQ-5D	Low–High	SD	SF-36	Low–High	SD
Spica cast pre	81%	52–100	16	65%	37–94	24	85%	72–97	9
Spica cast post1	64%	36–78	14	45%	35–68	10	74%	66–80	5
diff		17%	4		20%	7		9%	4
p		0.001			0.014			0.004	
	CP	low–high	SD	EQ-5D	low–high	SD	SF-36	low–high	SD
Foam splint pre	74%	50–100	22	60%	24–100	26	80%	63–99	11
Foam splint post1	73%	58–89	13	53%	38–81	15	78%	73–87	5
diff		1%	4		7%	6		2%	2
p		0.965			0.269			0.437	

Six weeks after surgery, values for CPCHILD (Figure 4), EQ-5D, and SF-36 were lower in the spica cast group than in the foam splint group, despite the fact that the difference did not reach the level of statistical significance (CPCHILD 73% vs. 64%, $p = 0.147$). The difference between the two groups decreased until the 12-week follow-up, still without statistical significance.

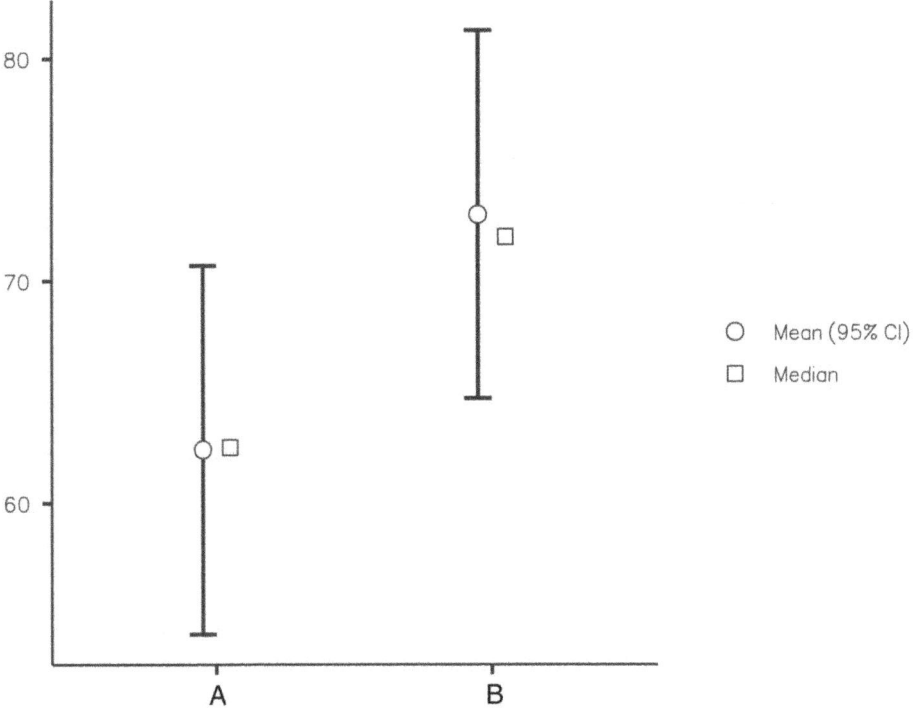

Figure 4. CPCHILD score at the 6-week follow-up for spica cast (A) and foam splint (B).

4. Discussion

Clinical trials on children and handicapped persons need to be carried out under sound ethical and scientific standards, considering their personal and legal independency.

Participation in a clinical trial needs in-depth discussion with the legal guardian and appropriate discussion with the child, depending on age and capacity.

Dysplasia of the hip must be treated prior to the ability to give informed consent to prevent deterioration or even loss of gait and posture. Therefore, it must be clarified to the patient and the guardian that hip reconstructive surgery is not only a measure to improve function, but also the quality of life for many years.

There is evidence that hip reconstructive surgery has a positive effect on the quality of life of children with cerebral palsy: DiFazio et al. were able to show the positive effect of hip reconstructive surgery in children with cerebral palsy in 2016 [15].

Despite the decades-long history of surgical correction of the hip and pelvis, there is no final consensus about the ideal modality or duration of postoperative immobilization, although the discussion is vivid and controversial [9].

Complications associated with spica cast immobilization are known, and recent publications have shown adverse events in 4.5% to 13.4% of cases in hip reconstructive surgery and up to 28of in cases in femoral fractures treated with spica casts [11,20]. The study group of Pisecky et al. presented a complication rate of 27.3% using spica cast immobilization in hip reconstructive surgery. Complications were more common in patients with NDH (35%) than DDH (22%). Nine out of twenty-three adverse events were considered to be cast-associated [21].

Aiming for the reduction of superficial skin lesions, Murgai et al. presented data for foam padding of the spica cast in 920 patients with 2481 immobilizations. It was possible to show a decrease in the complication rate in A-frame casts from 13.4% to 4.5%. Patients with neurologic disorders had the lowest complication rate with 0.7%, and neurovascular deficits were described in none of the cases with foam padding, in contrast to 4.5% in patients without additional measures [11].

DiFazio et al. presented a complication rate of 28% in cases treated with spica cast immobilization for femoral fractures. Thirty-one percent of the patients needed a readmission for recasting [20]. In a prospective trial, the same group was able to show a reduction of the complication rate from 13.6 to 6.6 cases per 1000 castings by using foam pads to enhance the cast [12].

As a study group with a large amount of experience in the usage of foam splints, Gather, Dreher et al. established a straightforward immobilization protocol with early physiotherapeutical remobilization and full weight bearing four weeks postoperatively after immobilization. According to the results of the study, no device-associated complication was seen. Therefore, it can be assumed that foam splinting is as safe as spica casting concerning the postoperative immobilization for the fixation of the osseous result [10].

Nevertheless, these reports are retrospective case series, and high-quality prospective randomized clinical trials are lacking. A broad variety of feasible aftercare procedures is known and, in most institutions, the surgeon's preference, personal experiences, or just tradition is the reason given for a type of postoperative immobilization. It is thought to be a compromise to protect the result of the surgical procedure on one hand and to prevent superficial skin lesions or worse complications on the other. The fear from loss of correction stands in contrast to a short and complication-free period of immobilization, as desired by the patient and the caretaker. Mostly, minor adverse events, such as skin lesions, superficial wound healing problems, and hygienic challenges, are responsible for many unscheduled outpatient contacts. These unplanned contacts bind medical professionals to time-consuming procedures and lead to rising costs in the health care system. More severe complications, such as deeper lesions of the skin, may need unplanned readmission to hospital, and in some cases surgical revision, with the risk of further adverse events. Interfering with the patient's autonomy and the caretaker's independence, readmissions and surgical procedures should be avoided by averting the underlying complication. Apart from the patient-related drawbacks, the financial burden of unplanned readmissions to hospital and recasting is enormous. In 2011, DiFazio calculated expenses of USD 12,719 for readmission and recasting in the operating room under sedation [20]. Furthermore, unplanned procedures take up necessary time in the operating room and, in the worst case, postpone planned surgical procedures.

In order to improve evidence relating to postoperative treatment, this is the first prospective randomized clinical trial comparing spica casts and foam splints for postoperative immobilization in patients who received hip reconstructive surgery. The purpose of this ongoing study is to evaluate quality of life and complication rates between these two different immobilization devices, and the preliminary data show promising results.

Until today, spica cast immobilization is still a widely used regimen of aftertreatment following pelvic surgery in children. It is necessary to provide criteria for the usage of a foam splints instead of casting in immobilization after hip reconstructive surgery.

Strengths and Limitations

Providing the first prospective randomized clinical trial on the topic of foam splinting and casting in immobilization after hip reconstructive surgery, the obtained data may support decision making in postoperative care concerning the safety and satisfaction of patients and caretakers. This clinical trial was planned under high ethical and legal standards and has passed the ethical review committees. At this point, the main limitation to achieve statistical significance may be the small number of participants of 10 patients in each group. The present data show the necessity to include at least 17 patients in each group to reach levels of statistical significance. More patients must be included in the study and further trials may be needed to obtain reliable data.

5. Conclusions

The data suggest higher patient and caretaker satisfaction in the foam splint group. The preliminary results of this clinical trial show an improvement of the QOL scores when using a foam splint compared to the conventionally used spica cast. Nevertheless, the values do not show statistical significance, most likely because of the low number of patients included and the relatively small difference. The conduction of the clinical trial is necessary.

Author Contributions: Conceptualization, L.P., G.G., M.C.M.K. and T.G.; methodology, L.P. and M.C.M.K.; software, L.P.; validation, S.S., C.S. and L.P.; formal analysis, C.H. and L.P.; investigation, L.P., G.G., C.H. and C.S.; resources, L.P. and T.G.; data curation, M.G. and L.P.; writing—original draft preparation, L.P., M.G. and C.H.; writing—review and editing, L.P., G.G., M.C.M.K. and T.G.; visualization, L.P.; supervision, M.C.M.K. and T.G.; project administration, L.P.; funding acquisition, L.P. All authors have read and agreed to the published version of the manuscript.

Funding: The trial is publicly funded by a competitive grant from the Medical Society of Upperaustria, Dinghoferstraße 4, 4020 Linz, Austria; the funder has no role in the collection, management, analysis, and interpretation of data; the writing of the report; and the decision to submit the report for publication.

Institutional Review Board Statement: The study was conducted according to the guidelines of the Declaration of Helsinki and approved by the Institutional Review Board 'Ethikkommission des Landes Oberösterreich' EK Nr: 1183/2018, February 12th 2019; the trial was registered at the German Clinical Trials Register DRKS-ID: DRKS00016861.

Informed Consent Statement: Informed consent was obtained from all subjects involved in the study. All participants and their legal guardians must understand and subscribe to the written informed consent form, including the consent for publication, including potentially identifiable images.

Data Availability Statement: The data presented in this study are available on request from the corresponding author. The data are not publicly available due to data protection policy involving children and patronized subjects.

Acknowledgments: The ethical review committee supported this protocol with ethical and legal advice; special thanks to the medical society of Upper Austria for the generous financial support of our clinical research; Open Access Funding by the University of Linz.

Conflicts of Interest: The authors declare no conflict of interest.

References

1. Huser, A.; Mo, M.; Hosseinzadeh, P. Hip Surveillance in Children with Cerebral Palsy. *Orthop. Clin. N. Am.* **2018**, *49*, 181–190. [CrossRef] [PubMed]
2. Chan, G.; Miller, F. Assessment and treatment of children with cerebral palsy. *Orthop. Clin. N. Am.* **2014**, *45*, 313–325. [CrossRef]
3. Root, L. Surgical treatment for hip pain in the adult cerebral palsy patient. *Dev. Med. Child Neurol.* **2009**, *51* (Suppl. S4), 84–91. [CrossRef] [PubMed]
4. Lloyd-Roberts, G.C.; Catterall, A.; Salamon, P.B. A controlled study of the indications for and the results of femoral osteotomy in Perthes' disease. *J. Bone Jt. Surg. Br.* **1976**, *58*, 31–36. [CrossRef] [PubMed]
5. Poussa, M.; Hoikka, V.; Yrjonen, T.; Osterman, K. Early signs of poor prognosis in Legg-Perthes-Calve disease treated by femoral varus osteotomy. *Rev. Chir. Orthop. Reparatrice Appar. Mot.* **1991**, *77*, 478–482.
6. Thompson, G.H. Salter osteotomy in Legg-Calve-Perthes disease. *J. Pediatr. Orthop.* **2011**, *31*, S192–S197. [CrossRef] [PubMed]
7. Onimus, M.; Manzone, P.; Allamel, G. Prevention of hip dislocation in children with cerebral palsy by early tenotomy of the adductor and psoas muscles. *Ann. Pediatr.* **1993**, *40*, 211–216.
8. Braatz, F.; Eidemuller, A.; Klotz, M.C.; Beckmann, N.A.; Wolf, S.I.; Dreher, T. Hip reconstruction surgery is successful in restoring joint congruity in patients with cerebral palsy: Long-term outcome. *Int. Orthop.* **2014**, *38*, 2237–2243. [CrossRef]
9. Emara, K.; Kersh, M.A.A.; Hayyawi, F.A. Duration of immobilization after developmental dysplasia of the hip and open reduction surgery. *Int. Orthop.* **2019**, *43*, 405–409. [CrossRef]
10. Gather, K.S.; von Stillfried, E.; Hagmann, S.; Muller, S.; Dreher, T. Outcome after early mobilization following hip reconstruction in children with developmental hip dysplasia and luxation. *World J. Pediatr.* **2018**, *14*, 176–183. [CrossRef]
11. Murgai, R.R.; Compton, E.; Patel, A.R.; Ryan, D.; Kay, R.M. Foam Padding in Postoperative Lower Extremity Casting: An Inexpensive Way to Protect Patients. *J. Pediatr. Orthop.* **2018**, *38*, e470–e474. [CrossRef]
12. Difazio, R.L.; Harris, M.; Feldman, L.; Mahan, S.T. Reducing the Incidence of Cast-related Skin Complications in Children Treated with Cast Immobilization. *J. Pediatr. Orthop.* **2017**, *37*, 526–531. [CrossRef] [PubMed]
13. Moher, D.; Schulz, K.F.; Altman, D.G. The CONSORT statement: Revised recommendations for improving the quality of reports of parallel-group randomised trials. *Lancet* **2001**, *357*, 1191–1194. [CrossRef]
14. Clark, M.P.; Westerberg, B.D. Holiday review. How random is the toss of a coin? *CMAJ* **2009**, *181*, E306–E308. [CrossRef]
15. DiFazio, R.; Shore, B.; Vessey, J.A.; Miller, P.E.; Snyder, B.D. Effect of Hip Reconstructive Surgery on Health-Related Quality of Life of Non-Ambulatory Children with Cerebral Palsy. *J. Bone Jt. Surg. Am.* **2016**, *98*, 1190–1198. [CrossRef] [PubMed]
16. Brazier, J.E.; Harper, R.; Jones, N.M.; O'Cathain, A.; Thomas, K.J.; Usherwood, T.; Westlake, L. Validating the SF-36 health survey questionnaire: New outcome measure for primary care. *BMJ* **1992**, *305*, 160–164. [CrossRef] [PubMed]
17. Wille, N.; Badia, X.; Bonsel, G.; Burstrom, K.; Cavrini, G.; Devlin, N.; Egmar, A.-C.; Greiner, W.; Gusi, N.; Herdman, M.; et al. Development of the EQ-5D-Y: A child-friendly version of the EQ-5D. *Qual. Life Res.* **2010**, *19*, 875–886. [CrossRef]
18. Rosenbaum, P.L.; Palisano, R.J.; Bartlett, D.J.; Galuppi, B.E.; Russell, D.J. Development of the Gross Motor Function Classification System for cerebral palsy. *Dev. Med. Child Neurol.* **2008**, *50*, 249–253. [CrossRef]
19. Difazio, R.L.; Vessey, J.A.; Zurakowski, D.; Snyder, B.D. Differences in health-related quality of life and caregiver burden after hip and spine surgery in non-ambulatory children with severe cerebral palsy. *Dev. Med. Child Neurol.* **2016**, *58*, 298–305. [CrossRef]
20. DiFazio, R.; Vessey, J.; Zurakowski, D.; Hresko, M.T.; Matheney, T. Incidence of skin complications and associated charges in children treated with hip spica casts for femur fractures. *J. Pediatr. Orthop.* **2011**, *31*, 17–22. [CrossRef]
21. Pisecky, L.; Grossbotzl, G.; Gahleitner, M.; Haas, C.; Gotterbarm, T.; Klotz, M.C. Results after spica cast immobilization following hip reconstruction in 95 cases: Is there a need for alternative techniques? *Arch. Orthop. Trauma Surg.* **2021**, 1–9. [CrossRef] [PubMed]

MDPI
St. Alban-Anlage 66
4052 Basel
Switzerland
Tel. +41 61 683 77 34
Fax +41 61 302 89 18
www.mdpi.com

Children Editorial Office
E-mail: children@mdpi.com
www.mdpi.com/journal/children

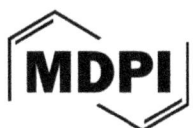

www.ingramcontent.com/pod-product-compliance
Lightning Source LLC
LaVergne TN
LVHW070505100526
838202LV00014B/1794